Atlas of
INFECTIOUS DISEASES

Volume VI

PLEUROPULMONARY AND BRONCHIAL INFECTIONS

Atlas of
INFECTIOUS DISEASES

Volume VI

PLEUROPULMONARY AND BRONCHIAL INFECTIONS

Editor-in-Chief

Gerald L. Mandell, MD

Professor of Medicine
Owen R. Cheatham Professor of the Sciences
Chief, Division of Infectious Diseases
University of Virginia Health Sciences Center
Charlottesville, Virginia

Editor

Michael S. Simberkoff, MD

Chief, Infectious Diseases Section
New York Veterans Affairs Medical Center
Associate Professor of Medicine
New York University School of Medicine
New York, New York

With 20 contributors

Churchill
Livingstone

DEVELOPED BY CURRENT MEDICINE, INC.
PHILADELPHIA

CURRENT MEDICINE

400 MARKET STREET, SUITE 700
PHILADELPHIA, PA 19106

Library of Congress Cataloging-in-Publication Data

Pleuropulmonary and bronchial infections / editor-in-chief, Gerald L. Mandell; editor, Michael S. Simberkoff; developed by Current Medicine, Inc.
      p. cm. – (Atlas of infectious diseases ; v. 6)
  Includes bibliographical references and index.
  ISBN 0-443-07740-1 (hard cover)
  1. Bronchi–Infections–Atlases. I. Mandell, Gerald L.
II. Simberkoff, Michael S., 1936– . III. Current Medicine, Inc. IV. Series.
  [DNLM: 1. Lung Diseases–diagnosis–atlases. 2. Lung Diseases–microbiology–atlases.
WF 17 P726 1996]
RC778.P54 1996
616.2'407–dc20
DNLM/DLC
for Library of Congress   95-45642
                                                      CIP

Development Editors: ....Lee Tevebaugh and Michael Bokulich
Editorial Assistant: ....Elena Coler
Art Director: ....Paul Fennessy
Design and Layout: ....Patrick Whelan and Patrick Ward
Illustration Director: ....Ann Saydlowski
Illustrators: ....Weislawa Langenfield, Beth Starkey,
                                        Lisa Weischedel, and Gary Welch
Production: ....David Myers and Lori Holland
Typesetting Director: ....Colleen Ward
Managing Editor: ....Lori J. Bainbridge

Printed in Hong Kong by Paramount Printing Group Limited.

10 9 8 7 6 5 4 3 2 1

PREFACE

The diagnosis and management of patients with infectious diseases are based in large part on visual clues. Skin and mucous membrane lesions, eye findings, imaging studies, Gram stains, culture plates, insect vectors, preparations of blood, urine, pus cerebrospinal fluid, and biopsy specimens are studied to establish the proper diagnosis and to choose the most effective therapy. The *Atlas of Infectious Diseases* will be a modern, complete collection of these images. Current Medicine, with its capability of superb color reproduction and its state-of-the-art computer imaging facilities, is the ideal publisher for the atlas. Infectious diseases physicians, scientists, microbiologists, and pathologists frequently teach other health-care professionals, and this comprehensive atlas with available slides is an effective teaching tool.

Dr. Michael Simberkoff is an expert with the broad overview of one who studies the interface of infectious diseases and pulmonary medicine. He has brought together a distinguished group of authors who have prepared superb chapters. The conditions displayed range from the very common to those that are amazingly rare. The images are instructive and comprehensive. This volume will be a valuable resource for clinicians caring for patients and teachers of pulmonary medicine.

Gerald L. Mandell, MD

CONTRIBUTORS

Donald Armstrong, MD
Chief, Infectious Diseases Service
Department of Medicine
Memorial Sloan-Kettering Cancer Center
Professor of Medicine
Cornell University Medical College
New York, New York

Robert F. Betts, MD
Professor of Medicine
Director, Educational Programs
University of Rochester School of Medicine and Dentistry
Strong Memorial Hospital
Rochester, New York

Roger C. Bone, MD
Professor of Medicine
President/Chief Executive Officer
Medical College of Ohio
Toledo, Ohio

Richard E. Bryant, MD
Director, Infectious Diseases Section
Oregon Health Sciences University
Portland, Oregon

Scott F. Davies, MD
Professor of Medicine
University of Minnesota
Director, Division of Pulmonary and Critical Care Medicine
Hennepin County Medical Center
Minneapolis, Minnesota

Ann R. Falsey, MD
Assistant Professor of Medicine
University of Rochester School of Medicine and Dentistry
Rochester General Hospital
Rochester, New York

Jay A. Fishman, MD
Assistant Professor of Medicine
Harvard Medical School
Associate Chief and Clinical Director
Infectious Disease for Transplantation
Massachusetts General Hospital
Boston, Massachusetts

John Froude, MB, BS, MRCP
Clinical Professor
Department of Medicine
New York University
Bellevue Hospital Medical Center
New York, New York

Caroline B. Hall, MD
Professor of Pediatrics
University of Rochester School of Medicine and Dentistry
Strong Memorial Hospital
Rochester, New York

James J. Herdegen, MD
Assistant Professor
Pulmonary and Critical Care Medicine
Rush-Presbyterian-St. Luke's Medical Center
Chicago, Illinois

Jaishree Jagirdar, MD
Associate Professor of Pathology
New York University Medical Center
Chief of Surgical Pathology
Bellevue Hospital
New York, New York

Howard L. Leaf, MD
Assistant Professor of Clinical Medicine
New York University School of Medicine
Infectious Diseases Section
New York Veterans Affairs Medical Center
New York, New York

Melanie J. Maslow, MD, FACP
Assistant Chief, Infectious Diseases Section
New York Veterans Affairs Medical Center
Clinical Assistant Professor of Medicine
New York University School of Medicine
New York, New York

Herbert Y. Reynolds, MD
J. Lloyd Huck Professor of Medicine
Chairman, Department of Medicine
The Milton S. Hershey Medical Center
The Pennsylvania State University
Hershey, Pennsylvania

Richard B. Roberts, MD
Professor and Vice-Chairman, Department of Medicine
The New York Hospital–Cornell Medical Center
New York, New York

Robert H. Rubin, MD
Osborne Chair in Health Sciences and Technology
Harvard Medical School
Chief, Infectious Disease for Transplantation
Massachusetts General Hospital
Boston, Massachusetts

Christopher J. Salmon, MD
Assistant Professor of Radiology
Director, Thoracic Imaging
Oregon Health Sciences University
Portland, Oregon

George A. Sarosi, MD
Professor of Medicine
Standford University School of Medicine
Standford, California
Chairman, Department of Medicine
Santa Clara Valley Medical Center
San Jose, California

Michael S. Simberkoff, MD
Chief, Infectious Diseases Section
New York Veterans Affairs Medical Center
Associate Professor of Medicine
New York University School of Medicine
New York, New York

John J. Treanor, MD
Associate Professor of Medicine
University of Rochester School of Medicine and Dentistry
Strong Memorial Hospital
Rochester, New York

Contents

Chapter 8
Protozoan and Helminthic Infections of the Lungs

John Froude

Chapter 9
Pleural Effusion and Empyema

Christopher J. Salmon and Richard E. Bryant

Chapter 10
Pneumonias in Cancer Patients

Donald Armstrong

Chapter 11
Respiratory Infections in Transplant Recipients

Jay A. Fishman and Robert H. Rubin

Chapter 12
Pulmonary Manifestations of Extrapulmonary Infection

James J. Herdegen and Roger C. Bone

Chapter 13
Acute and Chronic Bronchitis and Bronchiolitis

Herbert Y. Reynolds and Michael S. Simberkoff

Index

CHAPTER 1

Gram-Positive Bacterial Infections of the Lungs

Richard B. Roberts

PATHOGENESIS AND ETIOLOGY

Etiologic determinants for pneumonia

Host characteristics
  Age
  State of health
  Immunocompetence

Environmental exposure
  Geographic location
  Community acquired vs nosocomial
  Closed population settings (daycare centers, military camps,
    nursing homes)
  Unusual exposures (*eg*, animals)

Pathogen characteristics
  Virulence
  Inoculum size

FIGURE 1-1 Etiologic determinants for pneumonia. Determinants may be classified on the basis of the host, environmental exposures, and the pathogen. A detailed history from the patient is important in the consideration of each of these determinants and therefore the possible etiologic agent. For example, exposure to animals has been associated with the following causes of pneumonitis: anthrax, brucellosis, plague, tularemia, psittacosis, and leptospirosis. Inoculum size of the pathogen may be determined by the number of organisms inoculated or by the inability of the host to reduce the infecting inoculum, such as *Mycobacterium tuberculosis* in gastrectomy patients.

Pathogenic mechanisms and pathogens of pneumonia

Mechanisms	Pathogens
Inhalation	*Streptococcus pneumoniae,** S. pyogenes** *Mycobacterium, Legionella* Influenza virus, measles virus, adenovirus *Coccidioides, Histoplasma, Cryptococcus Coxiella burnetti* (Q fever)
Aspiration	Anaerobes, *Streptococcus pneumoniae,** Staphylococcus aureus,** Haemophilus influenzae,* gram-negative bacilli
Hematogenous	*Staphylococcus aureus,** gram-negative bacilli (*Pseudomonas aeruginosa*) *Candida Strongyloides, Ascaris*
Contiguous spread	Anaerobes, gram-negative bacilli *Entamoeba histolytica*
Reactivation	*Mycobacterium* Cytomegalovirus *Coccidioides, Histoplasma, Blastomyces Toxoplasma, Strongyloides Pneumocystis carinii*

*Gram-positive organisms.

FIGURE 1-2 Pathogenic mechanisms and pathogens of pneumonia. Pneumonia develops by five different mechanisms. Identifying the mechanism may be helpful in directing empiric antimicrobial therapy to a specific etiologic agent. The general mechanisms and most likely pathogens are listed in the figure. Certain bacteria, such as *Streptococcus pneumoniae* and *Staphylococcus aureus* may cause pneumonia by more than one mechanism.

Gram-positive bacteria associated with pneumonia

Gram-positive cocci
Streptococcus
  S. pneumoniae (pneumococcus)
  S. pyogenes (group A)
  S. agalactiae (group B)
  Group C and G streptococci
  Anaerobic streptococci (peptostreptococci)
  S. anginosus (*S. milleri*)

Gram-positive bacilli
Bacillus
  B. anthracis
  B. cereus
Corynebacterium
  Rhodococcus equi (*C. equi*)

FIGURE 1-3 Gram-positive bacteria associated with pneumonia. The most common gram-positive cocci associated with pulmonary infections are pneumococci and *Staphylococcus aureus.* Anaerobic streptococci and *Streptococcus anginosus* are pulmonary pathogens in patients with aspiration of oral contents. Gram-positive bacilli are uncommon etiologic agents, although necrotizing pneumonia due to *Rhodococcus equi* has been observed in HIV-infected individuals.

PNEUMOCOCCAL PNEUMONIA

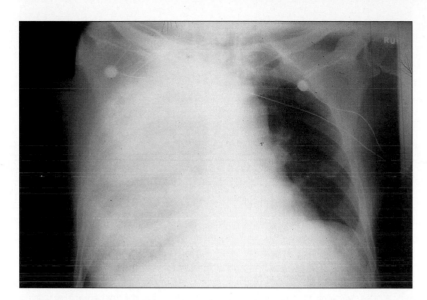

FIGURE 1-4 Chest radiograph showing multilobar consolidation in pneumococcal pneumonia. A 64-year-old man presented with a 6-day history of fever, shaking chills, chest pain, and cough productive of rust-cultured sputum. One day before admission, he developed dyspnea and confusion. His past medical history was remarkable for mild hypertension and a 150-pack-year smoking history. The patient had not received pneumococcal vaccination. An admission chest film revealed consolidation of the right upper, middle, and lower lobes.

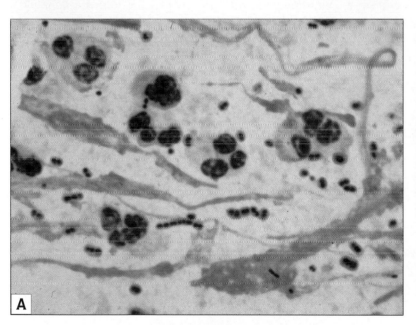

A

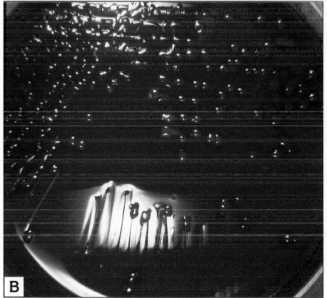

B

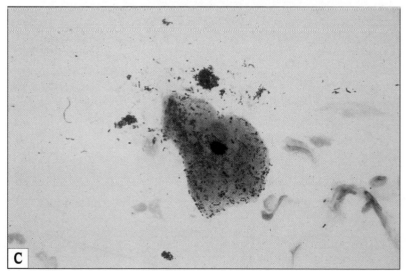

C

FIGURE 1-5 Microbiologic studies in pneumococcal pneumonia. **A.** Sputum Gram stain from the patient in Figure 1-4. Many polymorphonuclear leukocytes with lancet-shaped, gram-positive cocci in pairs and chains can be seen, indicative of *Streptococcus pneumoniae*. To be adequate for evaluation, a sputum sample must have ≥ 25 leukocytes per low-power field. **B,** Cultures from sputum, blood, and spinal fluid grew type-3 *S. pneumoniae* as mucoid colonies on blood agar. **C,** A high-power view reveals the presence of epithelial cells, suggesting that the specimen is from the upper respiratory tract.

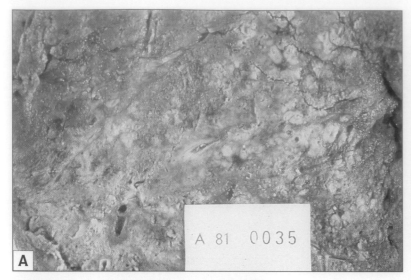

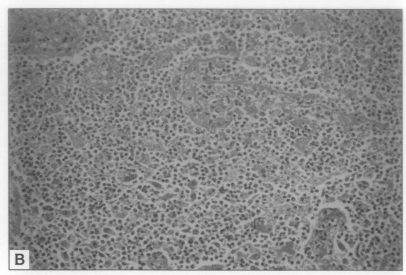

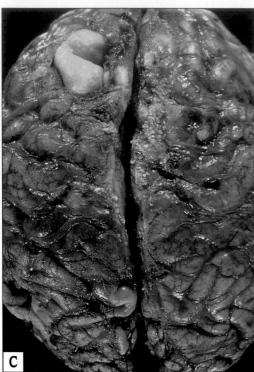

FIGURE 1-6 End-organ damage in pneumococcal pneumonia. The patient (*see* Figs. 1-4 and 1-5) developed respiratory failure, hypotension, and renal failure. He died on the third hospital day. **A**, Postmortem examination of the right lung revealed marked consolidation with many yellow-green, 0.2- to 1.0-cm abscesses. **B**, Microscopic examination of lung tissues showed a diffuse alveolar infiltrate with neutrophils, fibrin, and mononuclear cells. **C**, The leptomeninges were congested and opalescent, consistent with meningitis. The valvular endocardium was unremarkable.

Poor prognostic factors in pneumococcal pneumonia
Bacteremia
Type-3 pneumococci
Age (elderly)
Splenectomy or functional asplenia
Multilobe involvement
Leukopenia
Jaundice
Hypotension
Extrapulmonary complications
Meningitis
Endocarditis

FIGURE 1-7 Poor prognostic factors in pneumococcal pneumonia. As shown by the patient in Figure 1-4, mortality from pneumococcal pneumonia is associated with the presence of one or more risk factors. This patient had five risk factors (bacteremia, type-3 pneumococci, elderly, multilobe involvement, and an extrapulmonary complication).

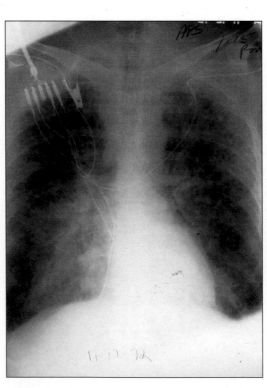

FIGURE 1-8 Chest radiograph showing pneumococcal bronchopneumonia of the right lower lobe in a patient with hypogammaglobulinemia. The pulmonary manifestations of pneumococcal infections can present in various forms and severity, including consolidation as well as bronchopulmonary involvement of one or more segments or lobes.

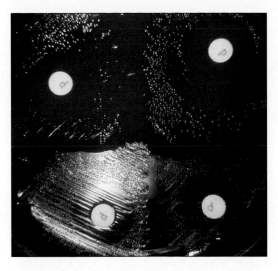

FIGURE 1-9 Optochin inhibition in pneumococcal cultures. Pneumococci are easily differentiated from other streptococci causing α-hemolysis on blood agar by their growth inhibition by optochin. As shown in this figure, a zone of inhibition surrounding an optochin disc (*P*) is demonstrated for three of the four α-hemolytic streptococcal isolates cultured in quadrants on a blood agar plate.

Clinical manifestations of pneumococcal pneumonia

Presenting symptoms
Sudden onset
Fever, rigors
Productive cough, with purulent, rust-colored sputum
Chest pain

Physical examination
Elevated temperature, high-grade
Tachypnea, tachycardia
Rales, possible consolidation

Laboratory examination
Leukocytosis
Chest radiograph: bronchopneumonic pattern or consolidation; may be segmental or lobar, involving one or more lobes
Sputum Gram stain: gram-positive cocci, often lancet-shaped with polymorphonuclear leukocytes

FIGURE 1-10 Clinical manifestations of pneumococcal pneumonia.

Risk factors for development of pneumococcal pneumonia

Defective antibody formation
  Primary: hypo- or agammaglobulinemia
  Secondary: multiple myeloma, chronic lymphocytic leukemia, HIV
Neutropenia
Splenic dysfunction: asplenia, sickle cell disease, thalassemia
Underlying medical conditions
  Alcoholism with cirrhosis
  Diabetes mellitus with acidosis
  Congestive heart failure
  Chronic obstructive pulmonary disease

FIGURE 1-11 Risk factors for development of pneumococcal pneumonia. Predisposing conditions for pneumococcal infections including pneumonia are 1) immunologic dysfunction related to antibody, leukocytes, or clearance by the reticuloendothelial system and 2) underlying medical conditions.

Indications for administration of pneumococcal vaccine

Chronic underlying diseases
  Congestive heart failure
  Alcoholism with cirrhosis
  Diabetes mellitus
  Chronic pulmonary disease
  Chronic renal disease
Age ≥ 60 years
Elderly residents of chronic care facilities
Patients ≥ 2 years with splenic dysfunction, (*eg,* sickle cell disease) or splenectomy
Outbreaks of multidrug-resistant pneumococci
Geographic outbreaks due to a known pneumococcal serotype

FIGURE 1-12 Indications for administration of pneumococcal vaccine. The known risk and poor prognostic factors associated with pneumococcal pneumonia (*see* Figs. 1-7 and 1-11) are reflected in the indications for vaccination. The pneumococcal vaccine consists of 23 immunologically distinct capsular polysaccharides, with these serotypes accounting for more than 90% of bacteremic pneumococcal disease in the United States. The estimated efficacy of this vaccine in patients aged < 55 years is > 85%. However, the efficacy decreases with advancing age and, possibly, in patients with certain underlying medical conditions. Like all polysaccharide vaccines, this vaccine is not immunogenic in children < 2 years of age, and efforts to develop a conjugate vaccine are underway. The availability of a conjugate vaccine is becoming more important in young children because of the alarming increase in multidrug-resistant pneumococci.

Complications of pneumococcal pneumonia
Pulmonary
Empyema
Bronchopleural fistula
Lung abscess
Pericarditis
Extrapulmonary
Meningitis
Endocarditis
Arthritis
Peritonitis

FIGURE 1-13 Complications of pneumococcal pneumonia. Complications may be associated with direct extension of the infection to the pleura or pericardium. Because, in general, pneumococci do not cause necrotizing pneumonitis, the presence of a lung abscess is due to either a serotype-3 organism, which is the most virulent of the 84 serotypes, or an endobronchial obstructing lesion with postobstructive pneumonia requiring bronchoscopy. Extrapulmonary complications are associated with bacteremic pneumococcal pneumonia, although in patients with spontaneous pneumococcal peritonitis, pneumonia may not be seen on chest radiographs and blood cultures may be negative. A significant mortality is observed in those patients with the triad of bacteremic pneumococcal pneumonia, meningitis, and endocarditis.

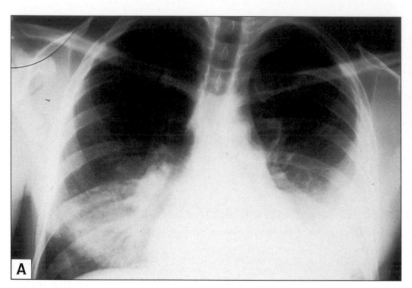

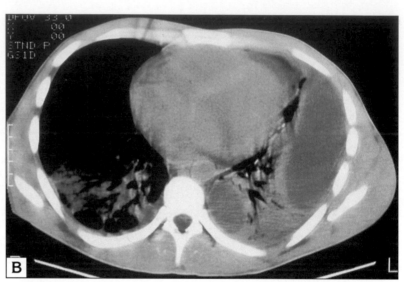

FIGURE 1-14 Pneumococcal pneumonia with empyema. A previously healthy 25-year-old man, presumably HIV positive with a CD+ count of 21/mm³, was hospitalized with a 4-day history of fever, productive cough, dyspnea, and pleuritic chest pain. **A,** Admission chest film revealed left lower, right lower, and right middle lobar consolidation with a left pleural effusion. Blood cultures were positive for type-14

Streptococcus pneumoniae. **B,** Six days after admission, computed tomography of the chest showed bibasilar infiltrates and a large loculated left pleural effusion. Radiographic-guided thoracentesis yielded 280 mL of cloudy fluid with a leukocyte count of 39,000/mm³ with 99% polymorphonuclear leukocytes, protein of 4.0 mg/dL, and glucose of 5 mg/dL, which are consistent with empyema.

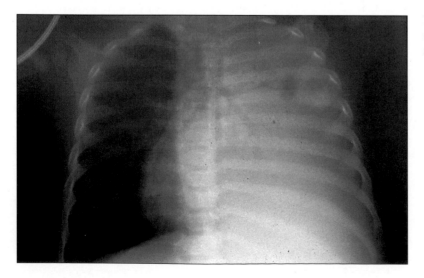

FIGURE 1-15 Pneumococcal pneumonia with empyema and bronchopleural fistula. Opacification of the entire left hemithorax is seen on the chest film.

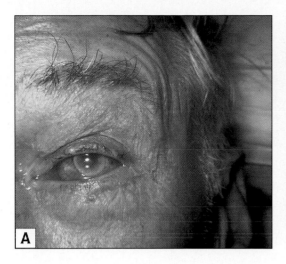

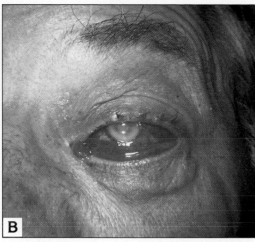

FIGURE 1-16 Pneumococcal endophthalmitis. **A**, A 63-year-old man was admitted for acute blindness in the left eye. Three weeks before admission, he developed fever, productive cough with rusty sputum, and pleuritic chest pain. On admission, the patient had left lower lobe pneumonia, mitral valve endocarditis, meningitis, and endophthalmitis secondary to a septic embolus. Cultures of blood, fluid from the anterior chamber of the left eye, and spinal fluid were positive for type-8 *Streptococcus pneumoniae*. **B**, Two weeks later, the endophthalmitis had worsened, necessitating eventual enucleation.

GROUP A STREPTOCOCCAL PNEUMONIA

Streptococcus pyogenes Pneumonia

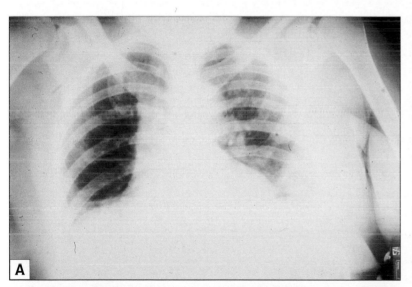

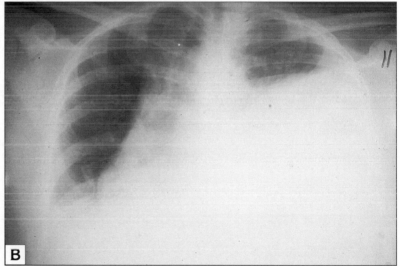

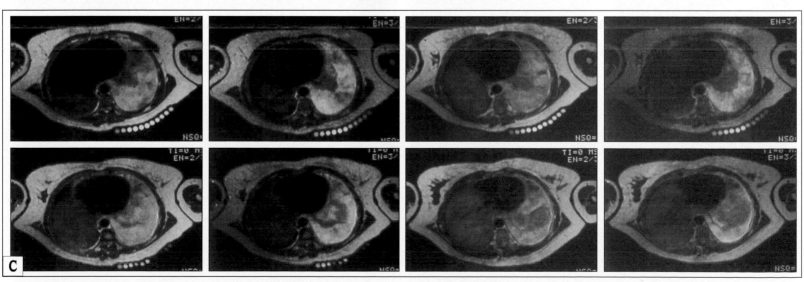

FIGURE 1-17 Group A streptococcal pneumonia with pleural effusion. A 48-year-old woman presented with 1-day history of fever, chills, dyspnea, and severe persistent pleuritic chest pain. Her past medical history included hypertension and adult-onset diabetes. **A**, An admission chest film revealed a left lower lobe infiltrate. **B**, Over the subsequent 6 days in the hospital, she was persistently febrile and short of breath, and a large left-sided pleural effusion accumulated. **C**, A magnetic resonance examination of the chest revealed a multiloculated left pleural effusion filled with debris, collapse of the left lower lobe with air bronchograms, and mediastinal shift to the right.

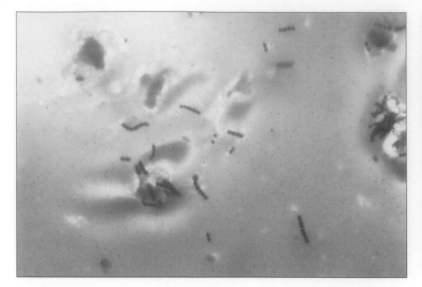

FIGURE 1-18 Gram stain of pleural fluid from patient in Figure 1-17. Thoracentesis revealed brownish viscid fluid with a leukocyte count of 10,500/mm^3 with 54% polymorphonuclear leukocytes, erythrocyte count of 8500/mm^3, protein of 5.5 mg/dL, glucose of 2.0 m/dL, and lactate dehydrogenase of 2460 U/L. Gram stain demonstrated gram-positive cocci in chains, and cultures grew group A streptococci (*Streptococcus pyogenes*).

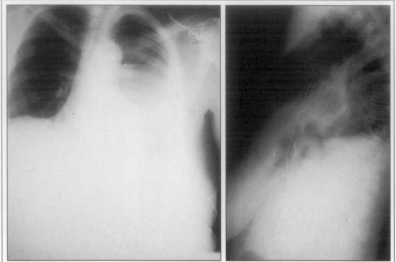

FIGURE 1-19 Chest radiographs showing partial resolution of group A streptococcal pneumonia. Following 2 weeks of chest tube drainage and antimicrobial therapy, partial resolution of the infiltrate and pleural fluid was noted on repeat posterior anterior and lateral chest films. Group A streptococcal pneumonia usually occurs in the clinical setting of either a previous viral respiratory tract infection or in closed population groups, such as military recruit installations, in which there is endemic streptococcal pharyngitis or colonization. Classically, the clinical presentation is acute, and patients appear extremely ill, often with marked pleuritic chest pain. On chest film, the combination of a pulmonary infiltrate, unilateral hilar adenopathy, and pleural effusion should alert the clinician to a possible streptococcal etiology. Pleural fluid is often hemorrhagic. Chest tube drainage and immediate antimicrobial therapy are necessary because the clinical course, as in this patient, may be protracted.

Streptococcal Toxic Shock Syndrome

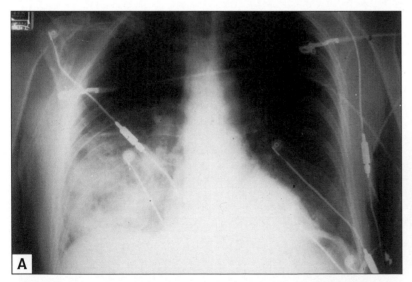

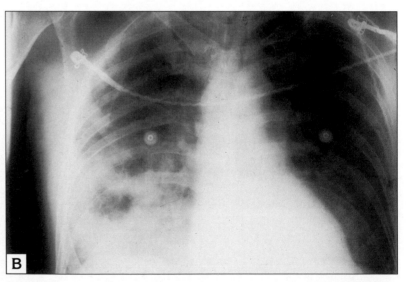

FIGURE 1-20 Progression of chest radiographic abnormalities in streptococcal toxic shock syndrome. A 53-year-old man walked into the emergency department with dyspnea and palpitations for 12 hours. He had been well until 3 days before admission when he noted an influenza-like syndrome, followed by blood-tinged sputum, drenching sweats, and dyspnea on the day of admission. **A,** An admission chest film showed right lower and middle lobe infiltrates with hyperlucent areas. By 4 hours after admission, he developed metabolic acidosis (arterial pH, 7.24; serum lactate, 9.5 mmol/L), renal insufficiency (blood urea nitrogen, 5.5 mg/dL; creatinine, 3.9 mg/dL), and refractory hypotension (systolic blood pressure < 90 mm Hg despite pressors; pulmonary capillary wedge pressure, 18 mm Hg; systemic vascular resistance, 1100 dynes ^{dot} sec/cm^{-5}; cardiac output, 3.2 L/min; left ventricular stroke work index, 11.0 g^{dot} m/m^2). **B,** Repeat chest film revealed progression of the infiltrates and two radiolucencies in the right lower lung field. (*continued*)

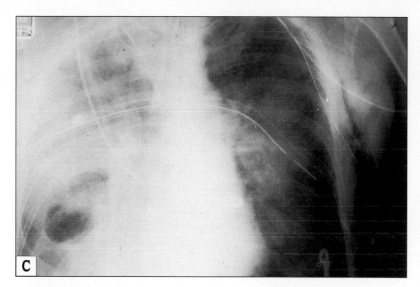

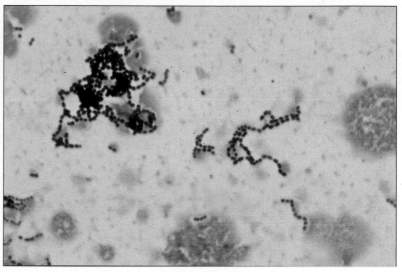

FIGURE 1-20 (*continued*) **C,** By 12 hours after admission, he had had two spontaneous pneumothoraces, and chest films now revealed bilateral infiltrates consistent with adult respiratory distress syndrome. He developed disseminated intravascular coagulation (platelets, 32,000/mm^3; prothrombin time, 18.3$_0$; partial thromboplastin time, 87.7; fibrinogen, 300 mg/dL). He died 8 hours later.

FIGURE 1-21 Cultures in streptococcal toxic shock syndrome (TSS). Blood, sputum, and pleural fluid cultures grew M type-1, T type-1 group A streptococci (*Streptococcus pyogenes*). M protein types 1 and 3 account for > 50% of group A streptococci associated with streptococcal TSS.

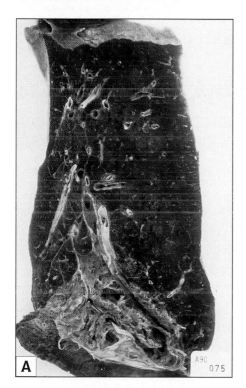

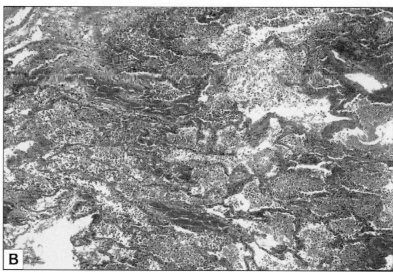

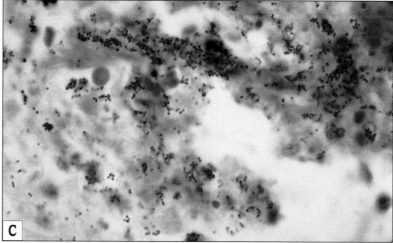

FIGURE 1-22 Postmortem examination in streptococcal toxic shock syndrome. **A,** Autopsy revealed a multiloculated, necrotic area in the right lower lung. **B,** Microscopically, both lungs contained numerous hemorrhagic abscesses, which were filled with acute inflammatory cells. **C,** Many gram-positive cocci were also seen in the hemorrhagic abscesses. Many alveoli were filled with polymorphonuclear leukocytes, and an intense vasculitis was observed adjacent to the abscesses.

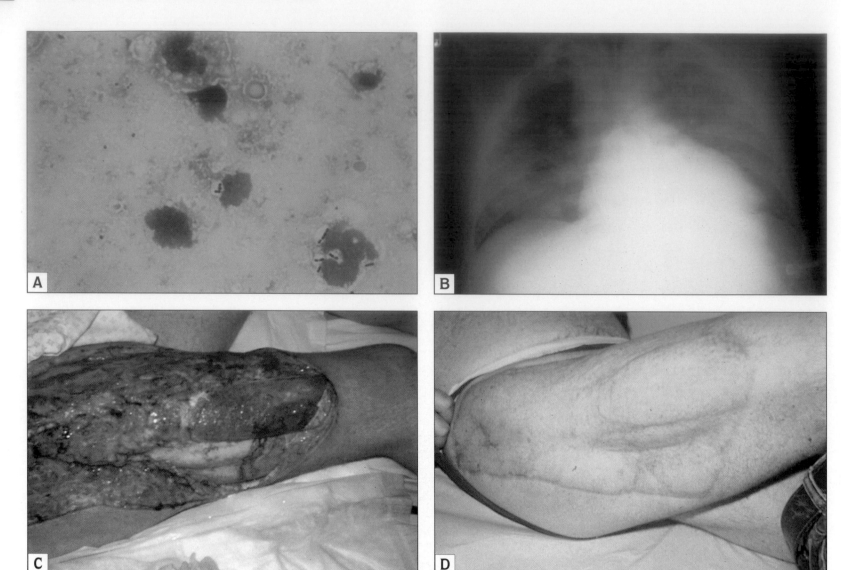

FIGURE 1-23 Group A streptococcal toxic shock syndrome (TSS) associated with necrotizing fasciitis. A resurgence of severe group A streptococcal (GAS) infections has been noted in the United States and Europe. The clinical entity of shock and multiorgan system failure associated with GAS bacteremia or with nonbacteremic, rapidly progressive, soft-tissue infection has become known as streptococcal TSS. The clinical manifestations of the syndrome may be mediated by one or more streptococcal exotoxins. Streptococcal TSS usually develops following an innocuous superficial injury, although other primary sites of infection may be the lungs or female genital tract (puerperal fever). A 36-year-old man walked into our emergency department with a painful thigh, where 3 days previously he had injected cocaine. On examination, his upper anterior thigh was very tender, erythematous, and indurated, and a 1-cm eschar was noted. **A**, Gram stain of a needle aspirate of the thigh demonstrated gram-positive cocci in chains, and the patient was placed on appropriate intravenous antibiotics. **B**, Despite therapy, the patient developed hypotension and oliguria, and the chest film showed bilateral diffuse infiltrates consistent with adult respiratory distress syndrome (oxygen partial pressure of 60 mm Hg). **C**, An extensive fasciotomy for necrotizing fasciitis was performed. Cultures from the surgical wound grew group A streptococcus that was nontypable. Blood cultures were negative. **D**, He received multiple skin grafts to the right thigh and was discharged 6 weeks later.

Proposed case definition for streptococcal toxic shock syndrome

I. Isolation of group A streptococci (*Streptococcus pyogenes*)
  A. From a normally sterile site (*eg*, blood; cerebrospinal, pleural, or peritoneal fluid; tissue biopsy; surgical wound; etc)
  B. From a nonsterile site (*eg*, throat, sputum, vagina, superficial skin lesion, etc)

II. Clinical signs of severity
  A. Hypotension: systolic blood pressure ≤ 90 mm Hg in adults or < 5th percentile for age in children
    and
  B. Two or more of the following signs:
    1. Renal impairment: Creatinine ≥ 177 μmol/L (≥ 2 mg/dL) for adults or ≥ 2 × ULN for age, (preexisting renal disease, ≥ twofold elevation over baseline level)
    2. Coagulopathy: Platelets ≤ 100 × 10^9/L (≤ 100,000/mm³) or DIC (defined by prolonged PT/PTT, low fibrinogen level, and presence of FDPs)
    3. Liver involvement: ALT, AST, or total bilirubin levels ≥ 2 × ULN for age (in preexisting liver disease, ≥ twofold elevation over baseline level)
    4. ARDS: Defined by acute onset of diffuse pulmonary infiltrates and hypoxemia in absence of cardiac failure; evidence of diffuse capillary leak manifested by acute onset of generalize edema; or pleural or peritoneal effusions with hypoalbuminemia
    5. Generalize erythematous macular rash that may desquamate
    6. Soft-tissue necrosis, including necrotizing fasciitis/myositis or gangrene

ALT—alanine aminotransferase; ARDS—acute respiratory distress syndrome; AST—aspartate aminotransferase; DIC—disseminated intravascular coagulation; FDP—fibrin degradation product; PT/PTT—prothrombin time/partial thromboplastin time; ULN—upper limit of normal.

FIGURE 1-24 Proposed case definition for streptococcal toxic shock syndrome. (*Adapted from* the Working Group on Severe Streptococcal Infections [1]; with permission.)

Streptococcal Aspiration Pneumonia

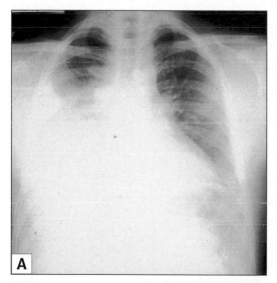
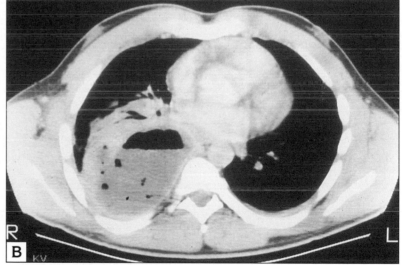
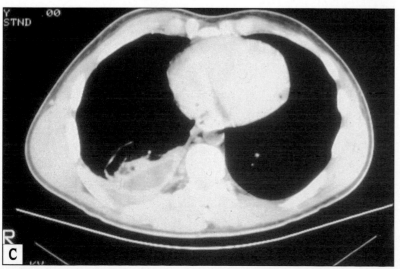

FIGURE 1-25 Aspiration pneumonia and pleural effusion due to *Streptococcus anginosus*. A 33-year-old man with posttraumatic epilepsy and nocturnal seizures since childhood was admitted with a 3-week history of fever, cough, dyspnea, and pleuritic chest pain that did not respond to oral erythromycin therapy. **A**, Admission chest film revealed right lower lobe pneumonia with a pleural effusion and possible air-fluid level. **B**, Computed tomography (CT) of the chest confirmed a loculated posterior fluid collection with an air-fluid level and right lower lobe pneumonia with compressive atelectasis. Under CT guidance, 50 mL of turbid yellow fluid was removed, which showed a pH of 7.07, leukocyte count of 13,200/mm³ with 30% polymorphonuclear leukocytes, protein of 5.3 mg/dL, glucose of 0 mg/dL, and lactate dehydrogenase of 7200 U/L. Gram stain demonstrated gram-positive cocci in pairs and chains, and cultures grew *Streptococcus anginosus*. **C**, Following 16 days of chest-tube drainage and antibiotic therapy, a repeat CT scan showed marked reduction in loculated fluid in the right posterior pleural space, and complete resolution of the pneumonia and atelectasis.

Predisposing conditions for oropharyngeal aspiration

Impaired consciousness
  Alcoholism
  Drug abuse
  Diabetic coma
  Seizures
  General anesthesia
  Cerebrovascular accident
Esophageal dysfunction
  Achalasia
  Scleroderma
  Strictures
  Carcinoma
  Neurologic deficits
Protective barrier disruption
  Tracheostomy
  Endotracheal intubation

FIGURE 1-26 Predisposing conditions for oropharyngeal aspiration. Aspiration pneumonia may occur due to numerous predisposing conditions. The etiologic agents are those that predominate as oropharyngeal flora. Many factors in addition to those listed determine the bacterial flora, including adequate dentition, antibiotic use, and hospitalization of the patient. *Streptococcus anginosus* are microaerophilic viridans streptococci that require anaerobiosis, or carbon dioxide for growth in the diagnostic laboratory. This viridans streptococcal species is responsible for suppurative infections in many organ systems, including the central nervous system and pulmonary, abdominal, and pelvic regions. Other anaerobic streptococci (peptostreptococci) are also associated with necrotizing pneumonia and empyema following aspiration of oropharyngeal bacteria.

STAPHYLOCOCCAL PNEUMONIA

Predisposing conditions for staphylococcal pneumonia

Primary (inhalation, aspiration)
  Age—neonate and elderly
  Previous viral infection—especially influenza
  Chronic granulomatous disease
  Hospitalized and nursing home patients
  Hospital personnel
  Underlying medical illnesses—alcoholism, chronic lung
    disease, diabetes, renal failure, malignancy
  Therapeutic modalities—antibiotics, steroids, chemotherapy

Secondary (hematogenous, metastatic)
  Suppurative phlebitis—usually catheter-related
  Intravenous drug abuse—usually associated with right-sided
    endocarditis
  Dermatologic disorders, including burns
  Cellulitis or other localized infected sites

FIGURE 1-27 Predisposing conditions for staphylococcal pneumonia.

Primary Staphylococcal Pneumonia

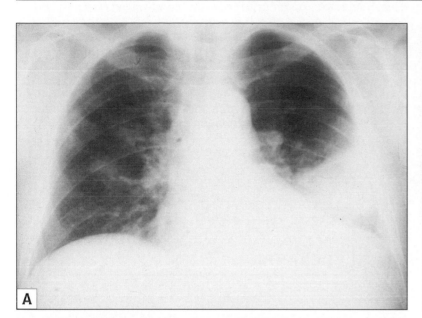

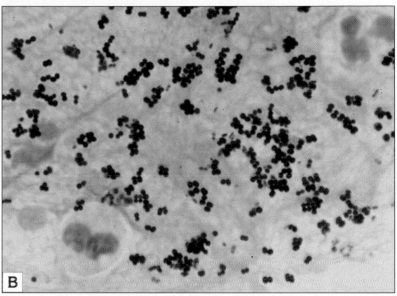

FIGURE 1-28 Primary staphylococcal pneumonia following influenza. A 52-year-old man was admitted after 10 days of an influenza-like illness (fever, malaise, arthralgias), for which he received 5 days of tetracycline therapy with no response. One day previously, he developed increased fever, cough, dyspnea, and pleuritic chest pain. **A**, Admission chest film revealed an alveolar infiltrate of the left lower lobe. **B**, Sputum Gram stain demonstrated numerous gram-positive cocci in clumps. Blood and sputum cultures grew *Staphylococcus aureus*. Influenza A serum titers on admission were 1:128, and at discharge 6 weeks later, 1:16.

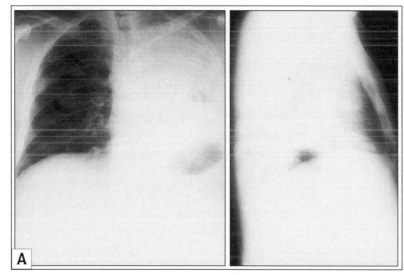

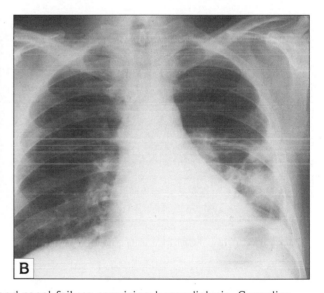

FIGURE 1-29 Chest radiograph showing atelectasis and mucous plugging complicating primary staphylococcal pneumonia. **A**, The patient in Figure 1-28 had a 6-week hospital course that was complicated by left lung collapse due to mucous plugging. **B**, The lung re-expanded 1 week later. Other complications included a myocardial infarction, and renal failure requiring hemodialysis. Complications are not uncommon in primary staphylococcal pneumonia. Other complications include cavity (abscess) formation (*see* Fig. 1-30), empyema necessitating adequate drainage, and formation of pneumatoceles, which occur predominantly in children.

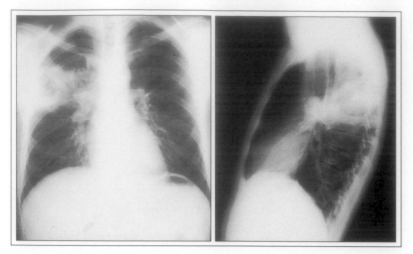

FIGURE 1-30 Posteroanterior and lateral chest films demonstrating staphylococcal aspiration pneumonia. A 27-year-old man developed fever, cough productive of blood-tinged sputum, and pleuritic chest pain 2 days following an episode of acute emesis. Admission chest film revealed consolidation of the posterior segment of the right upper lobe with cavitation. Sputum cultures grew *Staphylococcus aureus*. His hospital course was complicated by desquamation of the palms and severe hemoptysis. Patients with primary staphylococcal pneumonia are usually very toxic and may respond more slowly to appropriate antimicrobial therapy than patients with other bacterial pneumonias.

Secondary Staphylococcal Pneumonia

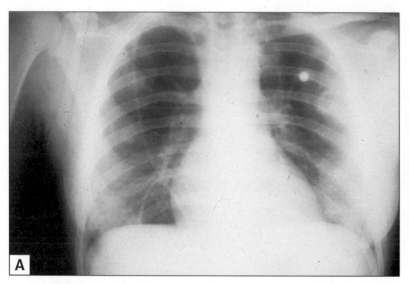

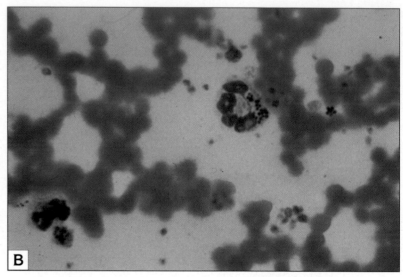

FIGURE 1-31 Hematogenous metastatic staphylococcal pneumonia secondary to catheter-related infection. A 20-year-old paraplegic man was hospitalized for possible sepsis. On examination, his temperature was 39° C and the site of his Broviac catheter was tender. **A**, Chest film showed multiple bilateral nodular lesions, one or two of which contained cavities. **B**, Sputum Gram stain showed mixed flora, but gram-positive cocci in clusters were demonstrated in the buffy coat of a peripheral blood smear. Two blood cultures grew *Staphylococcus aureus*. The Broviac catheter was removed, and the patient received antistaphylococcal therapy for 4 weeks.

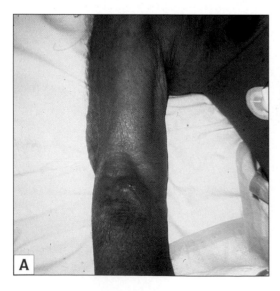

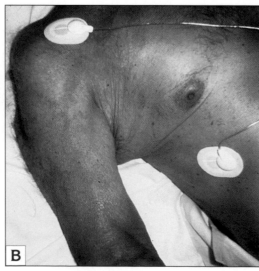

FIGURE 1-32 Suppurative phlebitis, metastatic pneumonia, and endocarditis due to intravenous catheter-related staphylococcal bacteremia. A 78-year-old man was transferred to the intensive care unit because of hypotension and obtundation several hours following a transurethral prostatic resection. An intravenous catheter was placed in the right cephalic vein to monitor central venous pressure. Fever subsequently developed, and blood cultures repeated over a 48-hour period grew *Staphylococcus aureus*. **A** and **B**, Phlebitis and surrounding cellulitis that extended to the anterior chest wall were noted. The intravenous catheter was removed, and 4 mL of purulent material was expressed from the puncture site. (*continued*)

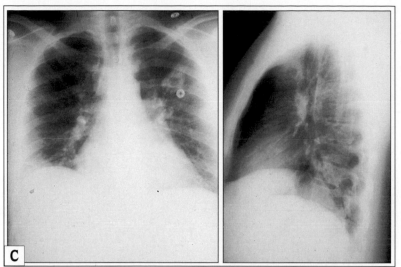

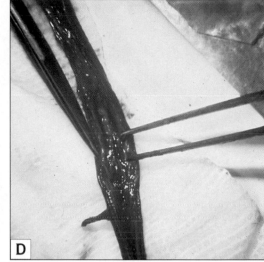

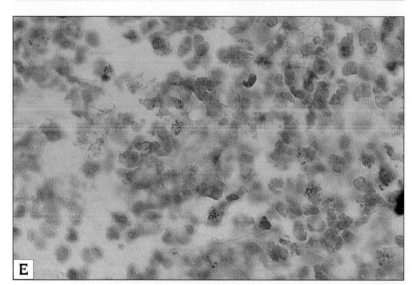

FIGURE 1-32 (*continued*) C, As seen on chest radiographs, multiple pulmonary infiltrates developed secondary to prolonged staphylococcal bacteremia. D, The entire cephalic vein was resected, which upon incising open revealed suppurative phlebitis. E, Gram stain of the purulent material demonstrated gram-positive cocci in clusters, and cultures grew *S. aureus*. Postoperatively, the patient deteriorated clinically and died 5 weeks later.

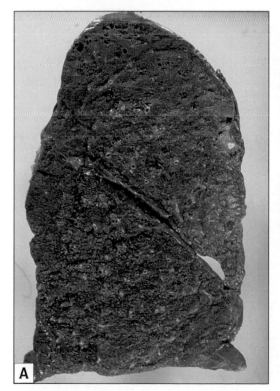

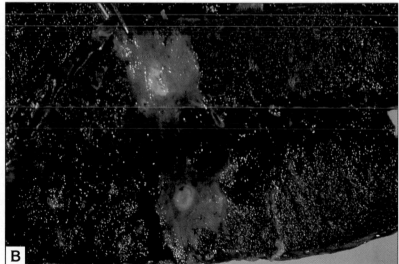

FIGURE 1-33 Autopsy examination in metastatic staphylococcal pneumonia and endocarditis. A and B, Postmortem examination of the lung from the patient in Figure 1-32 revealed multiple septic pulmonary thromboemboli with localized pneumonia and abscess formation. (*continued*)

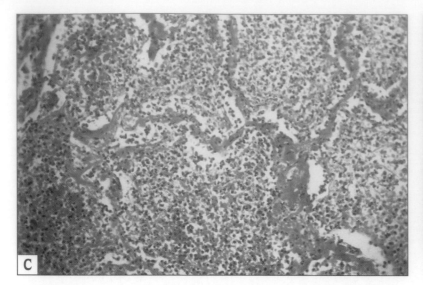

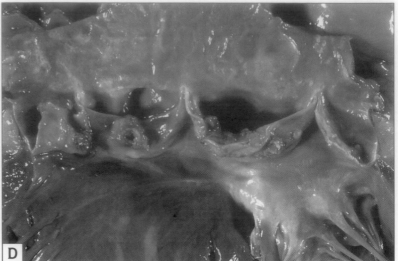

FIGURE 1-33 (*continued*) **C**, Microscopically, localized areas of acute and chronic inflammation with organized abscess formation were seen. **D**, All three cusps of the aortic valve displayed friable vegetations with a 3-mm perforation of the posterior cusp. Hematogenous staphylococcal pneumonia, unlike primary pneumonia, is characterized by multiple areas of bronchopneumonia with or without cavitation. Most commonly, this process is associated with an intravascular infection, either suppurative phlebitis in hospitalized patients with intravenous catheters or right-sided endocarditis in intravenous drug users. The pulmonary process in these latter patients may be due to prolonged bacteremia or septic embolization from infected vegetations on the tricuspid or pulmonary valve. Other less common associations are listed in Figure 1-27. In these patients, the sputum Gram stain and culture may not reveal staphylococci, although by definition, blood cultures are always positive. The most common complication in metastatic staphylococcal pneumonia is cavitation or abscess formation in the sites of necrotizing bronchopneumonia.

THERAPY FOR GRAM-POSITIVE PNEUMONIAS

A. Therapeutic options for gram-positive bacterial pneumonia: *Pneumococcal pneumonia*

Organism	Antibiotic	Dosage
Streptococcus pneumoniae	Procaine penicillin	600,000 U twice a day intramuscularly × 5–10 days
	Aqueous crystalline penicillin	1 MU every 4 hrs intravenously × 5–10 days
	Amoxicillin	250 mg every 8 hrs orally × 5–10 days
	Cefazolin	1.0 g every 8 hrs intravenously × 5–10 days
Penicillin-resistant	Vancomycin	0.5–1.0 g every 12 hrs intravenously × 5–10 days
	Ceftriaxone	1.0–2.0 g every 12–24 hrs intravenously × 5–10 days

B. Therapeutic options for gram-positive bacterial pneumonia: Group A streptococcal infections

Organism	Antibiotic	Dosage
Streptococcus pyogenes	Aqueous crystalline penicillin	1 MU every 4 hrs intravenously × 7–10 days
	Cefazolin	1.0–1.5 g every 6 hrs intravenously × 7–10 days
	Erythromycin	500 mg every 6 hrs intravenously × 7–10 days
Streptococcal toxic shock syndrome	Aqueous crystalline penicillin	2 MU every 4 hrs intravenously × 10–14 days
	Clindamycin	600–900 mg every 6–8 hrs intravenously × 10–14 days

FIGURE 1-34 Therapeutic options for gram-positive bacterial pneumonias. **A**, Pneumococcal pneumonia. **B**, Group A streptococcal infections. (*continued*)

C. Therapeutic options for gram-positive bacterial pneumonia: Streptococcal aspiration pneumonia

Organism	Antibiotic	Dosage
Anaerobic or microaerophilic streptococci	Aqueous crystalline penicillin Cefazolin Erythromycin	1 MU every 4 hrs intravenously × 7–10 days 1.0–1.5 g every 6 hrs intravenously × 7–10 days 500 mg every 6 hrs intravenously × 7–10 days

D. Therapeutic options for gram-positive bacterial pneumonia: Staphylococcal pneumonia

Organism	Antibiotic	Dosage
Staphylococcus aureus	Nafcillin Oxacillin Cefazolin	1.5–2.0 g every 4–6 hrs intravenously × 10–14 days 1.0–2.0 g every 4–6 hrs intravenously × 10–14 days 1.0–1.5 g every 4–6 hrs intravenously × 10–14 days
Methicillin-resistant	Vancomycin	0.5–1.0 g every 12 hrs intravenously × 10–14 days

FIGURE 1-34 *(continued)* **C,** Streptococcal aspiration pneumonia.
D, Staphylococcal pneumonia.

REFERENCE

1. Working Group on Severe Streptococcal Infections: Defining the group A streptococcal toxic shock syndrome: Rationale and consensus definition. *JAMA* 1993, 269:390–391.

SELECTED BIBLIOGRAPHY

Forni AL, Kaplan EL, Schlievert PM, Roberts RB: Clinical and microbiological characteristics of severe group A streptococcus infections and streptococcal toxic shock syndrome. *Clin Infect Dis* 1995, 21:333–340.

Musher DM: *Streptococcus pneumoniae.* In Mandell GL, Bennett JE, Dolin R (eds.): *Principles and Practice of Infectious Diseases*, 4th ed. New York: Churchill Livingstone; 1995:1811–1826.

Shlaes DM, *et al.*: Infections due to Lancefield group F and related streptococci (*S. milleri, S. anginosus*). *Medicine* 1981, 60:197–207.

Stevens DL: Invasive group A streptococcus infections. *Clin Infect Dis* 1992, 14:2–13.

Weinstein L, Fields BN: Staphylococcal pneumonia. *Semin Infect Dis* 1983, 5:47–55.

CHAPTER 2

Gram-Negative Bacterial Infections of the Lungs

Melanie J. Maslow

ETIOLOGY AND PATHOGENESIS

Etiologic agents of gram-negative bacillary pneumonia

Haemophilus influenzae	*Morganella morganii*	*Pseudomonas pseudomallei*
Klebsiella pneumoniae	*Salmonella* spp	*Providencia* spp
Escherichia coli	*Enterobacter* spp	*Pasteurella multocida*
Pseudomonas aeruginosa	*Serratia marcescens*	*Brucella* spp
Acinetobacter baumannii	*Moraxella catarrhalis*	*Francisella tularensis*
Citrobacter spp	*Pseudomonas cepacia*	*Yersinia pestis*
Proteus spp	*Xanthomonas maltophilia*	

FIGURE 2-1 Etiologic agents of gram-negative bacillary pneumonia. Gram-negative bacilli have been recognized as a cause of pneumonia for decades. Since the 1960s, this group of bacteria has assumed increasing importance in lower respiratory tract infection. Gram-negative bacilli cause both community-acquired and nosocomial pneumonia.

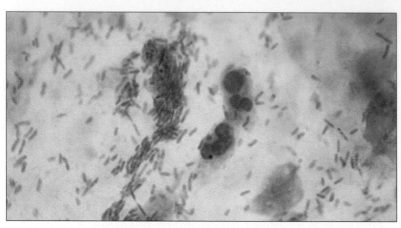

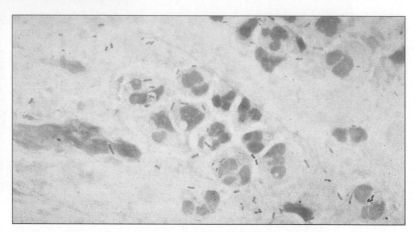

FIGURE 2-2 Sputum Gram stain showing polymorphonuclear leukocytes and numerous gram-negative bacilli. Gram-negative aerobic bacteria account for approximately 60% of cases of nosocomial pneumonia and are estimated to cause between 6% and 20% of community-acquired bacterial pneumonia. The mortality rate from gram-negative pneumonia ranges from 30% to 50%. This high rate is a function of both underlying host factors and the special virulence factors associated with these organisms [1].

FIGURE 2-3 Sputum Gram stain demonstrating intracellular gram-negative bacilli. Confirming that gram-negative bacilli are responsible for pneumonia is often a difficult clinical problem because these organisms may colonize the proximal airways. Gram-negative aerobic bacilli may be cultured from 2% to 11% of normal people, and *Haemophilus influenzae* may colonize up to 80% of the population. Correlation between culture results and sputum Gram stain results may provide supportive evidence that the organism is responsible for infection. (*Courtesy of* H. Murray, MD.)

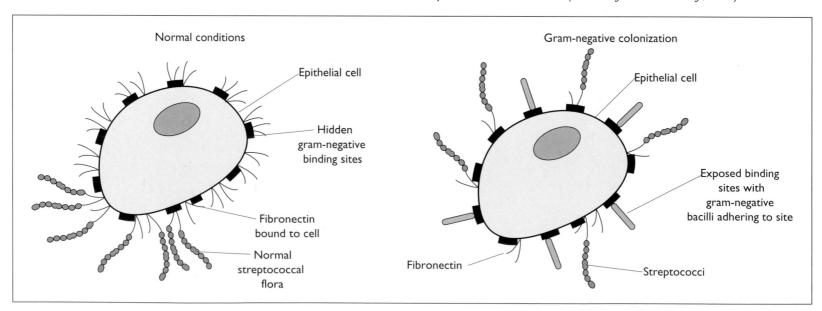

FIGURE 2-4 Mechanisms of adherence of gram-negative bacteria to epithelial cells. Colonization of the oropharynx by *Pseudomonas aeruginosa* and enteric gram-negative bacilli is uncommon in healthy people but develops frequently in acutely ill patients and those with chronic illnesses. The ability of cells to resist adherence by gram-negative bacilli is related to the concentration of fibronectin, a high-molecular-weight fibrous glycoprotein, on the cell surface.

Fibronectin on the surface of oral epithelial cells has binding sites for gram-positive organisms, such as *Staphylococcus aureus* and streptococci, but blocks the binding sites of gram-negative bacilli. Colonization of the respiratory tract is accompanied by increased protease levels in salivary secretions and a decreased amount of fibronectin on the cell surface. This decrease exposes gram-negative binding sites and results in colonization by gram-negative bacilli [2].

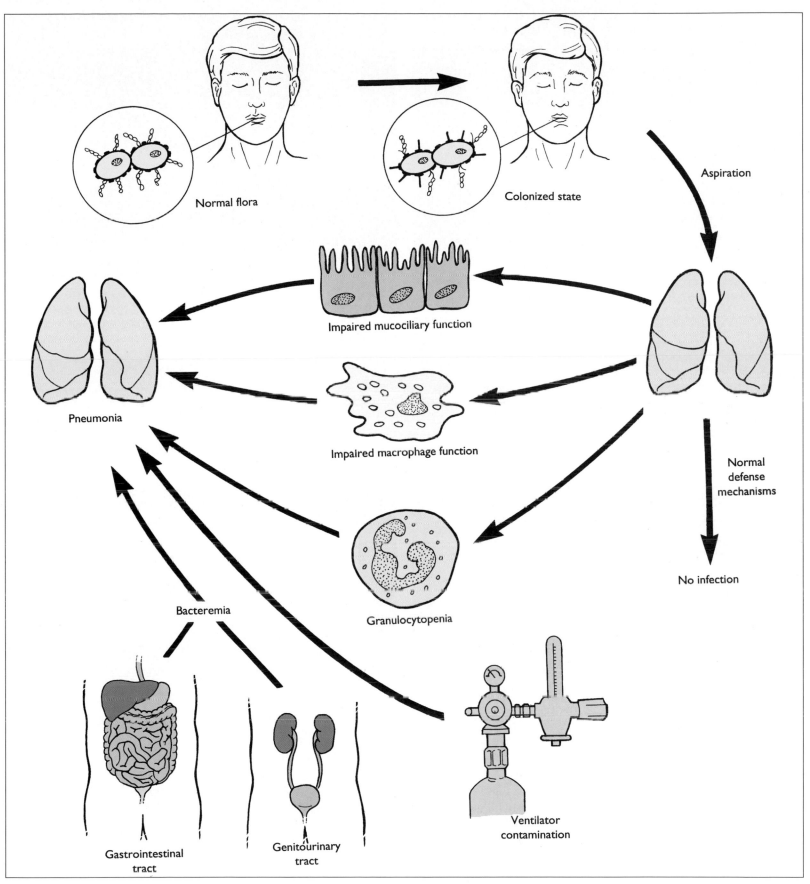

FIGURE 2-5 Pathogenesis of gram-negative pneumonia. Once gram-negative bacilli have established colonization, multiplication results in high bacterial concentrations in oral secretions. Secretions are then aspirated in small liquid boluses into the lungs. Pneumonia results if the pulmonary defense mechanisms are impaired by various mecha-nisms, including alveolar hypoxia, decreased mucociliary clearance, decreased phagocyte migration associated with alcoholism, and neutropenia. Other less frequent routes of infection are bacteremic spread to the lung from other foci of infection and aerosol contami-nation through respiratory equipment.

Predisposing factors to gram-negative pneumonia

Alcoholism
Cardiac disease
Chronic lung disease
Diabetes mellitus
Renal disease
Malignancy
Immunosuppressive therapy
AIDS
Institutionalization
Age > 60 years
Prior antibiotic therapy
Hospitalization
Neutropenia
Assisted ventilation
Burns
Postoperative state

FIGURE 2-6 Predisposing factors to gram-negative pneumonia. The risk factors predisposing to colonization and infection of the respiratory tract by gram-negative bacilli are listed. Specific factors may predispose to community-acquired and/or nosocomial infection. Often, multiple factors coexist within the same individual.

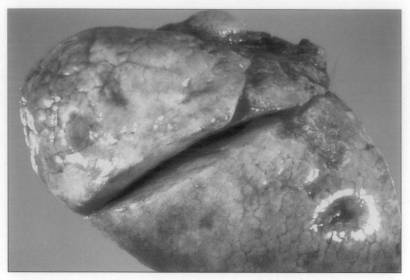

FIGURE 2-7 Pleural surface of the lung in gram-negative pneumonia. A gross photograph of the right lung shows white discoloration involving all three lobes, which represents consolidation. Microscopically, there is accumulation of fibrin and neutrophils in the alveolar space.

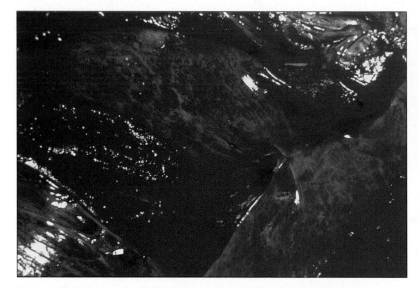

FIGURE 2-8 Lung surface early in the course of gram-negative pneumonia. On this close-up photograph, consolidation is first evident in the red hepatization stage in which the involved areas of lung are red, wet, and firm, grossly resembling the liver. Extensive extravasation of erythrocytes and fibrin occurs, and neurotrophils begin to fill alveolar spaces. The fibrin present has not yet contracted, and necrosis has not developed.

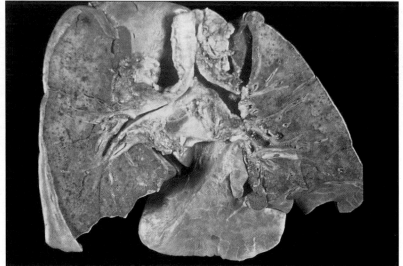

FIGURE 2-9 Gross pathology of diffuse bronchopneumonia commonly seen with the Enterobacteriaceae and *Pseudomonas aeruginosa*. The tan areas represent the gray hepatization stage of consolidation. Massive numbers of neutrophils and macrophages fill the alveolar spaces, and cellular degeneration is beginning. The fibrinous exudate is starting to contract, but necrosis is not yet visible.

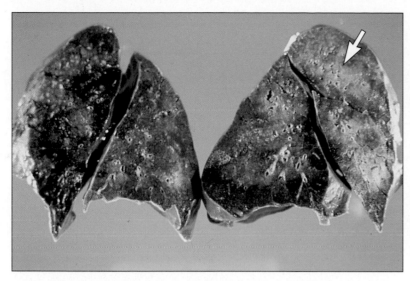

FIGURE 2-10 Diffuse bronchopneumonia on the cut surface of both lungs. The right lung is primarily involved (*arrow*). The tan areas represent gray hepatization or the late stage of consolidation. Necrosis has not occurred.

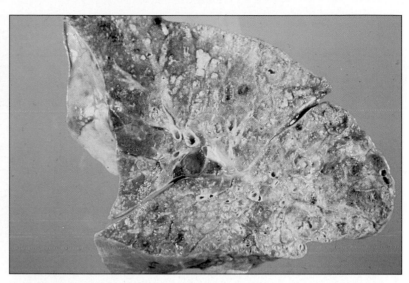

FIGURE 2-11 Cut surface of a lung specimen from a patient with necrotizing pneumonia. The white areas represent necrosis. The tan and gray areas show the later stage of consolidation. This pattern of infection is seen with several gram-negative bacteria, including *Pseudomonas*, *Serratia*, and *Acinetobacter*.

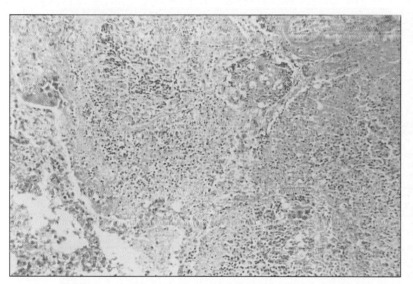

FIGURE 2-12 Photomicrograph of lung tissue in *Pseudomonas* pneumonia. The alveolar spaces are filled with neutrophils and fibrin. At this later stage of infection, the fibrinopurulent exudate has been partially removed by macrophages.

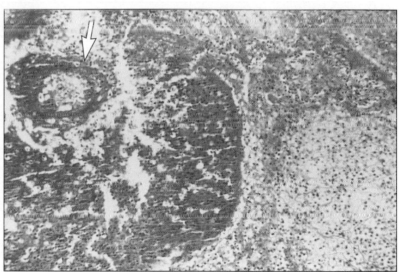

FIGURE 2-13 Photomicrograph of lung demonstrating a blood vessel with necrosis and inflammation. This picture of necrotizing vasculitis is typical of *Pseudomonas* pneumonia. Ischemia and necrosis of the pulmonary parenchyma supplied by the involved vessel (*arrow*) will eventually occur.

FIGURE 2-14 Photomicrograph of a lung with acute necrotizing pneumonia. The purple areas are necrotic material. The alveolar spaces are filled with neutrophils and fibrin.

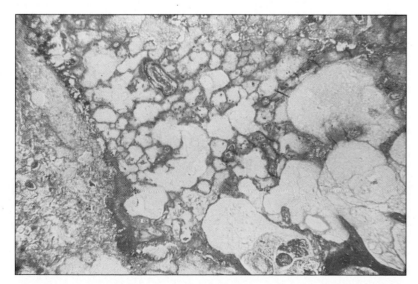

HAEMOPHILUS INFLUENZAE PNEUMONIA

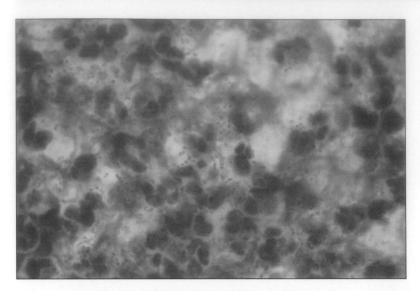

FIGURE 2-15 Sputum Gram stain from a patient with *Haemophilus influenzae* pneumonia demonstrating numerous polymorphonuclear leukocytes and small gram-negative coccobacilli. *H. influenzae* is a small (1 × 0.3 μm), nonmotile, non–spore-forming, gram-negative bacterium indigenous only to humans. Stained organisms vary microscopically from small coccobacilli to long filaments (pleomorphic), and these may stain inconsistently. *H. influenzae* is estimated to cause between 4% and 15% of cases of acute community-acquired pneumonia. The true incidence of infection is hard to determine accurately due to difficulty in growing the organism and the high degree of colonization [3].

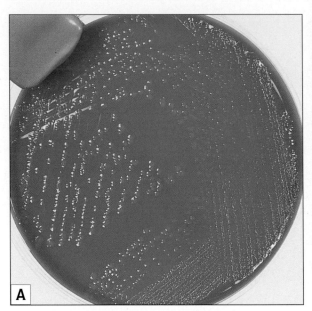

A

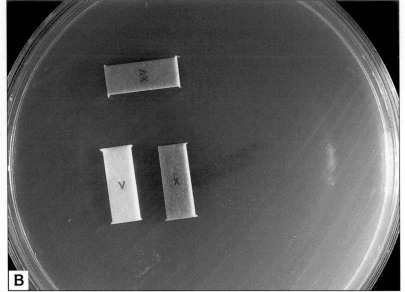

B

FIGURE 2-16 Colonies of *Haemophilus influenzae* on chocolate media. **A,** Culture plate showing typical colony morphology of unencapsulated *H. influenzae*. Most clinical isolates of *H. influenzae* are unencapsulated. These colonies are granular, transparent to slightly opaque, circular, and dome-shaped. Colonies of encapsulated isolates are larger, mucoid, and iridescent in oblique or ultraviolet light. *H. influenzae* is a facultative anaerobe. Although not a strict requirement, some strains grow best in 5% to 10% carbon dioxide. Viability is lost rapidly, requiring immediate inoculation of clinical specimens onto appropriate media. **B,** Aerobic growth of *H. influenzae* requires two supplements, factors X and V. A faint halo of growth is seen between the X and V strips and surrounding the XV strip. The requirement for both factors differentiates *H. influenzae* from *H. parainfluenzae*, which requires only V factor for growth. X factor is supplied by heat-stable iron-containing pigments that supply protoporphyrins essential for catalases, peroxidases, and cytochromes. V factor, which is heat-liable, is a coenzyme that can be supplied by NAD, NADP, or nicotinamide nucleoside. Chocolate media, often preferred for isolation, is prepared by adding sheep blood to an enriched agar base medium at a high enough temperature to lyse the red cells and release X and V factors.

Carriage rates and pathogenicity of *Haemophilus influenzae*

Strains	Carriage rates	Pathogenicity
Unencapsulated	50%–80%	Exacerbations of chronic bronchitis, otitis media, sinusitis, and conjunctivitis Bacteremia rare Patients commonly adults
Encapsulated, type b	2%–4%	Meningitis, epiglottitis, pneumonia, empyema, septic arthritis, cellulitis, osteomyelitis, pericarditis, and bacteremia Rarely glossitis, tenosynovitis, peritonitis, endocarditis, and ventriculitis (associated with shunts)
Encapsulated, types a, c–f	1%–2%	Rarely pathogenic

FIGURE 2-17 Carriage rates and pathogenicity of *Haemophilus influenzae*. *H. influenzae* is normally found in the pharynx. From infancy onward, carriage of one or more strains for days to months is common, and up to 80% of the population may be carriers. Most carriers harbor unencapsulated strains, but 3% to 5% have encapsulated strains. Of the six encapsulated serotypes (a–f), the majority of invasive disease is caused by serotype b. A natural or acquired deficiency of immunity to encapsulated strains leads to tissue invasion, with a high frequency of bacteremia and metastatic foci. Failure of local pulmonary defense mechanisms leads to pneumonia with unencapsulated strains and a low frequency of bacteremia. Routine vaccination of young children in the United States with a conjugate type b vaccine has resulted in a dramatic decline in invasive type b disease in this population. (*Adapted from* Turk [4]; with permission.)

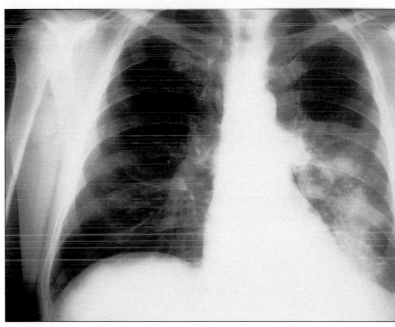

FIGURE 2-18 Chest radiograph from an alcoholic man with left lower lobe pneumonia due to *Haemophilus influenzae*. Predisposing factors to *H. influenzae* pneumonia in adults include chronic lung disease, diabetes, neoplasm, alcoholism, and immunodeficiency states. Adults with chronic bronchitis are at increased risk of both community-acquired and nosocomial *H. influenzae* pneumonia. The clinical presentation of pneumonia is similar to that of *Streptococcus pneumoniae* except that *Haemophilus* infection may have a slower clinical onset. The spectrum of radiologic findings includes segmental, lobar, bronchopneumonic, and interstitial infiltrates. Pleural effusion occurs in one half of cases.

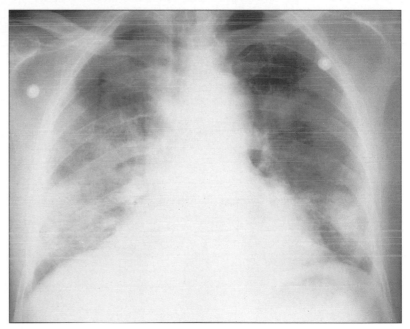

FIGURE 2-19 Chest radiograph of fulminant *Haemophilus influenzae* pneumonia in an elderly patient with gastric carcinoma showing bilateral infiltrates. Fulminant infection with respiratory failure has been described in older patients with serious underlying medical conditions as well as in normal individuals. Treatment of *H. influenzae* pneumonia requires knowledge of resistance patterns. Resistant strains of *H. influenzae* have been recognized in the United States since 1973 and are now common. Ampicillin resistance is mediated by β-lactamase production and varies by geographic area. Resistance to chloramphenicol, tetracycline, trimethoprim-sulfamethoxazole, rifampin, erythromycin, and older cephalosporins has been documented. Resistance has not been demonstrated to the third-generation cephalosporins and fluoroquinolones [5,6].

PSEUDOMONAS PNEUMONIA

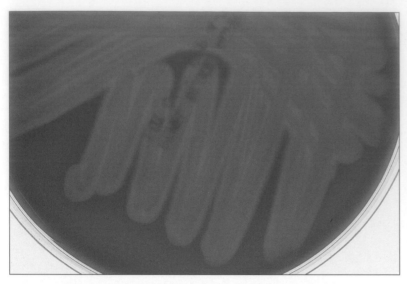

FIGURE 2-20 *Pseudomonas aeruginosa* colonies on blood agar demonstrating strong hemolysis. The organism forms flat spreading colonies with irregular edges. Mucoid strains are frequently isolated from the respiratory tract of patients with cystic fibrosis. *P. aeruginosa* is an obligate aerobe that grows readily on a wide range of media and has a characteristic grapelike odor. The ability to use simple organic molecules as a carbon and energy source allows multiplication in solutions such as weak antiseptics, saline, and soaps.

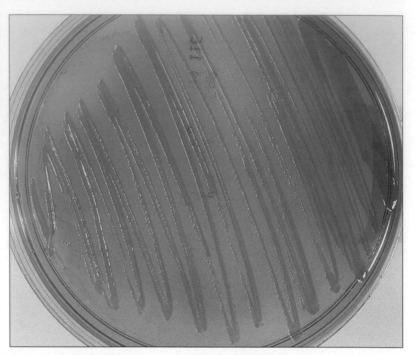

FIGURE 2-21 Colonies of *Pseudomonas aeruginosa* on MacConkey agar. *P. aeruginosa* produces a fluorescent water-soluble pigment, pyoverdin, and a second blue nonfluorescent pigment called *pyocyanin*. The pigments diffuse around colonies and aid in the initial identification. Pyocyanin suppresses growth of other bacteria and is toxic to the respiratory epithelium, facilitating *Pseudomonas* colonization.

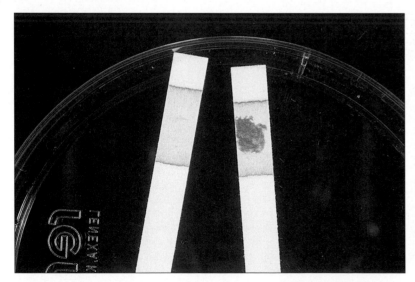

FIGURE 2-22 Oxidase test. The oxidase test indicates the presence of the enzyme cytochrome oxidase, which participates in both the electron transport and nitrate metabolism of some bacteria, including *Pseudomonas*. A purple-colored reaction results when a small portion of a colony is rubbed on to filter paper saturated with the oxidase reagent, yielding a positive result (*right*). A positive reaction excludes the organism from the family Enterobacteriaceae.

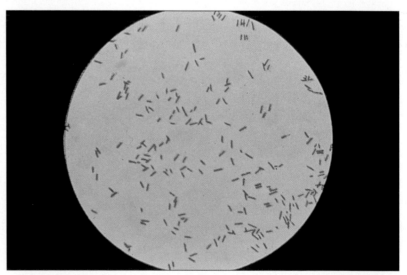

FIGURE 2-23 Typical morphology of *Pseudomonas* on Gram stain. The organism appears as a straight or slightly curved rod. Unlike the Enterobacteriaceae, *Pseudomonas* species have polar rather than peritrichous flagella. Clinical isolates may possess pili that act as adhesins to facilitate attachment to epithelial cells.

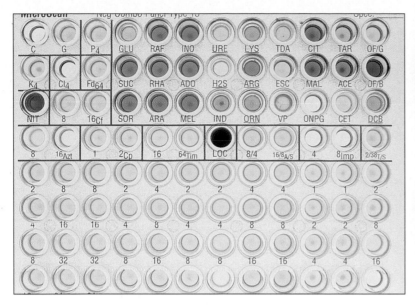

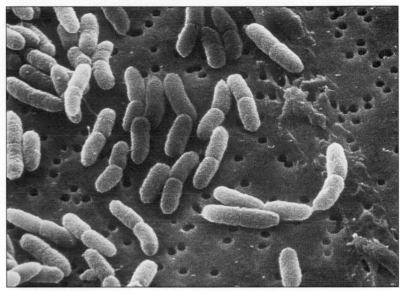

FIGURE 2-24 Microscan panel with *Pseudomonas aeruginosa*. This identification and susceptibility system uses wells that are incubated with a suspension of organisms for 15 to 18 hours (MicroScan Division, Baxter Healthcare Corp.). The identification and susceptibilities are interpreted visually or with an automated reader combined with a computer identification system. *P. aeruginosa* does not ferment lactose, is oxidase and catalase positive, oxidizes glucose in O–F carbohydrate base, and is unable to decarboxylase lysine or ornithine.

FIGURE 2-25 Scanning electron micrograph of *Pseudomonas aeruginosa*. This organism causes three distinct presentations of lower respiratory tract infection: nonbacteremic pneumonia, diffuse necrotizing infection with bacteremia, and chronic lower respiratory tract disease in patients with cystic fibrosis. The organism appears as rod-shaped bodies and measures 0.5 to 0.8 μm in width and 1.5 to 3.0 μm in length. Organisms can occur singly, in pairs, or in short chains. (*Courtesy of* N. Baker, PhD.)

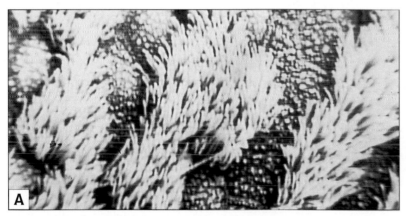

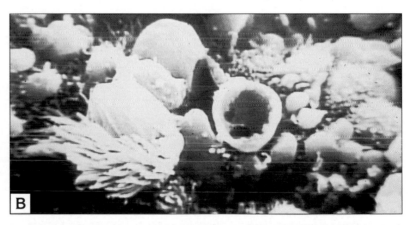

FIGURE 2-26 Scanning electron micrographs of normal and destroyed respiratory epithelium after *Pseudomonas* infection. **A,** Normal respiratory epithelium. **B,** The same tissue, after 12 to 16 hours of infection with exotoxin-A– and protease-producing *Pseudomonas*, shows tissue necrosis and cell death. *P. aeruginosa* possesses many substances, including extracellular

toxins (exotoxin A), proteolytic factors (elastase and collagenase) that cause necrosis of alveolar septa, hemolytic factors that destroy surfactant causing atelectasis, leukocidin, and endotoxin. Under certain conditions, a polysaccharide capsule, or slime, is produced that inhibits phagocytosis by alveolar macrophages. (*Courtesy of* N. Baker, PhD.)

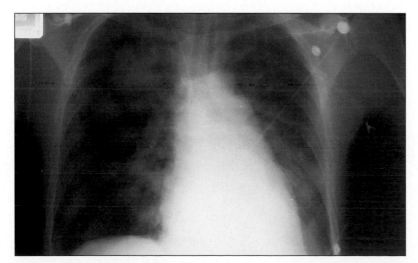

FIGURE 2-27 Chest radiograph in nonbacteremic *Pseudomonas aeruginosa* pneumonia showing multiple areas of confluent airspace disease bilaterally. Lower respiratory tract infection with *Pseudomonas* occurs almost exclusively in patients with compromised local or systemic defense mechanisms. Diffuse nonbacteremic bronchopneumonia occurs in patients with severe chronic cardiopulmonary disease and in hospitalized patients. This form of pneumonia can present as nodular infiltrates, often with cavitation, and as lobar consolidation.

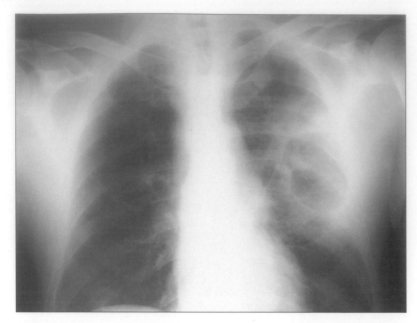

FIGURE 2-28 Chest radiography of a patient with oat cell carcinoma and a cavitary lesion in the left midlung field due to a *Pseudomonas* abscess. The patient also had blood cultures positive for *P. aeruginosa*. Bacteremic *Pseudomonas* pneumonia occurs primarily in patients with neutropenia or malignancy and is a fulminant disease with a high mortality. Bacteremic infection usually begins in the lung with bloodstream invasion and secondary sites of infection. There is usually a mixture of alveolar and interstitial infiltrates with coagulation necrosis or abscess formation.

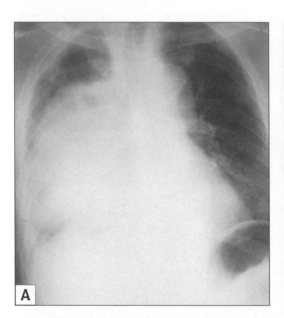
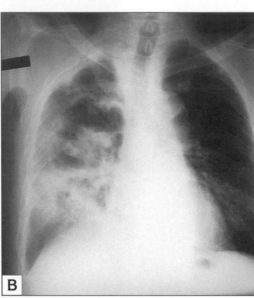

FIGURE 2-29 Chest radiographs of cavitary pneumonia due to *Pseudomonas aeruginosa*. **A**, A 75-year-old black man admitted with cavitary pneumonia involving the right upper, right middle, and right lower lobes. **B**, A follow-up chest radiograph 3 days later shows progression of infection with cavitary lesions and air-fluid levels in the right middle and right upper lobes. The abscesses slowly contracted and healed with scarring over 6 months.

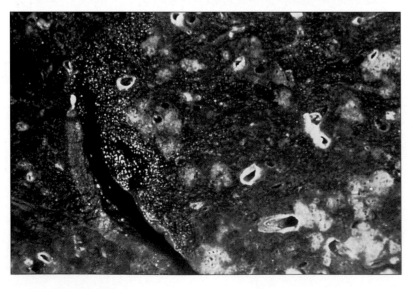

FIGURE 2-30 Autopsy sample of lung parenchyma from a patient with *Pseudomonas aeruginosa* pneumonia. A close-up photograph shows areas of hemorrhage with multiple yellow-white abscesses. Diffuse *Pseudomonas* bronchopneumonia may be associated with microabscess or macroabscess formation, necrosis of alveolar septa, and focal hemorrhage.

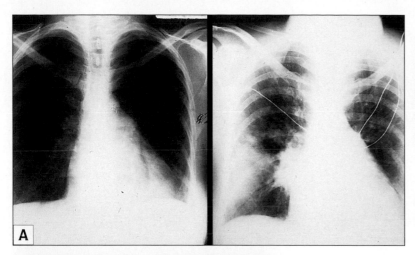

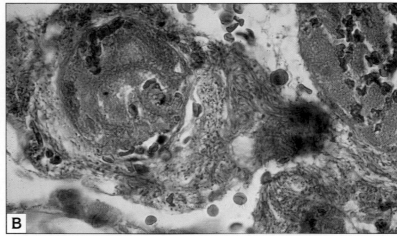

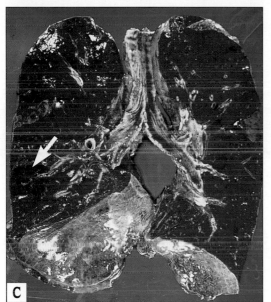

FIGURE 2-31 Fulminant necrotizing *Pseudomonas* with bacteremia. **A**, An immunocompromised woman presented with nonproductive cough, low-grade fever, and malaise (*left panel*). Three days later, she developed fulminant *Pseudomonas* bacteremia presenting clinically as pulmonary embolism with infarction and development of a wedge-shaped, pleural-based infiltrate of the right midlung field (*right panel*). This form of infection is characterized by invasion of vessels, vascular necrosis, necrotizing pneumonia, and hemorrhagic infarction. The lung involvement is the pulmonary counterpart of the skin lesion ecthyma gangrenosum. **B**, Microscopic pathology shows diffuse vessel wall necrosis of a small pulmonary artery with bacillary invasion of the media. The vessel lumen contains unclotted erythrocytes. Many bacilli were present in the media on higher magnification. The presence of massive numbers of bacteria within the vessel wall may give a basophilic discoloration with routine hematoxylin and eosin stain. **C**, Gross examination of the lungs showed areas of patchy consolidation throughout and numerous 2- to 4-mm gray-yellow nodules. There was a well-defined, wedge-shaped infarct in the middle lobe of the right lung (*arrow*). (*From* Soave *et al.* [7]; with permission.)

KLEBSIELLA PNEUMONIA

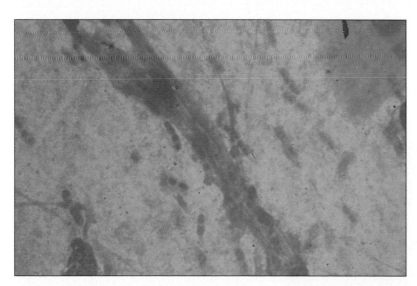

FIGURE 2-32 Sputum Gram stain of *Klebsiella pneumoniae*. *Klebsiella* organisms tend to be larger than other members of the Enterobacteriaceae. There are moderate numbers of large gram-negative–staining bacilli and inflammatory cells. *Klebsiella* has been recognized as a pathogen for humans from the time of Friedländer, when it was called the Friedländer bacillus. *K. pneumoniae* is often part of the normal flora of hospitalized patients, alcoholics, diabetics, and nursing home residents. *K. pneumoniae* is the *Klebsiella* species most commonly isolated from patients with pneumonia; *K. oxytoca* is isolated less frequently. The Friedländer bacillus probably represents *K. pneumoniae* types 1 through 6. (*Courtesy of* the Schering Corp.)

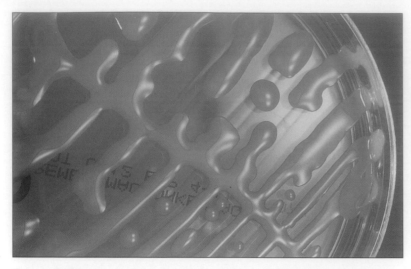

FIGURE 2-33 Lactose-fermenting colonies of *Klebsiella pneumoniae* on MacConkey agar. *Klebsiella* forms large mucoid colonies due to the prominent polysaccharide capsule. The capsule is a virulence factor in preventing phagocytosis and retarding leukocyte migration to the infected area. *K. pneumoniae* is the most frequent cause of community-acquired gram-negative pneumonia after *Haemophilus influenzae*.

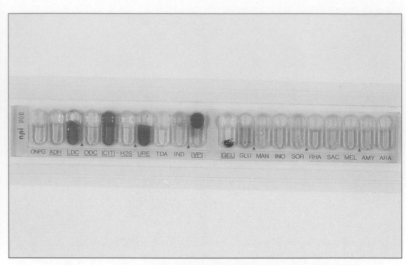

FIGURE 2-34 API 20E gram-negative panel after incubation with *Klebsiella pneumoniae*. The API system (bioMérieux Vitek, Inc.) uses dried reagents in plastic capsules into which a suspension of organisms is placed and incubated for 18 to 24 hours. This organism ferments lactose, does not produce hydrogen sulfide or indole, and produces a positive Voges-Proskauer reaction. The organism is intrinsically resistant to ampicillin and carbenicillin and has acquired R-plasmids mediating cephalosporin and aminoglycoside resistance. Treatment of nosocomial isolates requires knowledge of susceptibility patterns. Studies with the β-lactamase–stable cephalosporins, aztreonam, imipenem, and quinolones have yielded excellent cure rates.

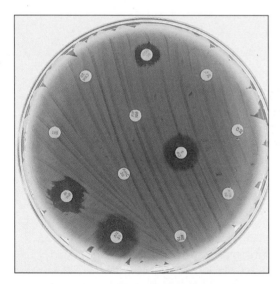

FIGURE 2-35 Kirby-Bauer susceptibility testing using a multidrug-resistant isolate of *Klebsiella pneumoniae*. This organism is sensitive only to imipenem, amikacin, and ciprofloxacin. Transferable plasmid-mediated resistance to late-generation cephalosporins in this genus has been increasingly reported in this country. Nosocomial outbreaks as well as sporadic cases have been reported [8].

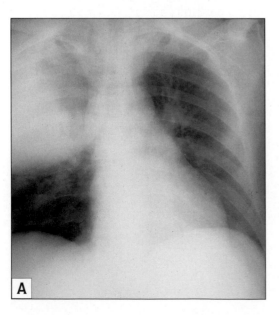

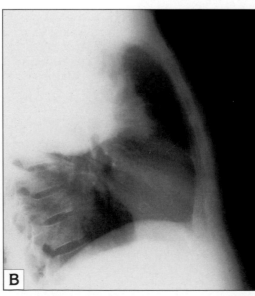

FIGURE 2-36 Chest radiographs of right upper lobe pneumonia due to *Klebsiella pneumoniae*, demonstrating the classic picture of infiltration with a bulging fissure. This radiologic finding occurs secondary to underlying necrotic inflammation and hemorrhage. Extensive scarring, necrosis, and abscess formation are characteristic of *Klebsiella* pneumonia. Microscopically, acute *Klebsiella* pneumonia is characterized by a diffuse intraalveolar inflammatory exudate that contains a large number of foamy macrophages in addition to neutrophils. Grossly, the lung is red to gray in color, and the cut surface may have a mucoid appearance. **A**, Posteroanterior view. **B**, Lateral view.

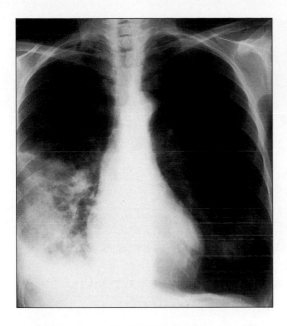

Figure 2-37 Chest radiograph from a 60-year-old woman with chronic obstructive pulmonary disease demonstrating a large right lower and middle lobe infiltrate secondary to *Klebsiella pneumoniae* infection. Lobar pneumonia is one of the primary infections caused by this organism. A frequent presentation is a lower lobe or segmental pneumonia that is indistinguishable radiographically from other gram-negative pneumonias. Sputum can be gray-green, blood-tinged, or currant jelly–like in consistency. Community-acquired infection is limited to compromised hosts and predominantly involves the elderly, diabetics, alcoholics, and patients with lung disease. Pneumonia is characteristically of acute onset, severe, and destructive.

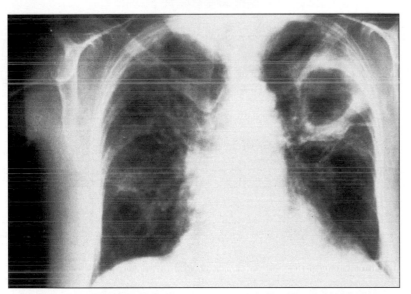

Figure 2-38 Chest radiograph showing chronic cavitary left upper lobe pneumonia secondary to *Klebsiella pneumoniae*. This unusual form of infection follows the acute disease and is characterized by abscess formation, anemia, and weight loss. The radiographic picture may mimic that of tuberculosis with formation of a thick-walled cavity. Chronic cavitary pneumonia is rarely reported today, and a review of cases raises the question of whether these patients had concomitant anaerobic infection [9].

ESCHERICHIA COLI PNEUMONIA

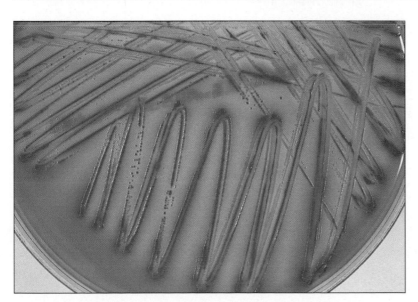

Figure 2-39 Lactose-fermenting *Escherichia coli* colonies on MacConkey agar. The acid products formed from metabolic processes lower the pH of the medium near the colony, turning the indicator red. *E. coli* is the best known and most common member of the Enterobacteriaceae and the bacterial species most commonly recovered in the clinical laboratory. This genus is motile and has peritrichous flagella.

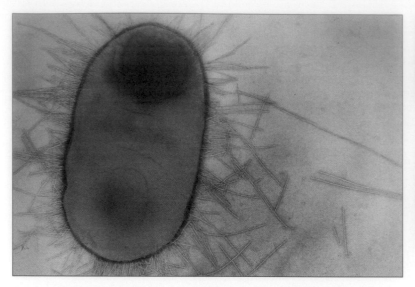

FIGURE 2-40 Scanning electron micrograph of *Escherichia coli* demonstrating the peritrichous flagella. The outermost border of *E. coli* displays fimbrae, fibrils, and/or colonizing factors that are indispensable in promoting adherence to mucosal surfaces. Strains that have the capacity to cause opportunistic infection generally have one or more virulence factors, including hemolysin production, serum resistance, and enhanced iron-uptake systems. No specific virulence factor in *E. coli* is known to be associated with respiratory tract disease.

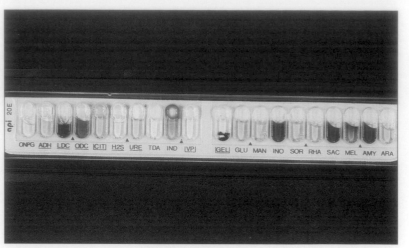

FIGURE 2-41 API 20E panel after incubation with *Escherichia coli*. In addition to lactose fermentation, *E. coli* is recognized by the positive indole, lysine, and methyl red reactions, negative Voges-Proskauer reaction, absent urease and phenylalanine deaminase activity, and absence of hydrogen sulfide production.

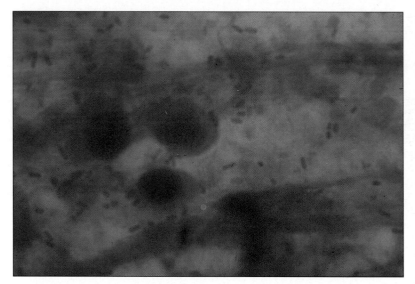

FIGURE 2-42 Sputum Gram stain in *Escherichia coli* pneumonia. On Gram stain, there are inflammatory cells with a moderate number of uniformly staining, small, gram-negative bacilli. *E. coli* ranks second after *Klebsiella pneumoniae* as the cause of community-acquired gram-negative aerobic pneumonia and ranks fourth as the cause of gram-negative nosocomial infections. Patients with community-acquired *E. coli* pneumonia are usually middle-aged to elderly with underlying diseases including diabetes, urinary tract infections, cirrhosis, and chronic cardiac or lung disease. (*Courtesy of* J.J. Rahal, Jr, MD.)

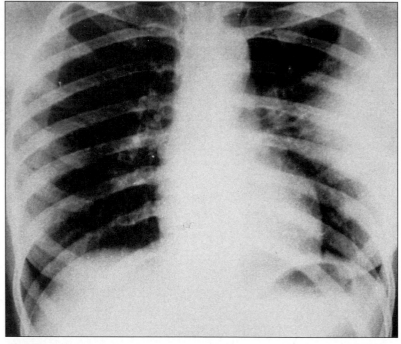

FIGURE 2-43 Chest radiograph of *Escherichia coli* pneumonia. Pneumonia develops after microaspiration of colonized upper airway secretions. *E. coli* infection causes bronchopneumonia involving the lower lobes and may result in empyema in one third of cases and bacteremia in one third of cases. On histologic section, the alveoli are filled with serum and moderate numbers of mononuclear cells. The mortality may exceed 50%. *E. coli* bacteremia from a gastrointestinal or urologic source results in pneumonia more commonly than bacteremia from other Enterobacteriaceae [10].

PROTEUS PNEUMONIA

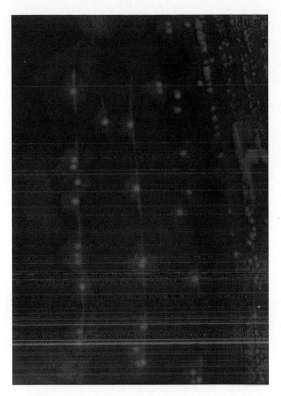

FIGURE 2-44 *Proteus mirabilis* on blood agar. *Proteus* species are lactose-negative, motile bacilli that produce abundant urease and are distinguishable by their ability to elaborate phenylalanine deaminase. *P. mirabilis* (indole negative) and *Proteus vulgaris* (indole positive) form a thin spreading growth, or swarm, from the original inoculum on the surface of moist agar media because of active motility.

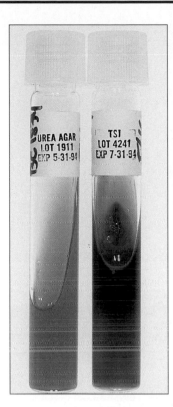

FIGURE 2-45 Urea agar slant and triple sugar iron agar inoculated with *Proteus mirabilis*. The ability of an organism to hydrolyze urea to ammonia and carbon dioxide is determined by inoculating it on a urea-containing agar slant. Urease-producing organisms produce alkaline products, which turn the phenol red indicator red to purple. Triple sugar irons (TSI) agar detects the ability to produce gas from the fermentation of sugars, to produce hydrogen sulfide gas, and to ferment lactose and sucrose. Production of hydrogen sulfide turns the medium black due to formation of an iron-containing precipitate.

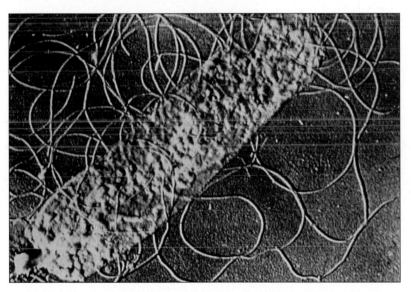

FIGURE 2-46 Scanning electron micrograph of *Proteus mirabilis* demonstrating hundreds of flagella per cell. This organism and other species are predominantly causes of nosocomial pneumonia but can cause community-acquired infection, especially in elderly patients with lung disease or alcoholism. Infection is acquired by aspiration of colonized pharyngeal secretions.

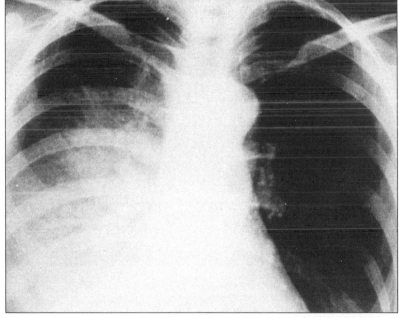

FIGURE 2-47 Chest radiograph of *Proteus mirabilis* pneumonia with a right lower lobe infiltrate. *Proteus* species produce a clinical picture similar to that of *Klebsiella* infection, with fever, chills, dyspnea, and purulent sputum. Dense infiltrates in the posterior segment of an upper lobe or superior segment of the right lower lobe are common. Progression to abscess formation or empyema may occur. Infection may be more insidious than with other gram-negative pneumonias, especially in patients with emphysema or chronic bronchitis, with patients complaining of worsening bronchitic symptoms for several weeks before the onset of pneumonia.

ENTEROBACTER PNEUMONIA

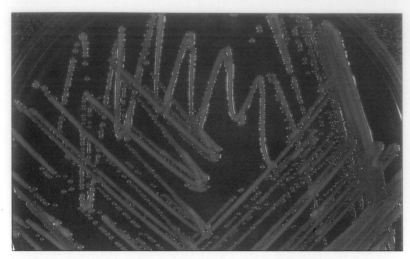

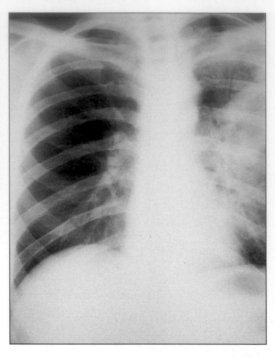

FIGURE 2-48 *Enterobacter aerogenes* colonies on MacConkey agar. This organism is a lactose fermenter and widely distributed in nature. It is similar to *Klebsiella* except that this genus is motile, ornithine positive, and less heavily encapsulated. There are 12 species, with *E. aerogenes* and *Enterobacter cloacae* the most common clinical isolates.

FIGURE 2-49 Chest radiograph of nosocomial pneumonia due to *Enterobacter aerogenes* showing a diffuse left upper and lower lobe bronchopneumonia. *Enterobacter* causes bronchopneumonia in elderly nursing-home residents and hospitalized patients. Community-acquired infection due to this organism is rare. Resistance mechanisms involve constitutive and inducible chromosomal mechanisms in addition to plasmids [11].

SERRATIA PNEUMONIA

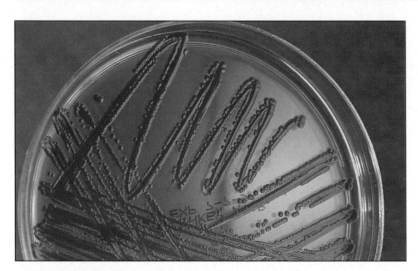

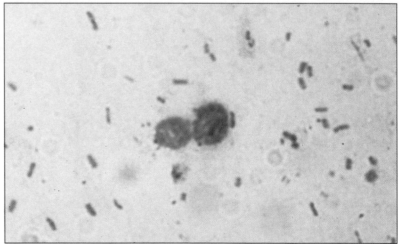

FIGURE 2-50 Pigmented colonies of *Serratia marcescens* on MacConkey agar. *Serratia* are motile organisms that ferment lactose slowly and are widely distributed in nature. *S. marcescens* is the most common species seen clinically. A minority of isolates produce a red pigment called *prodigiosin*. *Serratia* usually infects hospitalized patients with serious underlying illness or those receiving broad-spectrum antibiotics, causing an acute, necrotizing bronchopneumonia with abscess formation. Infection resembles other gram-negative pneumonias microscopically. Infection is sometimes associated with "pseudohemoptysis" when a pigmented strain is involved.

FIGURE 2-51 Sputum Gram stain of *Serratia marscescens* pneumonia. The Gram stain shows many polymorphonuclear leukocytes and multiple gram-negative bacilli. Vasculitis of scattered veins and arteries may be found in 75% of cases, but unlike that seen with *Pseudomonas aeruginosa*, intramural bacilli are not found [12]. (*Courtesy of* G. Owens, MD.)

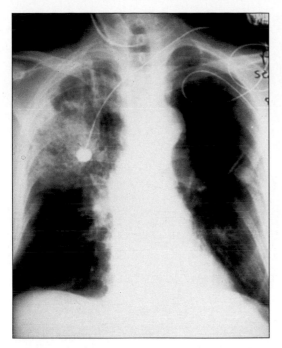

Figure 2-52 Chest radiograph showing necrotizing pneumonia due to *Serratia marcescens*. There is a patchy right upper lobe infiltrate with areas of necrosis in the upper lung zone. (*Courtesy of* G. Owens, MD.)

ACINETOBACTER PNEUMONIA

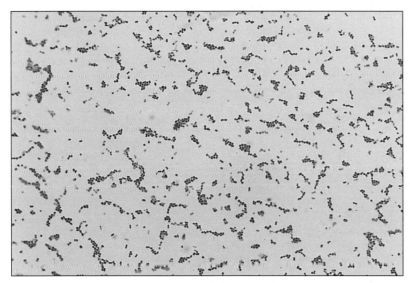

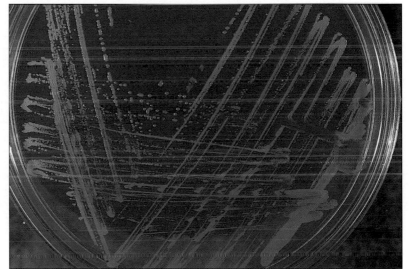

Figure 2-53 Gram stain of *Acinetobacter baumannii*. *Acinetobacter* demonstrate a unique morphology compared with other gram-negative bacilli. *Acinetobacter* are nonmotile, usually encapsulated, and oxidase negative and can be isolated from many environmental sources. They usually appear as coccobacillary cells, often appearing as diplococci, and may be confused with *Neisseria* and *Haemophilus* on Gram stain. Pneumonia due to *Acinetobacter* is primarily nosocomial, although community-acquired cases have been reported.

Figure 2-54 *Acinetobacter* colonies on MacConkey agar. This organism grows well on MacConkey agar, and gray-white colonies 2 to 3 mm in diameter are visible after 18 to 24 hours. Until recently, the genus *Acinetobacter* contained one species, *A calcoaceticus*, subdivided into two subspecies, *anitratus* and *lwoffi*. In 1986, the taxonomy of the genus was changed to include 12 different groups referred to as *genospecies*. *A. baumanii* accounts for most of the clinical isolates. These organisms are widely distributed in the environment.

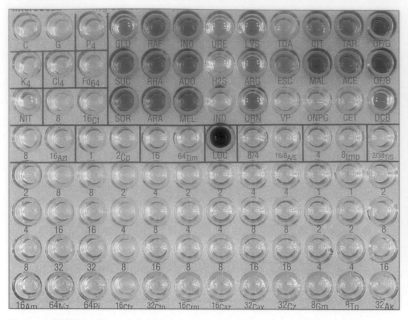

FIGURE 2-55 Microscan panel of *Acinetobacter baumanii*. This organism is oxidase negative and catalase positive, and it is differentiated from the Enterobacteriaceae by its failure to grow in the butt of triple sugar iron agar and its inability to reduce nitrate. The treatment of infections due to *Acinetobacter* species is complicated by the widespread multidrug resistance of the organism. Most strains are still susceptible to imipenem, amikacin, trimethoprim-sulfamethoxazole, quinolones, and third-generation cephalosporins [13].

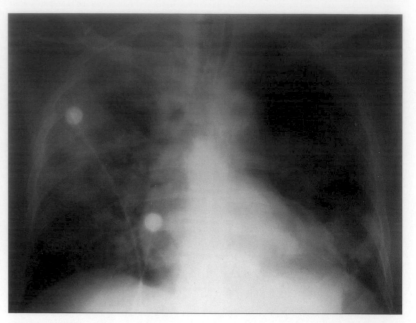

FIGURE 2-56 Chest radiography of community-acquired *Acinetobacter* pneumonia. This fulminant disease is often accompanied by positive blood cultures. It occurs in older persons with chronic diseases, especially alcoholism, and presents with respiratory distress and severe hypoxemia. The radiography findings are not distinctive and may include a lobar or bronchopneumonic pattern. The infiltrates may progress to bilateral involvement on therapy. Pleural effusion occurred in one half of the patients and the mortality rate was 43% in one study. A cluster of *Acinetobacter* pneumonia was reported in foundry workers, associated with chronic exposure to metallic dust [14].

THERAPY

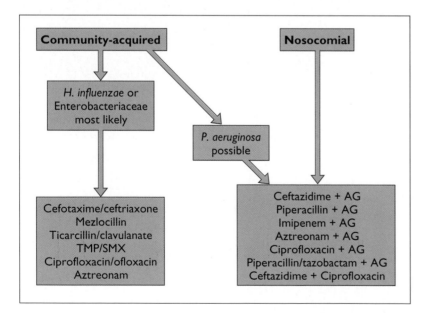

FIGURE 2-57 Treatment options for gram-negative bacillary pneumonia. Empiric treatment of gram-negative bacillary pneumonia should be selected with an awareness of the likely pathogens involved, antibiotic susceptibility patterns within the environment (community, nursing home, or hospital), and the patient's predisposing factors for infection. After the pathogen has been identified, therapy can be modified based on the *in vitro* susceptibility data. *Pseudomonas aeruginosa* pneumonia should be considered in patients with granulocytopenia, cystic fibrosis, and HIV infection, especially those on trimethoprim/sulfamethoxazole (TMP/SMX) prophylaxis. (AG—aminoglycoside.)

ACKNOWLEDGMENTS

The author thanks Herbert Koch and Anthony Morales for their excellent photography; Eli Lilly and Company for their contribution to this chapter; and Dr. K. Sandhu for her microbiologic expertise.

REFERENCES

1. Fang G, Fine M, Orloff J, *et al.*: New and emerging etiologies for community-acquired pneumonia with implications for therapy: A prospective multicenter study of 359 cases. *Medicine* 1990, 69:307–316.

2. Woods DE: Role of fibronectin in the pathogenesis of gram-negative bacillary pneumonia. *Rev Infect Dis* 1987, 9(suppl 4):S386–S390.

3. Moxon ER: *Haemophilus influenzae.* *In* Mandell GL, Bennett JE, Dolin R (eds.): *Principles and Practice of Infectious Diseases*, 4th ed. New York: Churchill Livingstone; 1995:2039–2045.

4. Turk DC: Clinical importance of *Haemophilus influenzae*—1981. *In* Sell SH, Wright PF (eds.): *Haemophilus influenzae: Epidemiology, Immunology, and Prevention of Disease*. New York: Elsevier; 1982:3–9.

5. Eveloff SE, Braman SS: Acute respiratory failure and death caused by fulminant *Haemophilus influenza* pneumonia. *Am J Med* 1990, 88:683–685.

6. Jorgensen JH: Update in mechanisms and prevalence of antimicrobial resistance in *Haemophilus influenzae. Clin Infect Dis* 1992, 14:1119–1123.

7. Soave R, Murray HW, Litrenta MM: Bacterial invasion of pulmonary vessels: *Pseudomonas* bacteremia mimicking pulmonary thromboembolism with infarction. *Am J Med* 1978, 65:864–867.

8. Meyer KS, Urban C, Eagan JA, *et al.*: Nosocomial outbreak of *Klebsiella* infection resistant to late-generation cephalosporins. *Ann Intern Med* 1993, 119:353–358.

9. Carpenter JL: *Klebsiella* pulmonary infections: Occurrence at one medical center and review. *Rev Infect Dis* 1990, 12:672–682.

10. Jonas M, Cunha BA: Bacteremic *E. coli* pneumonia. *Arch Intern Med* 1982, 142:2157–2159.

11. Karnad A, Alvarez S, Berk SL: *Enterobacter* pneumonia. *South Med J* 1987, 5:601–604.

12. Meltz DJ, Grieco MH: Characteristics of *Serratia marcescens* pneumonia. *Arch Intern Med* 1973, 132:359–364.

13. Seifert H, Baginski R, Schulze A, Pulverer G: Antimicrobial susceptibility of *Acinetobacter* species. *Antimicrob Agents Chemother* 1993, 38:750–753.

14. Rudin M, Michael J, Huxley E: Community-acquired *Acinetobacter* pneumonia. *Am J Med* 1979, 67:39–43.

SELECTED BIBLIOGRAPHY

Eisenstadt J, Crane LR. Gram-negative bacillary pneumonias. *In* Pennington JE (ed.): *Respiratory Infections: Diagnosis and Management*, 3rd ed. New York: Raven Press; 1994:369–406.

Karnad A, Alvarez S, Berk SL: Pneumonia caused by gram-negative bacilli. *Am J Med* 1985, 79(suppl 1A):61–67.

Levison ME, Kaye D: Pneumonia caused by gram-negative bacilli: An overview. *Rev Infect Dis* 1985, 7(suppl 4):S656–S665.

Neu HC: Antimicrobial therapy of gram-negative bacillary pneumonia. *In* Sande MA, Hudson LD, Root RK (eds.): *Respiratory Infections*. New York: Churchill Livingstone; 1986:235–251.

Sanders CC, Sanders WE: Beta lactam resistance in gram-negative bacteria: Global trends and clinical impact. *Clin Infect Dis* 1992, 15:824–839.

CHAPTER 3

Atypical Pneumonia and Pneumonia Due to Higher Bacteria

Melanie J. Maslow
Jaishree Jagirdar

MYCOPLASMA PNEUMONIA

Pathogens causing atypical pneumonia

Mycoplasma pneumoniae
Chlamydia psittaci
Chlamydia pneumoniae
Chlamydia trachomatis
Coxiella burnetii
Legionella spp
Francisella tularensis
Influenza A and B
Adenovirus
Parainfluenza virus
Respiratory syncytial virus

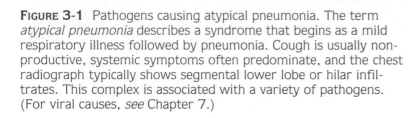

FIGURE 3-1 Pathogens causing atypical pneumonia. The term *atypical pneumonia* describes a syndrome that begins as a mild respiratory illness followed by pneumonia. Cough is usually non-productive, systemic symptoms often predominate, and the chest radiograph typically shows segmental lower lobe or hilar infil-trates. This complex is associated with a variety of pathogens. (For viral causes, *see* Chapter 7.)

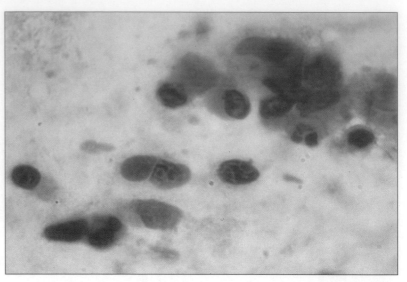

FIGURE 3-2 Sputum Gram stain under oil-immersion magnification in *Mycoplasma* pneumonia. Numerous mononuclear cells, including lymphocytes and immature macrophages, can be seen, with only rare bacteria. This appearance is fairly typical of the Gram stain seen with many of the atypical respiratory pathogens.

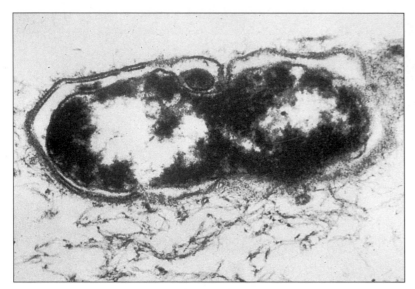

FIGURE 3-3 Electron photomicrograph of *Mycoplasma pneumoni-ae*. The trilaminar cell membrane, cytoplasm containing ribo-somes, and the characteristic prokaryotic nucleoid are visible. *Mycoplasma* are the smallest free-living cells in existence. They are pleomorphic organisms 0.3 to 0.8 μm in diameter, contain both RNA and DNA, and lack a cell wall. *Mycoplasma* reproduce by binary fission, with a mean generation time of 1 to 3 hours. *M. pneumoniae* is estimated to cause over 12 million cases of res-piratory tract infection yearly in the general population and 50% of pneumonia cases in closed populations. (*Courtesy of* Abbott Laboratories.)

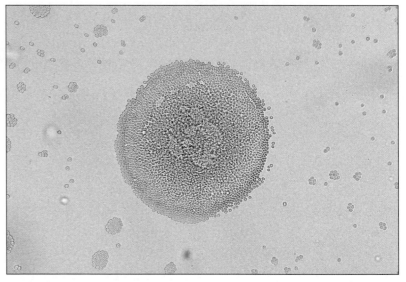

FIGURE 3-4 *Mycoplasma pneumoniae* colony on mycoplasma glucose agar to which sheep red blood cells have become adsorbed. *M. pneumoniae* is the only species that demonstrates the property of adsorption. Enriched media containing precursors for nucleic acid, protein, and lipid biosynthesis is essential for growth due to the small amount of genetic material in organisms of this genus. On solid media, colonies are small and can be seen only with magnifica-tion. Serologic techniques for diagnosis of *Mycoplasma* infection include complement fixation, indirect hemagglutination, and enzyme-linked immunoassay. Advances in diagnostic specificity have been obtained by using more defined protein antigen preparations of *M. pneumoniae* cells [1]. (Original magnification, × 50.)

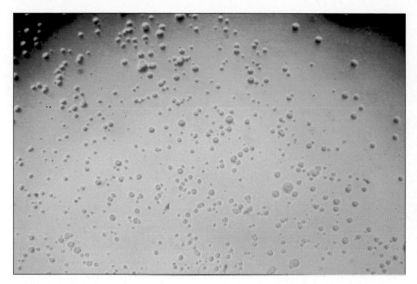

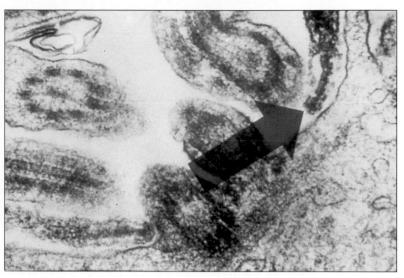

FIGURE 3-5 *Mycoplasma pneumoniae* recovered from respiratory secretions growing on selective mycoplasma agar. Growth begins with a granule that is drawn down by capillary action into the gel, followed by growth upward to the surface. On solid media, colonies are usually granular, as opposed to the "fried egg" appearance of other species. The direct identification of *Myco- plasma* colonies on agar by direct immunofluorescence is a rapid and specific new technique. Investigational techniques to identify the organism directly from respiratory secretions include antigen capture–enzyme immunoassay and polymerase chain reaction amplification of sequences within the P1 and 16S ribosomal RNA genes [2]. (*Courtesy of* Abbott Laboratories.)

FIGURE 3-6 Electron micrograph of a single *Mycoplasma* cell attached to an epithelial cell. *Mycoplasma pneumoniae* attach firmly to epithelial cells by a specialized terminal organelle (*arrow*) unique to the species, the P1 protein. *M. pneumoniae*, a filamen- tous organism, moves down the trachea and slips between cilia. The terminal tip facilitates attachment to a glycoprotein on the host cell, after which the organism produces hydrogen peroxide and superoxide resulting in cilial and epithelial damage. (*Courtesy of* Abbott Laboratories.)

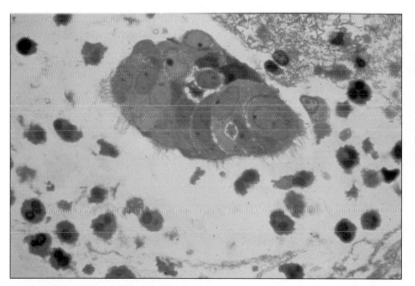

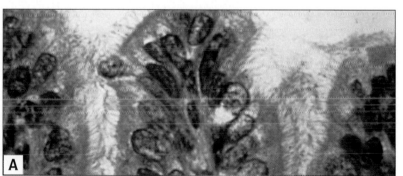
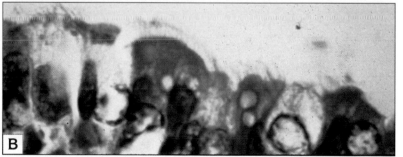

FIGURE 3-7 High-power magnification of cellular damage caused by *Mycoplasma pneumoniae* infection. A clump of desquamated epithelium and phagocytic cells is visible. Destroyed cells can sometimes be seen in sputum samples. Pathologic examination of infected tissue shows hyperplasia of type II pneumocytes and peri- bronchiolar septal widening with lymphocytes and plasma cells lin- ing bronchiolar walls. (*Courtesy of* Abbott Laboratories.)

FIGURE 3-8 Cell injury in *Mycoplasma* infection. **A**, Uninfected, ciliated epithelium are seen lining a tracheal ring after 48 hours in organ culture. **B**, The same epithelial cell is shown 48 hours after inoculation of the organ culture with *M. pneumoniae*. Cell injury is manifested by cytoplasmic eosinophilia and vacuolization and by nuclear swelling with chromatin margination. Immune-mediated mechanisms are thought to be involved in *M. pneumoniae* infec- tion. *M. pneumoniae* can stimulate mitogenic activity by B and T lymphocytes, result in interferon production, and depress cell- mediated immune reactions to unrelated antigens [3]. (*Courtesy of* Abbott Laboratories.)

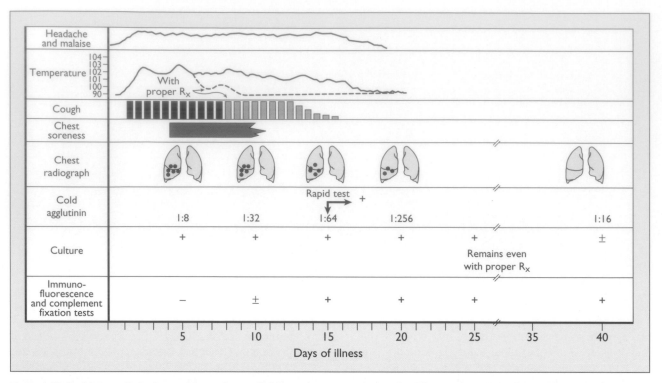

FIGURE 3-9 Major clinical manifestations of *Mycoplasma* pneumonia. The major clinical manifestations and serologic findings over the course of *Mycoplasma* pneumonia are outlined. Most *Mycoplasma pneumoniae* infections lead to clinically apparent (as opposed to subclinical) disease, usually involving only the upper respiratory tract. Disease develops after a 2- to 3-week incubation with the insidious onset of fever, malaise, headache, and cough. This insidious onset contrasts with the acute onset of respiratory symptoms in influenza or adenovirus infection. The cough progresses over 1 to 2 days and may become debilitating. (Rx—prescription.) (*From* Baum [4]; with permission.)

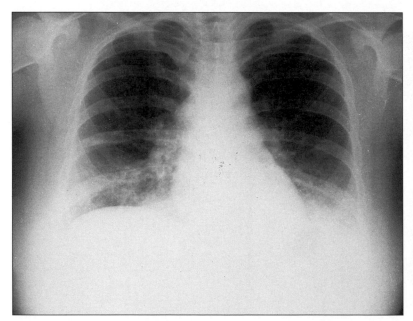

FIGURE 3-10 Chest radiograph of a young woman with *Mycoplasma pneumoniae* pneumonia showing bilateral patchy alveolar opacities of the lower lobes. There is a wide spectrum of radiographic presentations in *M. pneumoniae* pneumonia, including alveolar disease, interstitial disease, or combined interstitial/alveolar disease. Infiltrates are characteristically unilateral patchy areas of bronchopneumonia, usually involving the lower lobes; multilobar involvement, pleural effusion, and hilar adenopathy have been described. *M. pneumoniae* infection often begins insidiously with gradual onset of constitutional and pneumonic symptoms. As the disease progresses, fever and a hacking cough productive of mucoid or mucopurulent sputum develop. (*From* Marrie [5]; with permission.)

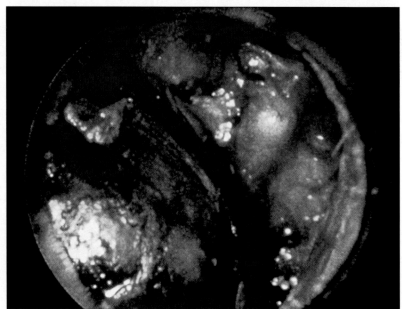

FIGURE 3-11 Bullous myringitis associated with *Mycoplasma pneumoniae* infection. Symptoms of sore throat, cervical adenopathy, and ear pain may coexist with respiratory symptoms. Although as many as one third of patients complain of earache, frank myringitis occurs in only about 15% of cases. When blebs or bullae are present, hemorrhage into the bleb usually occurs within 1 to 2 days. (*Courtesy of* Abbott Laboratories.)

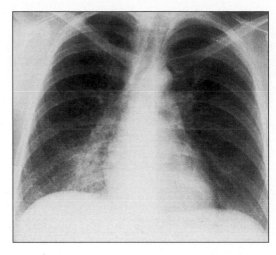

FIGURE 3-12 Chest radiograph of a young adult with severe cold-agglutinin-induced hemolytic anemia secondary to *Mycoplasma* pneumonia. Both alveolar and interstitial disease can be seen. Cold hemagglutinin is an IgM antibody that usually exhibits specificity for the I antigen of red cells. Approximately 50% of infected patients develop cold agglutinins, but significant intravascular hemolysis usually occurs only in patients with high titers (≥1:500), often during the recovery phase. Most patients recover from *M. pneumoniae* pneumonia without treatment, but the illness can be prolonged with symptoms for up to 6 weeks. Tetracycline and erythromycin are effective in reducing the duration of symptoms; newer therapeutic options include clarithromycin, azithromycin, and the fluoroquinolones [6]. (*From* Marrie [5]; with permission.)

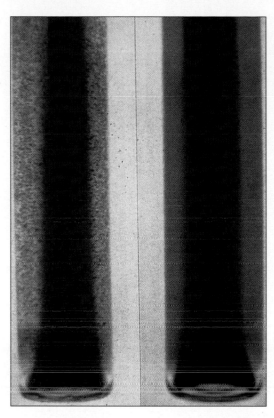

FIGURE 3-13 Bedside cold agglutinatinin test for *Mycoplasma* pneumonia. The bedside cold agglutinin test is less sensitive than laboratory testing, but a positive test is highly suggestive of *Mycoplasma* infection. Blood is drawn in a tube containing anticoagulant. Normally, there is smooth coating of the tube (*left*). The tube is then immersed in ice or refrigerated to 4° C and examined for the presence of macroscopic agglutination (*right*). This agglutination disappears on rewarming. (*Courtesy of* Abbott Laboratories.)

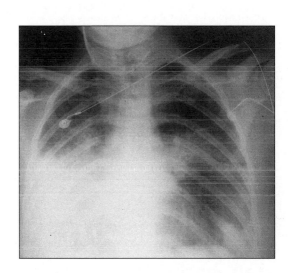

FIGURE 3-14 Chest radiograph of a 16-year-old girl who developed rapidly progressive pneumonia due to *Mycoplasma pneumoniae* after near-drowning. Antibody titers to *M. pneumoniae* rose from < 1:8 during the acute phase to 1:2048 in the convalescent phase. She recovered on erythromycin therapy. Fulminant mycoplasma disease occurs in 2% to 10% of hospitalized patients. Extensive involvement and lobar consolidation may lead to respiratory failure. Infection may involve the central nervous system, heart, skin (erythema multiforme), gastrointestinal tract, kidneys, and joints [3,7].

Extrapulmonary manifestations of *Mycoplasma infection*

Dermatologic	Musculoskeletal
Stevens-Johnson syndrome	Polyarthralgias
Erythema nodosum	Arthritis
Urticaria	Myalgias
Macular or morbilliform rash	Raynaud's phenomenon
Cardiac	Autoimmune hemolytic anemia
Arrhythmia	Renal failure
Chest pain	Hepatitis
Conduction defects	Bullous myringitis
Heart failure	
Neurologic	
Aseptic meningitis	
Meningoencephalitis	
Transverse myelitis	
Peripheral neuropathy	

FIGURE 3-15 Extrapulmonary manifestations of *Mycoplasma* infection. Virtually any organ system can be involved during the course of mycoplasma infection. *Mycoplasma pneumoniae* has been isolated from extrapulmonary lesions in some patients; immune mechanisms of damage have also been implicated.

Antimicrobial treatment of *Mycoplasma* pneumonia	
	Dosage
Adults	
Tetracycline	500 mg every 6 hrs
Erythromycin	500 mg every 6 hrs
Doxycycline	100 mg every 12 hrs
Clarithromycin	250 mg every 12 hrs
Azithromycin	250 mg every 24 hrs
Ciprofloxacin	500 mg twice a day
Ofloxacin	400 mg twice a day
Children	
Erythromycin	250 mg every 6 hrs
Erythromycin ethyl succinate	10 mg/kg every 6 hrs

FIGURE 3-16 Antimicrobial treatment of *Mycoplasma* pneumonia. Mycoplasma pneumonia is self-limited, but treatment with effective antibiotics shortens the duration of illness, thereby decreasing the risk of secondary infection. Organisms may be recovered from sputum for several weeks despite adequate treatment. (*From* Baum [8]; with permission.)

LEGIONELLOSIS

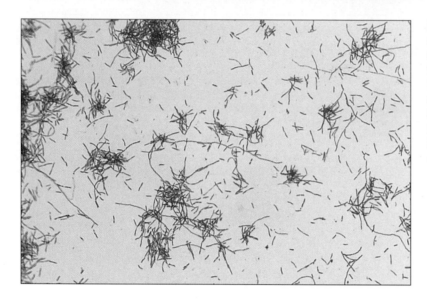

FIGURE 3-17 Gram stain of *Legionella pneumophila* from a colony, counterstained with carbol-fuchsin. *Legionella* are pleomorphic, aerobic bacilli that stain faintly gram negative. Longer filamentous forms are seen in pure culture; in clinical specimens, the organisms usually appear as small coccobacilli. *Legionella* species have a single polar flagella and multiple pili and share other ultrastructural features of gram-negative bacilli. The family Legionellaceae has more than 30 species. Twenty species have been implicated in human disease, but most cases of legionellosis are caused by *L. pneumophila* groups 1, 4, and 6 [9].

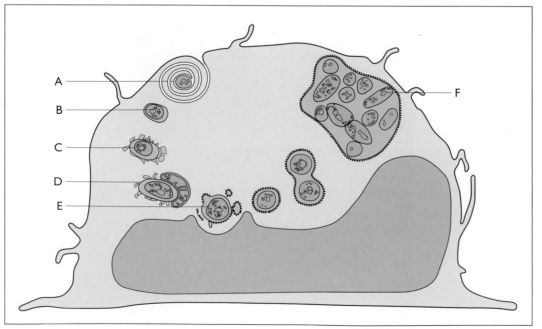

FIGURE 3-18 Replicative cycle of *Legionella pneumophila*. *L. pneumophila* is phagocytosed by a monocyte through formation of a pseudopod, which coils around the organism (*A*) as it is ingested and forms a vacuolar phagosome (*B*). The phagosome is surrounded first by smooth vesicles (*C*), then mitochondria (*D*), and finally ribosomes (*E*). The organism multiplies within the phagosome (*F*) until cell rupture occurs. (*From* Horowitz [10]; with permission.)

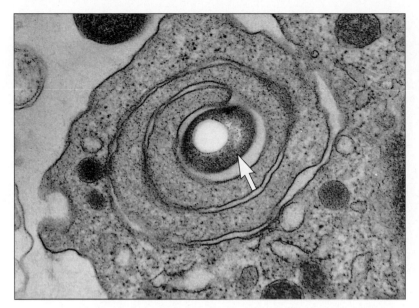

FIGURE 3-19 Electron micrograph of a human monocyte ingesting *Legionella pneumophila*. A pseudopod of the phagocytic cell is seen coiling around the *L. pneumophila* organism (*arrow*), which contains a lucent fat vacuole. (Original magnification, × 28,500.) (*From* Horowitz [11]; with permission.)

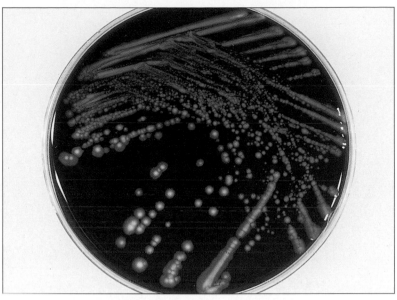

FIGURE 3-20 *Legionella pneumophila* colonies on charcoal yeast extract agar buffered to pH 6.9. *Legionella* are nutritionally fastidious and will not grow on standard media. The organism may take up to 5 days to form visible colonies, which are glistening, convex, and slightly irregular, ranging in size from pinpoint to 4 mm in diameter. The organisms's natural habitat is aquatic bodies such as lakes, streams, and ponds as well as man-made habitats such as cooling towers and potable water distribution systems.

Ecology and transmission of *Legionella pneumophila*

Habitats

Natural	Man-made
Rivers	Cooling towers
Freshwater lakes	Hot-water storage tanks
Streams	Evaporative condensers
Thermal effluent	Air conditioners
	Whirlpools

Transmission

Aerosols	Aspiration	Direct installation
Nebulizers	Contaminated water	Respiratory tract manipulation
Humidifiers	Nasogastric tubes	
Water faucets		
Whirlpool spas		
Excavation sites		

FIGURE 3-21 Ecology and transmission of *Legionella pneumophila*. *L. pneumophila* survives a wide range of environmental conditions, including temperatures of 0° to 68° C and water-treatment processes, to proliferate in both natural and man-made habitats. Transmission is predominantly via aerosol formulation, but aspiration and direct instillation of infected materials into the lower respiratory tract have been documented.

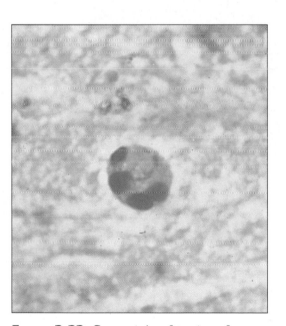

FIGURE 3-22 Gram stain of sputum from the orotracheal tube of a patient with *Legionella pneumophila* lung abscess. Intracellular, faintly staining, gram-negative rods are visible within neutrophils, documenting that *L. pneumophila* can sometimes be seen by Gram staining of clinical material. The Dieterle and Gimenez stains can be used to visualize the organism in tissues. (*From* Lewin *et al.* [12]; with permission.)

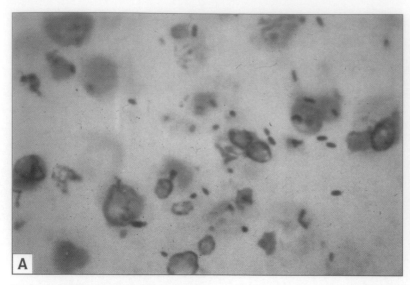

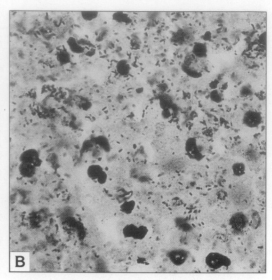

FIGURE 3-23 Dieterle silver impregnation stain of *Legionella pneumophila*. **A**, Sputum. **B**, Lung biopsy tissue. With the Dieterle silver impregnation stain, the organisms appear black to dark brown and coccobacillary. The silver stains, including Dieterle and Warthin-Starry, can be used for paraffin-fixed tissue sections.

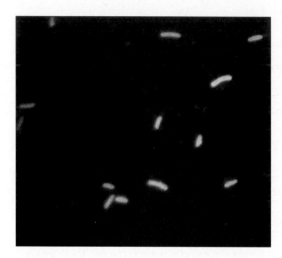

FIGURE 3-24 *Legionella pneumophila* stained with homologous direct fluorescent antibody conjugate. This stain uses specific fluorescein isothiocyanate–conjugated polyvalent antisera for the rapid detection of *Legionella* species from respiratory specimens and has a sensitivity ranging from 25% to 80%. A major problem is its cross-reactivity with other organisms, including some *Pseudomonas* species, *Xanthomonas maltophilia*, and some strains of *Bacteroides fragilis*. A new monoclonal antibody conjugate has decreased the incidence of false-positive reactions but is not recommended for use on potable or other water systems. A DNA probe is now commercially available that has a sensitivity of 70% to 75% and specificity of 99% to 100% [13]. (*Courtesy of* R. Schoentag, MD.)

Specialized laboratory tests for diagnosis of *Legionella* infection

Test	Sensitivity, %	Specificity, %
Culture		
Sputum	80	100
Transtracheal aspirate	90	100
Blood	20	100
Serology	40–60	96–99
Direct fluorescent antibody	50–70	96–99
Urinary antigen	80	100
DNA probe	60	95–99

FIGURE 3-25 Specialized laboratory test for diagnosis of *Legionella* infection. Sensitivity and specificity of the specialized laboratory tests used to establish the diagnosis of *Legionella* infection are shown. Isolation of the organism from respiratory secretions, preferably attained by bronchoscopy, is the gold standard test in diagnosis. (*From* Yu [14]; with permission.)

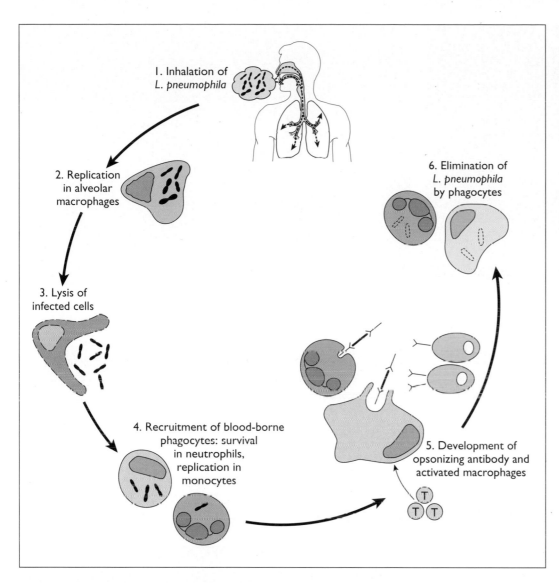

FIGURE 3-26 Pathogenesis of *Legionella* pneumonia. Most aerosolized bacilli entering the upper respiratory tract are cleared by the mucociliary process (*1*). Organisms evading this process are phagocytized by the alveolar macrophage, where they reside within a phagosome and thereby evade lysosomal fusion (*2*). Intracellular multiplication occurs until the cell ruptures (*3*). Polymorphonuclear leukocytes and monocytes are recruited but are unable to contain the infection (*4*). With the appearance of both cell-mediated and humoral immunity, an enhanced antimicrobial state enables macrophages and neutrophils to destroy the organism (*5* and *6*). (*Adapted from* Skerrett and Locksley [15]; with permission.)

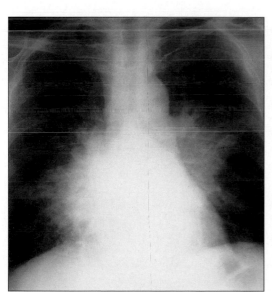

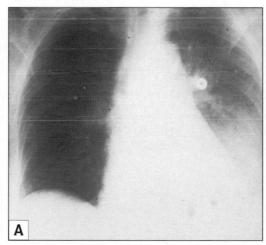

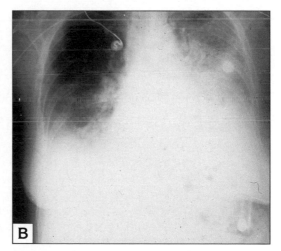

FIGURE 3-27 Chest radiograph of a patient with chronic lymphocytic leukemia demonstrating confluent right middle lobe and lingular infiltrates secondary to *Legionella pneumophila* pneumonia. Risk factors for *Legionella* infection include cigarette smoking, chronic obstructive pulmonary disease, steroid therapy, transplantation, and old age. *Legionella* species rank among the top three microbial agents of community-acquired pneumonia in several studies. (*Courtesy of* N. Ettinger, MD.)

FIGURE 3-28 Rapid progression of *Legionella* pneumonia from unilateral to bilateral involvement on chest radiographs. **A**, An admission in a patient with emphysema shows a left lower lobe infiltrate secondary to *Legionella*. **B**, A chest radiograph 2 days later demonstrates rapid progression to bilateral infiltrates with effusions. *Legionella* pulmonary infection ranges from a mild cough with low-grade fever to a rapidly progressive pneumonia with multiorgan failure. The typical radiographic finding is a unilateral alveolar infiltrate when first seen, with progression to bilateral involvement at the peak of disease. Cavitation and mass lesions have been described, and effusions develop in 22% to 63% of patients. Extrapulmonary manifestations include gastrointestinal and neurologic symptoms; abnormalities of other organ systems, including the liver, kidneys, and musculoskeletal system, may be noted on laboratory examination [16]. (*Courtesy of* R. Holzman, MD.)

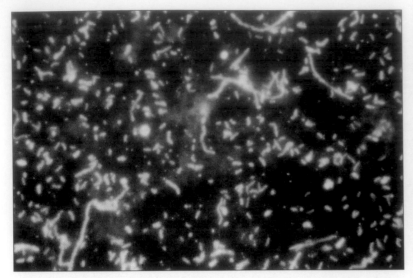

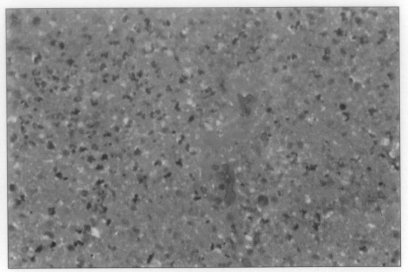

FIGURE 3-29 Lung biopsy specimen stained with fluorescein-conjugated polyvalent antisera directed against *Legionella* antigens. When *Legionella* antigen is present and reacts with antibody, the organisms fluoresce brightly. Specific antibody can be used to detect other *Legionella* species. The serum indirect immunofluorescent antibody test is often used to make the diagnosis of *Legionella* pneumonia. *In vitro* susceptibility testing is not standardized and does not correlate with *in vivo* response to infection. Erythromycin is the treatment of choice; other effective drugs include rifampin, the newer macrolide antibiotics, quinolones, and trimethoprim-sulfamethoxazole.

FIGURE 3-30 High-power hematoxylin-eosin stain of acute *Legionella* pneumonia demonstrating necrotizing inflammation, infiltration by macrophages, and nuclear dust. Microscopically, *Legionella* pneumonia is best described as an acute fibrinopurulent pneumonia. The inflammatory exudate consists of some neutrophils and abundant macrophages and fibrin, and it primarily involves the alveoli and small airways.

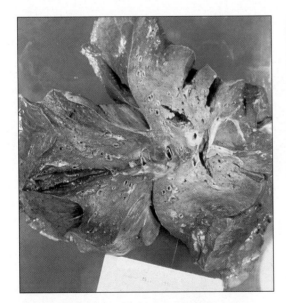

FIGURE 3-31 Autopsy specimen from a patient with *Legionella pneumophila* pneumonia. Multiple areas of consolidation involve the right half of the specimen. The typical gross appearance of *Legionella* pneumonia is that of a bronchopneumonia. More severe forms may resemble acute airspace pneumonia. Destruction of lung architecture is seen in severe cases, and visible abscesses were seen in 20% of autopsy cases in one series [17].

Legionella species causing pneumonia	
Strain	**Year isolated**
L. micdadei	1943
L. bozemanii	1959
L. pneumophila	1977
L. dumoffii	1978
L. longbeachae	1980
L. jordanis	1978
L. gormanii	1978
L. feeleii	1981
L. hackeliae	1981
L. maceachernii	1979
L. wadsworthii	1981
L. birminghamensis	1986
L. cincinnatiensis	1982
L. oakridgensis	1981
L. anisa	1981
L. sainthelensi	1981
L. tucsonensis	1984
L. lansingensis	1987

FIGURE 3-32 *Legionella* species causing pneumonia. Since the discovery of *L. pneumophila* in 1977, the family Legionellaceae has grown to include 34 species. Seventeen species in addition to *L. pneumophila* have been documented to cause human infection. (*From* Muder and Yu [18]; with permission.)

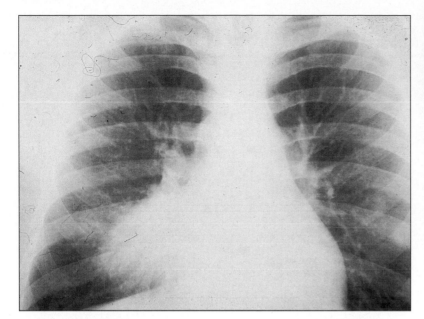

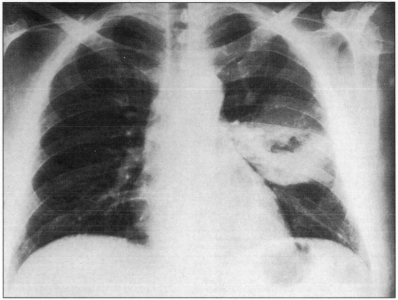

FIGURE 3-33 Chest radiograph from a renal transplant patient with right middle lobe pneumonia due to *Legionella micdadei* (Pittsburgh pneumonia). *L. micdadei* can stain weakly acid-fast in tissue with the Kinyoun and Fite stains and on sputum smears with the modified Ziehl-Neelsen stain. *L. micdadei* accounts for 6% of cases of *Legionella* infection in the United States and has a clinical and radiograph presentation similar to *L. pneumophila* infection. Disease due to *L. micdadei* occurs primarily in immuno-compromised hosts, particularly transplant patients, during steroid therapy, and in the elderly. Diagnosis is based on culture, serologic studies, and immunofluorescence assays [19].

FIGURE 3-34 Chest radiograph of an immunocompromised patient with *Legionella bozemanii* pneumonia. Cavitation seen within a left lower lobe infiltrate occurred despite treatment. The infiltrate resolved by 6 months. *L. bozemanii* causes approximately 3% to 5% of pneumonia caused by *Legionella* species. Nosocomial and community-acquired cases have been described. Risk factors for this infection include submersion in freshwater, serious underlying disease, and immunosuppressive therapy. The clinical and laboratory findings are similar to those of *L. pneumophila* infection [20]. (*From* Muder *et al.* [21]; with permission.)

Antibiotic therapy for *Legionella* infections	
Antimicrobial	**Dosage**
Erythromycin	1 g iv every 6 hrs
	500 mg orally every 6 hrs
Alternative agents	
Rifampin	600 mg orally every 12 hrs or 24 hrs
	600 mg iv every 12 hrs or 24 hrs
Trimethoprim-sulfamethoxazole	160/800 mg iv every 8 hrs
	160/800 mg orally every 12 hrs
Doxycycline	100 mg iv or orally every 12 hrs
Tetracycline	500 mg iv or orally every 6 hrs
Ciprofloxacin	400 mg iv every 8 hrs
	750 mg orally every 12 hrs
Azithromycin	500 mg orally every 24 hrs
Clarithromycin	500 mg orally every 12 hrs

iv—intravenously.

FIGURE 3-35 Antibiotic therapy for *Legionella* infections. Erythromycin has been the antibiotic of choice historically for treatment of legionelloses, but the newer macrolides and quinolones have superior *in vitro* activity and improved pharmacokinetics, although clinical trials of efficacy have not yet been done. Parenteral therapy should be given until there is demonstrated improvement before oral therapy is implemented. Duration of therapy is 10 to 14 days for normal hosts, with longer courses in immunocompromised patients. (*From* Muder and Yu [18]; with permission.)

CHLAMYDIA PNEUMONIA

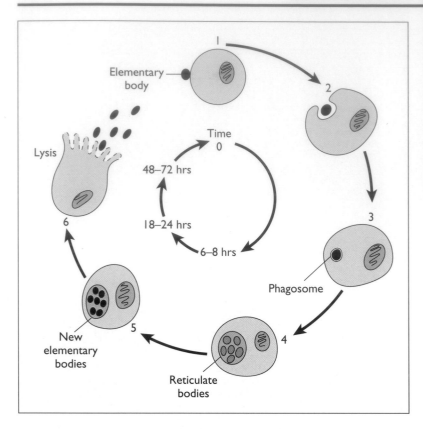

FIGURE 3-36 Life cycle of chlamydiae. Chlamydiae are obligate intracellular pathogens that are distinguished from other bacteria by a developmental cycle involving the elementary body, which survives extracellularly, and the reticulate body, which multiplies intracellularly. Elementary bodies attach to the surface of susceptible host cells (*1*), are ingested by endocytosis (*2*), and survive within a phagosome (*3*), somehow preventing lysosomal fusion. Within 6 to 8 hours after entering the cell, the elementary body reorganizes into the reticulate body (*4*), which divides by binary fission within the membrane-bound vacuole. After 18 to 24 hours from attachment, reticulate bodies reorganize into elementary bodies (*5*), which are released from vacuoles between 48 and 72 hours after initial infection (*6*).

Characteristics and properties of three pathogenic *Chlamydia* species

	C. pneumoniae	*C. trachomatis*	*C. psittaci*
Major diseases in humans	Pneumonia, bronchitis	Trachoma, STDs	Pneumonia, FUO
Natural hosts	Humans	Humans	Birds, lower mammals
No. of serovars	1 (TWAR)	18	Multiple
% DNA homology to TWAR	94%–100%	10%	5%
Elementary body by electron microscopy	Pear-shaped	Round	Round
Sensitive cell cultures	HL, HEp-2	HeLa 229, McCoy	Most
MOMP contains species-specific antigen	No	Yes	Yes
Inactivation of specific antigen by methanol	Yes	No	No

FUO—fever of unknown origin; MOMP—major outer membrane proteins; STD—sexually transmitted disease.

FIGURE 3-37 Characteristics and properties of three pathogenic *Chlamydia* species. Of the three species, *C. pneumoniae* is the most common cause of respiratory infection. *C. trachomatis* and *C. psittaci* also cause pneumonia, with *C. trachomatis* pneumonia occurring predominantly in infants. (*From* Grayston [22]; with permission.)

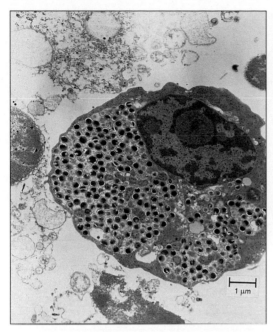

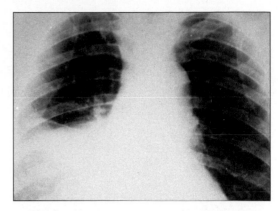

FIGURE 3-38 Transmission electron micrograph of *Chlamydia psittaci* isolated from a McCoy cell culture. The patient was a pigeon fancier hospitalized with pneumonia. *C. psittaci*, the etiologic agent of psittacosis, is a zoonositic pathogen transmitted to humans by inhalation of dried bird excreta. Parrots are the main reservoir, but almost any bird species can be infected. The elementary bodies are round with a narrow, uniformly distributed, periplasmic space that is characteristic of both *C. psittaci* and *C. trachomatis*. (*From* Oldach *et al.* [23]; with permission.)

FIGURE 3-39 Chest radiograph demonstrating right middle lobe consolidation in psittacosis. Owners of pet birds account for one half of psittacosis cases, but other occupational risks include pet-shop employees, veterinarians, zoo workers, and workers in poultry-processing plants. (*From* Schaffner [24]; with permission.)

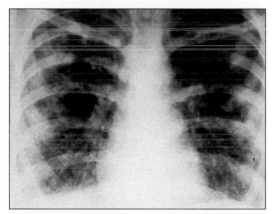

FIGURE 3-40 Chest radiograph of psittacosis demonstrating a patchy symmetrical interstitial infiltrate, especially involving the lower lobes. After the organism is inhaled, *Chlamydia psittaci* is taken up by the reticuloendothelial cells of the liver and spleen, where it replicates and spreads hematogenously to the lungs. Radiographic findings are varied. The most common presentation is as a patchy infiltrate radiating outward from the hilum; but miliary patterns, consolidation, and pleural effusion may be seen. (*From* Schaffner [24]; with permission.)

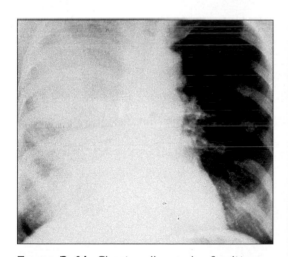

FIGURE 3-41 Chest radiograph of psittacosis showing progression of a right lower lobe consolidation to encompass the entire right lung. Psittacosis is a systemic illness that often begins suddenly with fever, chills, malaise, and severe headache. The cough is dry and hacking, may be productive, and is associated with dyspnea. Hepatosplenomegaly is often present. The infection is diagnosed serologically in most cases, because *in vitro* work with this organism is hazardous. The preferred treatment is tetracycline [25]. (*From* Schaffner [24]; with permission.)

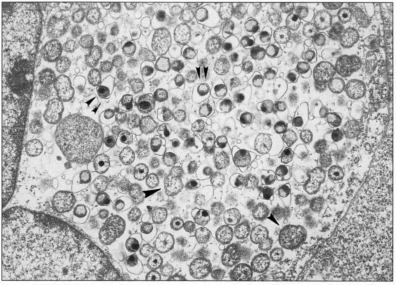

FIGURE 3-42 Electron micrograph of a *Chlamydia pneumoniae* inclusion after 72 hours of incubation in HEp-2 cells. The micrograph shows reticulate bodies (*single arrowheads*) and elementary bodies (*double arrowheads*) with the loose periplasmic membrane giving them a pear-shaped appearance. *C. pneumoniae* is a new chlamydial species that causes acute infection of the respiratory tract and may be responsible for 10% of hospitalized and outpatient cases of pneumonia. It differs from *C. trachomatis* and *C. psittaci* by its pear-shaped elementary body and shows little homology with the other species on DNA studies. The organism is also known as TWAR based on the first isolation in 1965 from a child with a trachoma-like illness in Taiwan (TW-183) and the first respiratory isolate from a college student in the United States in 1983 (AR-39) [26]. (*Courtesy of* M. Hammerschlag, MD.)

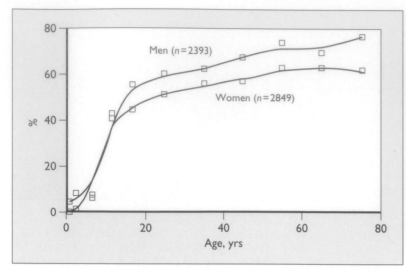

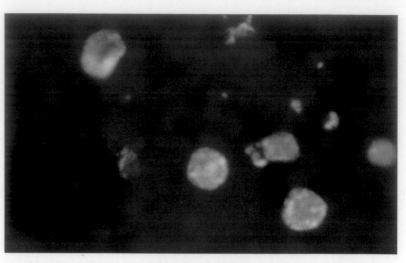

FIGURE 3-43 The prevalence of microimmunofluorescence antibody (IgG) to *Chlamydia pneumoniae* in 5242 persons in Seattle. The data demonstrate frequent infection in school-aged children and continuous exposure through adult life. Given the expected antibody decline after acute infection, these data suggest that an overwhelming majority of people are infected and that reinfection is common. (*From* Grayston [22]; with permission.)

FIGURE 3-44 Photomicrograph of *Chlamydia pneumoniae* in tissue culture demonstrating fluorescent staining of intracellular inclusions with monoclonal antibodies. *C. pneumoniae* is a fastidious grower and more difficult to isolate in tissue culture than other chlamydiae. Specific serologic tests are available for its diagnosis using complement fixation and microimmunofluorescence techniques. Polymerase chain reaction is a new investigational technique used to identify *C. pneumoniae*-specific DNA [27]. (*Courtesy of* M. Hammerschlag, MD.)

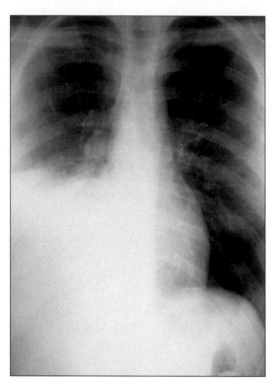

FIGURE 3-45 Chest radiograph from a 19-year-old man with *Chlamydia pneumoniae* infection and pleural effusion. The patient presented with fever, cough, and dyspnea and showed a moderate-sized right pleural effusion on chest radiography. *C. pneumoniae* was isolated from the pleural fluid and a nasopharyngeal culture. The illness often presents with sore throat and hoarseness, followed by cough in several days to a week. Most respiratory disease due to *C. pneumoniae* is mild, responding to outpatient therapy, but cough and malaise may be slow to resolve. The spectrum of *C. pneumoniae* infection includes bronchitis, primary pharyngitis, laryngitis, otitis, and sinusitis. No clinical controlled trials of treatment have been reported, but suggested therapy is tetracyline or erythromycin for 10 to 14 days. The newer macrolide antibiotics are active *in vitro* against this organism and have been studied *in vivo* in adults and children with *C. pneumoniae* pneumonia [28]. (*From* Augenbraun *et al.* [29]; with permission.)

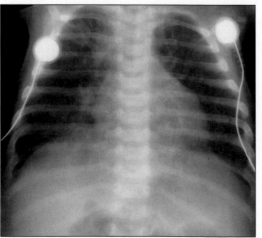

FIGURE 3-46 Chest radiograph of a 3-month-old boy with *Chlamydia trachomatis* pneumonia showing paracentral interstitial infiltrates and hyperaeration. *C. trachomatis* causes a distinct clinical syndrome in infants aged 4 to 24 weeks that is characterized by cough, congestion, tachypnea, and diffuse interstitial or alveolar infiltrates on chest radiographs. The infant is usually afebrile, and the illness is chronic, lasting 1 or more months. Approximately half of the patients have concomitant or previous conjunctivitis. Diagnosis is supported by isolation of *C. trachomatis* from tracheal aspirates and by elevated titers of IgM antibodies to *C. trachomatis*. Infection with this species has been reported in adults, usually in the setting of immunocompromise, but also in normal hosts [30]. (*Courtesy of* K. Roche, MD.)

Antibiotic treatment of *Chlamydia* pneumonia	
	Daily dose
Tetracycline	2 g
Doxycycline	200 mg
Erythromycin	2 g
Azithromycin	500 mg
Clarithromycin	1 g

FIGURE 3-47 Antibiotic treatment of *Chlamydia* pneumonia. The traditional and newer agents for treating *Chlamydia* pneumonia are listed. Duration of therapy ranges from 10 to 21 days and is dependent on the species, severity of infection, and underlying host factors. Studies with azithromycin and clarithromycin are currently underway.

COXIELLA BURNETII PNEUMONIA (Q FEVER)

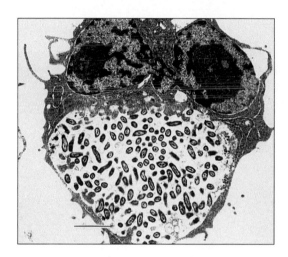

FIGURE 3-48 Transmission electron micrograph of *Coxiella burnetii* within a phagocyte. *C. burnetii*, the etiologic agent of Q fever, is a pleomorphic, obligate, intracellular coccobacillus with a gram-negative cell wall. The major reservoirs for this organism are sheep, goats, cattle, and ticks. Infection occurs by inhalation of aerosol particles containing the organism or through consumption of contaminated raw milk. The actual incidence of pneumonia caused by this pathogen ranges from 0% to 90%. Pulmonary infection exists in three forms: atypical pneumonia, rapidly progressive pneumonia, and asymptomatic infiltrates in a febrile patient [31]. (*From* Baca *et al.* [32]; with permission.)

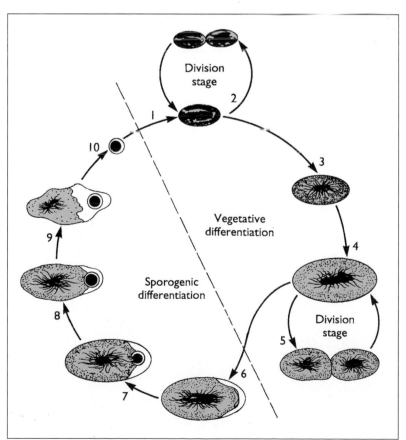

FIGURE 3-49 Developmental cycle of *Coxiella burnetii* within the phagolysosome of a eucaryotic cell. Engulfment of a spore or small cell variant (SCV) of *C. burnetii* by a phagocytic cell (*1*) leads to formation of a phagolysosome, within which the low pH activates the organism's metabolic pathways (*2*). The SVC may multiply by transverse binary fission (*3* and *4*) or differentiate into the vegetative cell variant (*5*). Further differentiation of the large cell variant (LCV) may proceed to a binary division stage (*6*) or coincide with sporogenic differentiation, resulting in unequal cell division. Changes during progressive infection of the cell may lead to sporogenesis (*7, 8,* and *9*) and spore formation (*10*). (*From* McCaul and Williams [33]; with permission.)

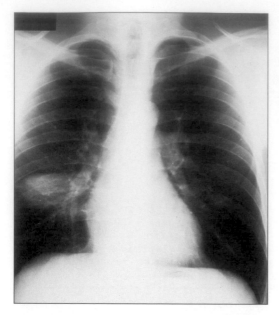

Figure 3-50 Chest radiograph of a right upper lobe segmental infiltrate secondary to *Coxiella burnetii* infection. Chest radiograph abnormalities in Q fever most resemble those seen with viral and *Mycoplasma pneumoniae* infection. There are usually single or multiple rounded segmental densities in the lower lobes; lobar consolidation, coin lesions, hilar adenopathy, atelectasis, and pleural effusions have been reported. The presence of a severe headache may be a clue to the diagnosis, which is confirmed serologically because isolation is difficult and hazardous to laboratory personnel. The treatment of choice for *C. burnetii* pneumonia is tetracycline. (*Courtesy of* T.J. Marrie, MD.)

Clinical manifestations of Q fever
Self-limited febrile illness
Flulike syndrome
Pneumonia
Endocarditis
Hepatitis
Osteomyelitis
Neurologic (encephalitis, aseptic meningitis)
Hematologic (bone marrow necrosis, hemolytic anemia, hypoplastic anemia)
Myocarditis
Optic neuritis
Arthritis
Thrombophlebitis

Figure 3-51 Clinical manifestations of Q fever. Coxiella burnetii infection has many clinical presentations. Infection is divided according to duration of symptoms into acute (< 6 months) and chronic (> 6 months). Endovascular infections and osteomyelitis are the most common manifestations of chronic Q fever [34].

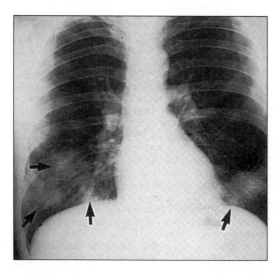

Figure 3-52 Chest radiograph from a patient who developed Q fever after his cat delivered kittens in the home. Multiple rounded opacities (*arrows*) can be seen on the chest film, which is a characteristic presentation of Q fever following exposure to infected cat placentas. The most common physical finding in the Q fever atypical pneumonia syndrome is inspiratory crackles. Patients with progressive pneumonia will have signs of pulmonary consolidation. (*From* Marrie [31]; with permission.)

NOCARDIOSIS

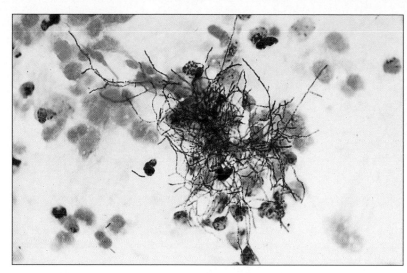

FIGURE 3-53 Sputum Gram stain from a patient with *Nocardia asteroides* pneumonia. The organism appears as thin, weakly gram positive, branching, often beaded filaments. *Nocardia* is a member of the order Actinomycetales, along with *Actinomyces* and *Streptomyces*, and was first described by Nocard in 1889 during an outbreak of bovine farcy. Although *Nocardia* exhibits the fungal characteristic of aerial hyphae, it is considered a higher bacterium because the cell wall consists of peptidoglycans and lacks chitin and cellulose. *Nocardia* is ubiquitous and is found primarily in soil and organic matter.

Pathogenic *Nocardia* species
Nocardia asteroides
Nocardia brasiliensis
Nocardia otitidiscavarium (caviae)
Nocardia farcinica
Nocardia transvalensis
Nocardia nova

FIGURE 3-54 Pathogenic *Nocardia* species. The organisms that cause nocardiosis in humans are listed. The taxonomy of *Nocardia* is currently evolving, and precise speciation within the genus is difficult. A new genus, *Actinomadura*, now designates those organisms that cause maduramycosis (madura foot).

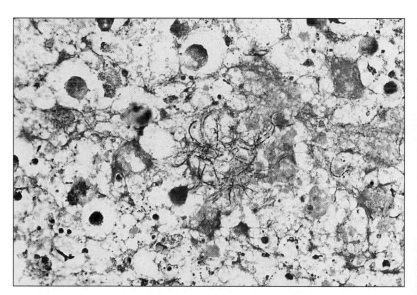

FIGURE 3-55 Modified sputum acid-fast stain of *Nocardia asteroides* from a patient with chronic alcoholism who presented with pneumonia and a multiloculated brain abscess. Many *Nocardia* species are acid-fast but retain fuchsin less avidly than *Mycobacterium* species. A modified Ziehl-Neelsen stain that decolorizes with 1% sulfuric acid instead of acid alcohol is best for demonstrating *Nocardia* in clinical specimens.

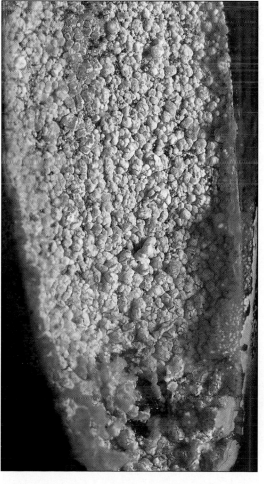

FIGURE 3-56 *Nocardia asteroides* colonies on a Sabouraud's glucose agar slant. *Nocardia* is an aerobe that can be cultivated on simple media. Colonies in pure culture may grow after 48 hours of incubation, but cultures from sputum take significantly longer to identify. Colony morphology is variable and ranges from orange, glabrous, and heaped to white, raised, and chalky with aerial hyphae. *N. asteroides* is the species most frequently associated with systemic disease, usually in immunocompromised hosts with lymphoreticular malignancies, transplants, underlying pulmonary disease, alcoholism, and HIV infection. *N. brasiliensis* usually causes cutaneous disease including mycetoma. *N. farcinica*, the species described by Nocard, has recently been added to the list of human pathogens.

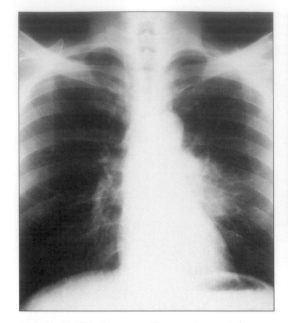

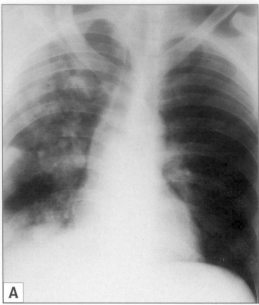

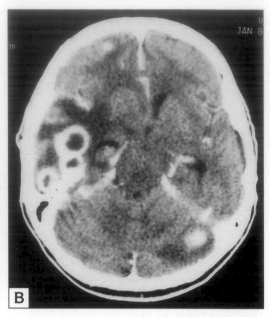

FIGURE 3-57 Chest radiograph revealing bilateral infiltrates secondary to *Nocardia asteroides* infection in a 49-year-old man with alcoholic liver disease. Infection with *Nocardia* typically begins in the lung, where it causes an acute, sometimes necrotizing, pneumonia. The infection may present radiographically as a nodule, abscess, pneumonia with empyema, or a miliary pattern. The indolent course may resemble tuberculosis or malignancy.

FIGURE 3-58 Hematogenous spread in *Nocardia asteroides* infection. **A**, A chest radiograph from a 57-year-old man with gastric lymphoma demonstrates a right-sided infiltrate secondary to *N. asteroides*. In the chronic pneumonia associated with *Nocardia* infection, multiple abscesses consisting of neutrophils and macrophages are separated by areas of fibrosis. **B**, A computed tomographic scan in the same patient demonstrates multiple brain abscesses. The organisms has a propensity for hematogenous spread, especially to the central nervous system, which is involved in one third of cases.

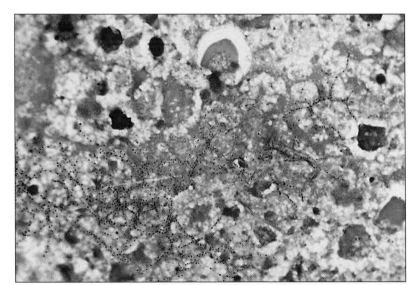

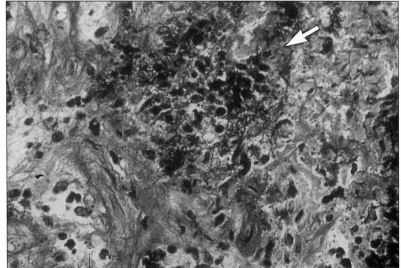

FIGURE 3-59 Gram stain of *Nocardia asteroides* brain abscess. Gram stain of samples of the brain abscess from the preceding case (*see* Fig. 3-58B) reveal the typical weakly gram-positive branching organisms. Sulfonamides have been the traditional antibiotic of choice for nocardiosis, with improvement usually within 7 to 10 days. Some *Nocardia* species are resistant to sulfonamides, and other treatment options include imipenem-cilastatin, ceftriaxone, amikacin, and minocycline. There is often poor correlation between *in vitro* susceptibility and response to therapy [35].

FIGURE 3-60 Gomori methenamine silver stain of *Nocardia asteroides* from necrotic brain tissue. The organisms appear as darkly staining networks (*arrow*). Hematoxylin-eosin and periodic acid–Schiff stains do not demonstrate this organism well histologically. Serologic diagnosis of *Nocardia* infection has been hampered by cross-reactivity with other organisms and lack of suitable antigens. An enzyme immunoassay using a 55-kD protein with specificity for *N. asteroides* has been used for rapid diagnosis [36].

Antibiotic treatment of *Nocardia* infection	
	Daily dose
Sulfadiazine	6–8 g
TMP/SMX	6 double-strength tablets*
Minocycline	200–400 mg
Amikacin	15 mg/kg
Imipenen	2 g
Ampicillin	8 g
Cefotaxime	6–8 g
Ceftriaxone	1–2 g
Fluoroquinolones	—
Amoxicillin/clavulanate	—

*Double-strength tablet contains 160 mg TMP/800 mg SMX.
TMP/SMX—trimethoprim/sulfamethoxazole.

FIGURE 3-61 Antibiotic treatment of *Nocardia* infection. Sulfonamides are the most-effective and best-studied drugs for treatment of nocardiosis. Use of other drugs must be supported by data from *in vitro* susceptibility testing. Combinations of amikacin and imipenem with cefotaxime and trimethoprim-sulfamethoxazole are synergistic *in vitro* for strains of *N. asteroides*. With fluoroquinolones, susceptibility varies according to the specific agent, but newer quinolones hold promise based on *in vitro* testing. Amoxicillin/clavulanate is an alternative for β-lactamase–producing strains of *N. brasiliensis*.

ACTINOMYCOSIS

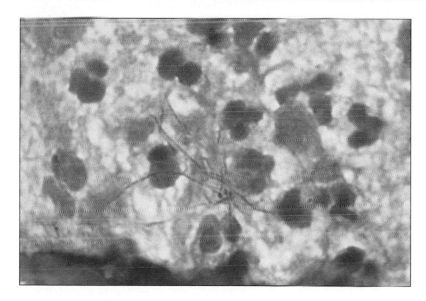

FIGURE 3-62 Sputum Gram stain of *Actinomyces israelii* demonstrating gram-positive branching organisms. Human actinomycosis is usually due to *A. israelii*, but three other species and the related genus of *Arachnia* can produce infection. *A. israelii* grows best anaerobically, but some strains are microaerophilic, and others can grow aerobically in carbon dioxide. *Actinomyces* are endogenous oral saprophytes and are not considered virulent pathogens. Thoracic infection usually follows aspiration of infected oral material.

Etiologic agents of actinomycosis
Actinomyces israelii
Actinomyces naeslundii
Actinomyces odontolyticus
Actinomyces viscosus
Actinomyces meyeri
Propionibacterium propionica

FIGURE 3-63 Etiologic agents of actinomycosis. Actinomycosis is most commonly caused by *Actinomyces israelii*. Advances in microbiologic techniques have identified additional species that also cause disease in humans.

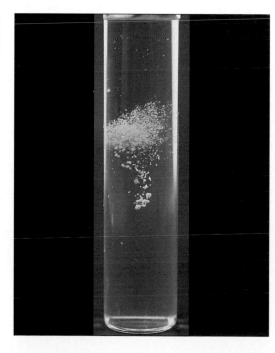

FIGURE 3-64 Colony morphology of *Actinomyces israelii* in thioglycolate broth. The organism requires rich media, such as blood or brain-heart infusion. Most strains form rough colonies on agar and grow at the bottom of broth tubes as aggregated clumps resembling bread crumbs. In anaerobic cultures, macroscopic colonies mature in about 1 week. Older colonies an agar are often raised, white, and irregular and are called *molar tooth colonies*.

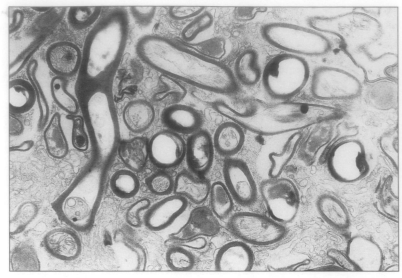

FIGURE 3-65 Transmission electron micrograph of *Actinomyces israelii* showing pleomorphic bacilliary forms with thick cell walls. The cells of *A. israelii* are usually l μm in diameter but extremely variable in length. The narrow filaments may fragment into bacilli. The organism is a prokaryotic bacteria that reproduces by fission. (*Courtesy of* G. Sidhu, MD.)

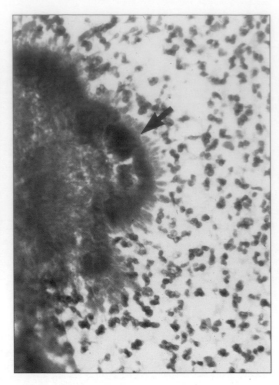

FIGURE 3-66 Hematoxylin-eosin section of an actinomycotic sulfur granule. Sulfur granules are distinctive masses of *Actinomyces* organisms cemented together and mineralized by calcium phosphate. The surface clubs (*arrow*) are normal filaments encapsulated within a polysaccharide–protein complex. When crushed, the granule becomes a mass of gram-positive branching filaments.

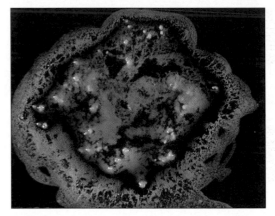

FIGURE 3-67 Macroscopic view of actinomycotic sulfur granules. Grossly, the granules are hard, gritty, and yellow to white, and they average 2 mm in diameter. These granules do not form *in vitro*. (*From* Lerner [37]; with permission.)

Clinical syndromes caused by *Actinomyces*

Oral–cervicofacial
Thoracic
Mediastinal
Abdominal
Pelvic
Central nervous system
Musculoskeletal
Dissemination

FIGURE 3-68 Clinical syndromes caused by *Actinomyces*. Actinomycosis can affect multiple organ systems. Factors predisposing to infection include disruption of mucosal barriers, aspiration, and, in the case of pelvic actinomycosis, the presence of a foreign body.

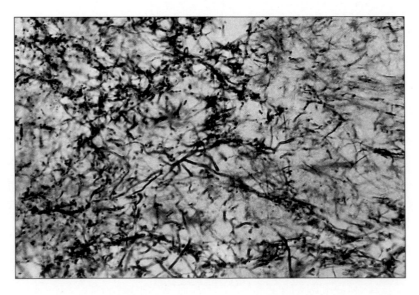

FIGURE 3-69 Gomori methenamine silver stain of an actinomycotic abscess. A pulmonary mass lesion, found to be an actinomycotic abscess at surgery, demonstrates the delicate, branched filaments of *Actinomyces*. Pulmonary actinomycosis can mimic carcinoma, tuberculous fibrocavitary disease, or a simple alveolar infiltrate. (*Courtesy of* G. Sidhu, MD.)

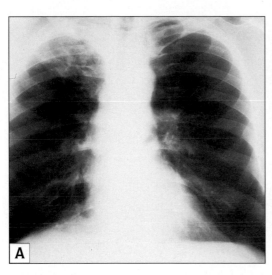
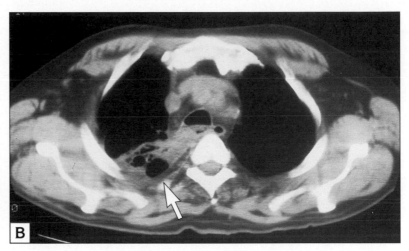

FIGURE 3-70 Pulmonary actinomycosis with fistula formation. **A** and **B**, A chest radiograph and computed tomography scan from a patient with diabetes show a chronic right upper lobe infiltrate with fistula formation to the right chest wall (*panel 70B; arrow*) secondary to actinomycosis. Radiographic findings in actinomycosis are nonspecific, but one or more small cavities are found in half of the cases. The typical pattern of acute infection is airspace pneumonia without segmental distribution, usually in the periphery of the lung. Without treatment, infection progresses to abscess, empyema, and chest wall involvement with inflammation of the soft tissues and rib destruction. Chronic infection leads to extensive fibrosis.

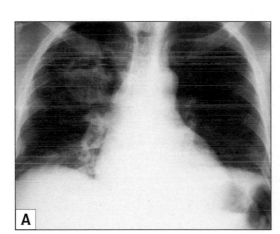
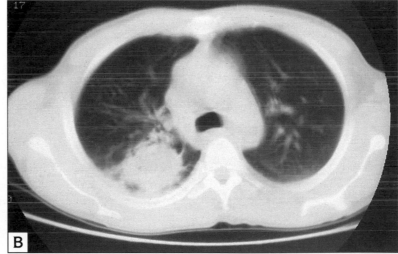

FIGURE 3-71 Cavitation and chest wall involvement in actinomycosis. **A** and **B**, A chest radiograph and computed tomography scan, from a 45-year-old severely retarded man with poor dentition, show a large right upper lobe infiltrate with cavitation that is invading the rib on computed tomography scan. Sputum Gram stain showed many gram-positive, beaded, branching organisms, and *A. israelii* was recovered from anaerobic cultures. Thoracic infection can involve the pleura, mediastinum, and chest wall in addition to the lungs. Clues to the presence of actinomycosis are lesions penetrating the chest wall, bony destruction, and infection traversing an interlobar fissure. Penicillin, in high intravenous doses, remains the drug of choice for treatment of *Actinomyces* infection at all sites. The organism is also susceptible to tetracycline, erythromycin, and clindamycin.

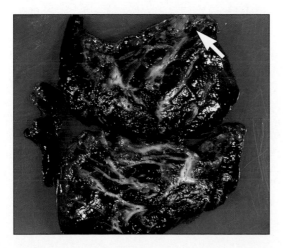

FIGURE 3-72 Autopsy specimen of chronic pulmonary actinomycosis. Extensive fibrosis is seen, primarily along the bronchi, with emphysema and a yellow area of consolidation (*arrow*). In chronic actinomycosis, healing by intense fibrosis occurs in one area, with acute suppuration in another location.

Antibiotic treatment of actinomycosis

	Daily dose
Aqueous penicillin	18–24 MU
Amoxicillin	1.5–3 g
Tetracycline	2 g
Doxycycline	200 mg
Erythromycin	2 g
Clindamycin	1.2–2.4 g
Imipenem	1.5–2 g

FIGURE 3-73 Antibiotic treatment of actinomycosis. Actinomycosis must be treated with high doses and for a prolonged period of time. Intravenous penicillin, 18 to 24 MU per day for 2 to 6 weeks, followed by oral penicillin or amoxicillin for 6 to 12 months, is a reasonable guideline. Duration of therapy is dependent upon the location and extent of disease and ranges from several weeks to 6 to 12 months.

ACKNOWLEDGMENTS

The authors thank Anthony Morales and Herbert Koch for their photography and Lederle Laboratories for their contribution to this chapter.

REFERENCES

1. Jacobs E: Serological diagnosis of *Mycoplasma pneumoniae* infections: A critical review of current procedures. *Clin Infect Dis* 1993, 17(suppl 1):S79–S82.

2. Marmion BP, Williamson J, Worswick DA, *et al.*: Experience with newer techniques for the laboratory detection of *Mycoplasma pneumoniae* infection: Adelaide, 1978–1992. *Clin Infect Dis* 1993, 17(suppl 1):S90–S99.

3. Cassell GH, Cole BC: Mycoplasmas as agents of human disease. *N Engl J Med* 1981, 304:80–89.

4. Baum SG: Mycoplasma infections. *In* Wyngaarden JB, Smith LH Jr, Bennett JC (eds.): *Cecil Textbook of Medicine*, 19th ed. Philadelphia: W.B. Saunders; 1992:1615.

5. Marrie TJ: Community-acquired pneumonia. *Clin Infect Dis* 1994, 18:501–515.

6. Bébéar C, Dupon M, Renaudin H, Barbeyrac B: Potential improvements in therapeutic options for mycoplasmal respiratory infection. *Clin Infect Dis* 1993, 17(suppl 1):S202–S207.

7. Koletsky RJ, Weinstein AJ: Fulminant *Mycoplasma pneumoniae* infection. *Am Rev Respir Dis* 1980, 122:491–496.

8. Baum SG: *Mycoplasma pneumoniae* and atypical pneumonia. *In* Mandell GL, Bennett JE, Dolin R (eds.): *Principles and Practice of Infectious Diseases*, 4th ed. New York: Churchill Livingstone; 1995:1704–1713.

9. Liu F, Wright DN: Gram stain in legionnaires' disease. *Am J Med* 1984, 77:549–550.

10. Horowitz MA: The legionnaires' disease bacterium (*Legionella pneumophila*) inhibits phagosome-lysosome fusion in human monocytes. *J Exp Med* 1983, 158:2108–2126.

11. Horowitz MA: Phagocytosis of the legionnaires' disease bacterium (*Legionella pneumophila*) occurs by a novel mechanism: Engulfment within a pseudopod coil. *Cell* 1984, 36:28.

12. Lewin S, Brettman LR, Goldstein EJC, *et al.*: Legionnaires' disease: A cause of severe abscess-forming pneumonia. *Am J Med* 1979, 76:339–342.

13. Koneman E, Allen S, Janda W, *et al.*: *Legionella*. *In* Koneman EW, Allen SD, Janda WM, *et al.* (eds.): *Color Atlas and Textbook of Diagnostic Microbiology*, 4th ed. Philadelphia: J.B. Lippincott; 1992:451–468.

14. Yu VL: *Legionella pneumophila* (legionnaires' disease). *In* Mandell GL, Bennett JE, Dolin R (eds.): *Principles and Practice of Infectious Diseases*, 4th ed. New York: Churchill Livingstone; 1995:2087–2097.

15. Skerrett SJ, Locksley RM: Legionellosis: Ecology and pathogenesis. *In* Sande MA, Hudson LD, Root RK (eds.): *Respiratory Infections*. New York: Churchill Livingstone; 1986:161–190.

16. Edelstein PH: Legionnaires' disease. *Clin Infect Dis* 1993, 16:741–749.

17. Winn WC, Myerowitz RL: The pathology of the *Legionella* pneumonias: A review of 74 cases and the literature. *Hum Pathol* 1981, 12:401–422.

18. Muder RR, Yu VL: Other *Legionella* species. *In* Mandell GL, Bennett JE, Dolin R (eds.): *Principles and Practice of Infectious Diseases*, 4th ed. New York: Churchill Livingstone, 1995:2097–2103.

19. Schwebke JR, Hackman R, Bowden R: Pneumonia due to *Legionella micdadei* in bone marrow transplant recipients. *Rev Infect Dis* 1990, 12:824–828.

20. Jaeger TM, Atkinson PP, Adams BA, *et al.*: *Legionella bozemanii* pneumonia in an immunocompromised patient. *Mayo Clin Proc* 1988, 63:72–76.

21. Muder RR, Yu VL, Parry MF: The radiologic manifestations of *Legionella* pneumonia. *Semin Respir Infect* 1987, 2:242–254.

22. Grayston JT: *Chlamydia pneumoniae* (TWAR). *In* Mandell GL, Bennett JE, Dolin R (eds.): *Principles and Practice of Infectious Diseases*, 4th ed. New York: Churchill Livingstone; 1995:1696–1701.

23. Oldach DW, Gaydos CA, Mundy LM, Quinn TC: Rapid diagnosis of *Chlamydia psittaci* pneumonia. *Clin Infect Dis* 1993, 17:338–343.

24. Schaffner W: *Chlamydia psittaci* (psittacosis). *In* Mandell GL, Bennett JE, Dolin R (eds.): *Principles and Practice of Infectious Diseases*, 3rd ed. New York: Churchill Livingstone; 1990:1440–1443.

25. Schachter J: *Chlamydia psittaci*—"reemergence" of a forgotten pathogen. *N Engl J Med* 1986, 315:189–191.

26. Grayston JT: Infections caused by *Chlamydia pneumoniae* strain TWAR. *Clin Infect Dis* 1992, 15:757–763.

27. Gaydos CA, Fowler CL, Gill VJ, *et al.*: Detection of *Chlamydia pneumoniae* by polymerase chain reaction–enzyme immunoassay in an immunocompromised population. *Clin Infect Dis* 1993, 17:1718–1723.

28. Hammerschlag MR: Antimicrobial susceptibility and therapy of infections caused by *Chlamydia pneumoniae*. *Antimicrob Agents Chemother* 1994, 38:1873–1878.

29. Augenbraun MH, Roblin PM, Mandel LJ, Hammerschlag MR: *Chlamydia pneumoniae* pneumonia with pleural effusion: Diagnosis by culture. *Am J Med* 1991, 91:437–438.

30. Samra Z, Pik A, Guidetti-Sharon A, Yaakov DB: Severe *Chlamydia trachomatis* pneumonia in a patient with no immune deficiency. *Arch Intern Med* 1988, 148:1345–1346.

31. Marrie TJ: *Coxiella burnetii* (Q fever). *In* Mandell GL, Bennett JM, Dolin R (eds.): *Principles and Practice of Infectious Diseases*, 4th ed. New York: Churchill Livingstone; 1995:1472–1476.

32. Baca OG, Akporiaye ET, Rowatt JD: Possible biochemical adaptations of *Coxiella burnetti* for survival within phagocytes: Effect of antibody. *In*

Schlessinger D (ed.): *Microbiology 1984*. Washington, DC: American Society for Microbiology; 1984:269–272.

33. McCaul TF, Williams JC: Developmental cycle of *Coxiella burnetii*: Structure and morphogenesis of vegetative and sporogenic differentiations. *J Bacteriol* 1981, 147:1063–1076.

34. Raoult D, Marrie T: Q fever. *Clin Infect Dis* 1995, 20:489–496.

35. Gombert ME, Aulicino TM, DuBouchet L, *et al.*: Therapy of experimental cerebral nocardiosis with imipenem, amikacin, trimethoprim-sulfamethoxazole, and minocycline. *Antimicrob Agents Chemother* 1986, 30:270–273.

36. Angeles AM, Sugar AM: Rapid diagnosis of nocardiosis with an enzyme immunoassay. *J Infect Dis* 1987, 155:292–296.

37. Lerner PI: *Actinomyces* and *Arachnia* species. *In* Mandell GL, Douglas RG, Bennett JM (eds.): *Principles and Practice of Infectious Diseases*, 3rd ed. New York: Churchill Livingstone; 1990:1932–1942.

SELECTED BIBLIOGRAPHY

Baum SG: *Mycoplasma pneumoniae* and atypical pneumonia. *In* Mandell GL, Bennett JE, Dolin R (eds.): *Principles and Practice of Infectious Diseases*, 4th ed. New York: Churchill Livingstone; 1995:1704–1713.

Edelstein PH: Legionnaire's disease. *Clin Infect Dis* 1993, 16:741–749.

Grayston JT: The chlamydial pneumonias. *In* Remington JS, Swartz MN (eds.): *Current Clinical Topics in Infectious Diseases*, vol 11. Boston: Blackwell Scientific Publications; 1991:1–18.

Lerner PI: Diseases due to higher bacteria. *In* Mandell GL, Bennett JE, Dolin R (eds.): *Principles and Practice of Infectious Diseases*, 4th ed. New York: Churchill Livingstone; 1995, 2273–2288.

Tuazon CU, Murray HW: Atypical pneumonias. *In* Pennington JE (ed.): *Respiratory Infections: Diagnosis and Management*, 3rd ed. New York: Raven Press; 1994:407–433.

CHAPTER 4

Tuberculosis and Other Mycobacterial Infections of the Lungs

Melanie J. Maslow

Mycobacterial species pathogenic for humans	
Common pathogens	**Rare pathogens**
M. tuberculosis	M. africanis
M. bovis	M. gordonae
M. ulcerans	M. terrae
M. leprae	M. asiaticum
M. avium complex	M. gastri
M. kansasii	M. flavescens
M. marinum	M. thermoresistibile
M. simiae	M. smegmatis
M. scrofulaceum	
M. szulgai	
M. xenopi	
M. fortuitum	
M. chelonae	
M. malmoense	
M. hemophilum	

FIGURE 4-1 Mycobacterial species pathogenic for humans. Many species of mycobacteria are pathogenic for humans. Whereas the agents of tuberculosis and leprosy have been known for over a century, our knowledge of the role of other mycobacteria in human disease began in the 1950s and continues to expand today.

MYCOBACTERIUM TUBERCULOSIS

Epidemiology

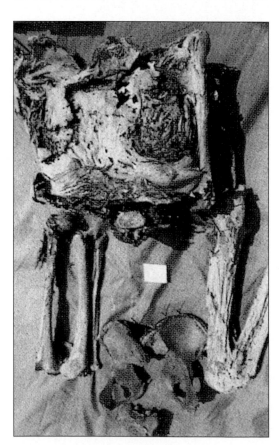

FIGURE 4-2 Tuberculosis in a 900-year-old Peruvian mummy. Tuberculosis was claimed by ethnohistorians to have been introduced into the Americas by the Europeans, causing devastating epidemics among the American Indians in the early 1600s. However, recent examination of a naturally mummified woman, who died approximately 900 years ago in southern Peru, revealed DNA specific to *Mycobacterium tuberculosis*, marking the first time DNA was recovered from an ancient sample of a disease-causing organism. Gross examination of the mummy revealed the right upper lobe to be adherent to the chest wall, a calcified 1.2-cm subpleural nodule, and two partly calcified right hilar masses. DNA was extracted from these lesions and subjected to polymerase chain reaction, targeting a segment of DNA unique to *M. tuberculosis*. A positive result was obtained from one lymph node, demonstrating the presence of tuberculosis in the New World in the pre-Columbus era [1]. (*From* Morell [2]; with permission.)

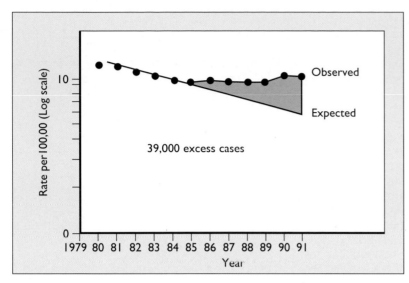

FIGURE 4-3 Observed: expected case rates for tuberculosis in the United States between 1980 and 1991. Until 1984, the morbidity rate from tuberculosis had been declining steadily in the United States. For the period 1985 to 1991, an excess of 39,000 cases of tuberculosis above expected numbers was observed. Factors contributing to this increase include homelessness, intravenous drug abuse, and, especially, the AIDS epidemic. (*From* American Thoracic Society [3]; with permission.)

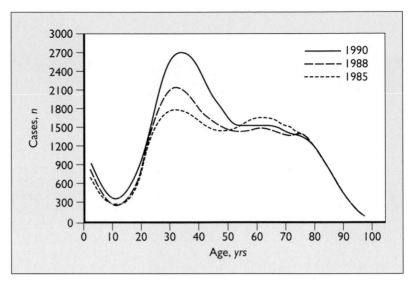

FIGURE 4-4 Age distribution of tuberculosis cases in the United States between 1985 and 1990. Tuberculosis had been most prevalent in the elderly, where it was due to reactivation of latent infection. Reports since 1985, however, indicate an increase in tuberculosis rates in younger persons, representing ongoing active transmission of new infection in the community. Active tuberculosis is now most often diagnosed in young adults, where HIV infection is most prevalent. (*From* Jereb *et al.* [4]; with permission.)

Estimated tuberculosis case rates in 1990 among WHO member states

Region	Cases, *n*	Percentage of all cases	Rate per 100,000 population
Africa	1,160,000	15%	220
Southeast Asia	2,470,000	31%	194
China	2,127,000	27%	191
Western Pacific*	420,000	5%	191
Eastern Mediterranean	594,000	7%	155
Americas (excluding USA and Canada)	534,000	7%	120
Europe, USA, Japan, Australia, New Zealand, Canada	392,000	5%	31
HIV-related	305,000	4%	6
Total	8,002,000	100%	152

*Excludes China, Japan, Australia, New Zealand.
WHO—World Health Organization.

FIGURE 4-5 Estimated worldwide case rates of tuberculosis, 1990. Estimated case rates of tuberculosis in different regions of the world are presented. HIV infection has become an important cofactor in tuberculosis infection. (*Adapted from* Sudre *et al.* [5]; with permission.)

High-risk populations to be screened for tuberculosis

Person infected with HIV or at risk
Close contacts of persons known or suspected to have TB, sharing the same household or other closed environments
Person with abnormal chest radiographs showing fibrotic lesions consistent with inactive TB
Persons with medical risk factors known to increase the risk of disease if infection has occurred:
Silicosis
Gastrectomy
Jejunoileal bypass
Weight of 10% or more below ideal body weight
Chronic renal failure
Diabetes mellitus
Conditions requiring prolonged high-dose corticosteroid therapy or other immunosuppressive therapy
Some hematologic disorders (*eg*, lymphoma, leukemia)
Other malignancies
Foreign-born persons from countries with high TB prevalence
Medically underserved low-income populations, including high-risk racial or ethnic minorities (*eg*, blacks, Hispanics, Native Americans), migrant workers, and the homeless
Alcoholics and intravenous drug users
Residents of long-term-care facilities, correctional institutions, mental institutions, shelters, nursing homes/facilities, other long-term residential facilities

TB—tuberculosis.

FIGURE 4-6 High-risk populations to be screened for tuberculosis. The risk of developing active tuberculosis once a person is infected is determined by multiple factors. Persons in high-risk groups should be aggressively screened for tuberculosis because of a high prevalence of infection and increased risk of disease following infection. (*Adapted from* Centers for Disease Control and Prevention [6]; with permission.)

Bacteriology

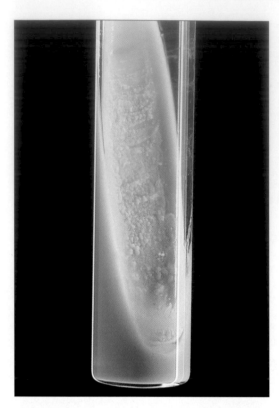

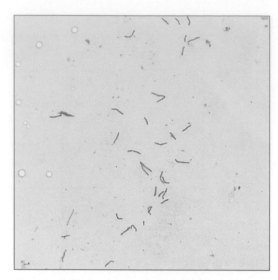

FIGURE 4-7 *Mycobacterium tuberculosis* colonies on Löwenstein-Jensen media. The organism grows in culture as slowly developing, rough colonies with a characteristic buff color. Under optimal conditions, colonies are recognizable in 3 weeks, but some strains may require 4 to 6 weeks. Löwenstein-Jensen media, an egg-based media containing malachite green to inhibit growth of contaminating bacteria, is commonly used in clinical laboratories. Other mycobacterial isolation media include Middlebrook 7H11, Middlebrook 7H10 (used predominantly for susceptibility testing), Mycobactosel, and Middlebrook 7H9 broth. For optimal recovery, a combination of liquid and solid media is recommended.

FIGURE 4-8 Typical cell morphology of *Mycobacterium tuberculosis* on acid-fast staining. The organism under oil-immersion microscopy is a thin, slightly curved bacillus, 2 to 4 µm long and 0.2 to 0.5 µm wide, that is deeply red stained and beaded in appearance. Organisms frequently appear as aggregates or in parallel strands. Acid-fast staining of clinical material, using either the Ziehl-Neelsen (hot stain) or Kinyoun (cold stain) method, is a rapid and inexpensive diagnostic tool, but the sensitivity is dependent on the number of acid-fast bacilli in the specimen. (Original magnification, × 250.)

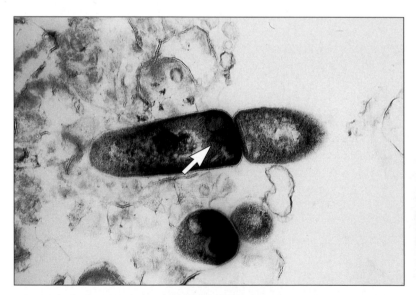

FIGURE 4-9 Transmission electron micrograph of *Mycobacterium tuberculosis*. Multiple mycobacteria with intracytoplasmic lipid droplets (*arrow*) and complex cell walls are evident. *M. tuberculosis* is an aerobic, non–spore-forming, nonmotile bacillus with a large content (25%) of high-molecular-weight lipids comprising the cell wall that give this genus the ability to bind fuchsin dye without decolorizing by alcohol. Mycolic acid is the main component of the complex lipids of mycobacteria, including mycosides, wax D, cord factor, and sulfolipids. Growth is slow, with a generation time of 15 to 20 hours. (*Courtesy of* G. Sidhu, MD.)

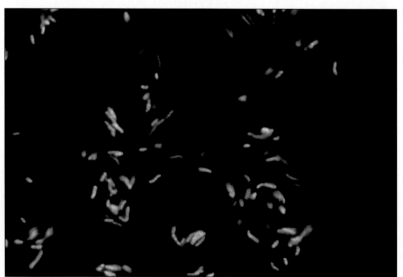

FIGURE 4-10 Fluorochrome-stained *Mycobacterium tuberculosis* with auramine O. Mycobacteria stain bright yellow against a dark background. This technique allows the slide to be scanned under lower magnification without sacrificing sensitivity. Fluorescent microscopy is more sensitive than standard acid-fast staining without loss of specificity. Modifications of this technique include the addition of rhodamine or acridine orange as counterstains. (Original magnification, × 1000.) (*Courtesy of* J. Jagirdar, MD.)

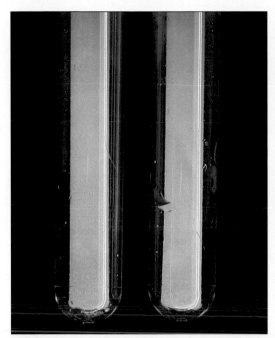

FIGURE 4-11 Niacin test for *Mycobacterium tuberculosis*. A positive niacing test is seen in the left tube, and a negative test on the right. The key identifying characteristic for *M. tuberculosis* is the accumulation of niacin on special media due to absence of the enzyme that converts free niacin to niacin ribonucleotide. An extract of mycobacteria is placed in the bottom of a tube to which a reagent-impregnated strip is added. A yellow color in the fluid within 12 to 15 minutes indicates niacin accumulation. Certain strains of *M. bovis*, *M. simiae*, and some *M. marinum* strains may also be niacin positive, but these species can be distinguished by other reactions.

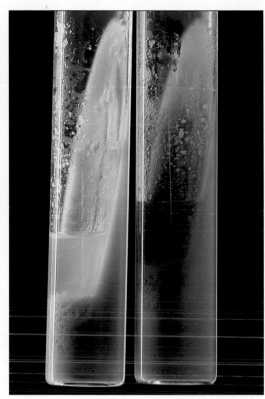

FIGURE 4-12 Nitrate reduction by *Mycobacterium tuberculosis*. *M. tuberculosis* is one of the few species of mycobacteria that produce nitroreductase, which catalyzes the reduction of nitrate to nitrite. An emulsion of mycobacteria is added to a test tube containing buffered sodium nitrate. A pink to red color, as seen in the right tube, indicates that nitrates have been reduced to nitrites.

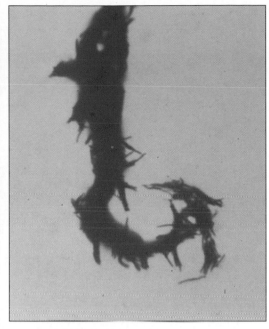

FIGURE 4-13 *Mycobacterium tuberculosis* demonstrating rope or "cording" phenomenon. Virulent strains of *M. tuberculosis* grown on the surface of liquid or solid media characteristically form strands or cords from production of cord factor, reliably differentiating these colonies from non-tuberculous mycobacteria. The role cord factor plays in the pathogenesis of tuberculosis is unknown. (*Courtesy of Becton Dickinson.*)

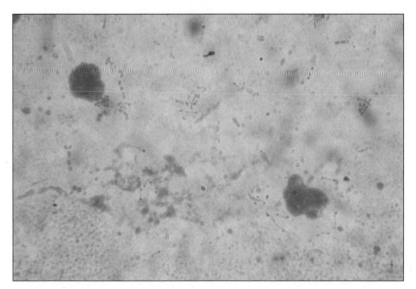

FIGURE 4-14 Kinyoun stain of sputum demonstrating numerous acid-fast bacilli. Approximately 10,000 acid-fast bacilli are needed per milliliter of sputum to be detected microscopically. Sputum for culture must first be treated by decontamination and digestion to reduce bacterial overgrowth and release trapped mycobacterial cells from liquefied mucus. The specimen then undergoes high-speed centrifugation to concentrate the organisms in the sediment.

Susceptibility Testing

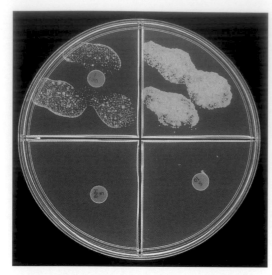

FIGURE 4-15 Mycobacterial susceptibility testing by the agar diffusion method. Testing demonstrates that a strain of *Mycobacterium tuberculosis* is resistant to isoniazid (INH) at the 0.2-µg/mL concentration (INH 1, *upper right quadrant*) but susceptible to 1 µg/mL (INH 5, *upper left quadrant*). Quadranted plates containing Middlebrook agar (one control quadrant and three quadrants containing specified antibiotic concentrations) are inoculated with a standard concentration of organisms; susceptibility is determined by comparing the number of colonies growing in the drug-containing quadrants with the control quadrant. Results are reported in terms of the percentage resistant, with 5% to 10% or greater resistance indicating clinical resistance.

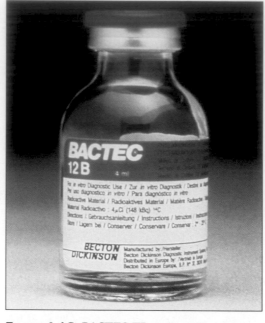

FIGURE 4-16 BACTEC TB radiometic system. The BACTEC TB system (Becton Dickinson, Sparks, MD) is an automated radiometric system based on the detection of radiolabeled $^{14}CO_2$ released in the vial from ^{14}C-palmitic acid in the broth medium. This system can be used for detection, isolation, and drug susceptibility testing of *Mycobacterium tuberculosis* and has reduced the time of isolation and identification from 4 weeks to about 2 weeks. Sensitivity testing is performed by inoculating positive specimens into antibiotic-containing bottles, and results are often available within 3 weeks of processing. Genetic probes can be used to provide rapid identification from an actively growing culture. An ideal diagnostic procedure would detect and identify mycobacteria directly from clinical specimens. The polymerase chain reaction has great potential, but more experience is needed with this technique [7]. (*Courtesy of* Becton Dickinson.)

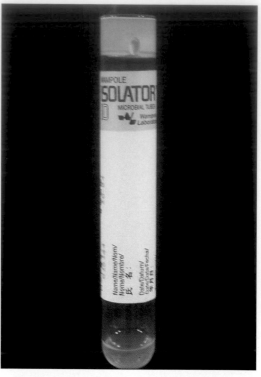

FIGURE 4-17 Lysis-centrifugation blood culture system. The lysis-centrifugation system (Isolator, Wampole Laboratories, Cranbury, NJ) for isolating mycobacteria from blood has increased the yield of cultures and shortened the recovery time. The lysis-centrifuge tube contains an anticoagulant and lysing agent that ruptures erythrocytes and neutrophils, releasing intracellular mycobacteria into the broth. After centrifugation, the eluate is discarded and 1.6 mL of the sediment is divided into 0.2-mL aliquots and plated on culture media.

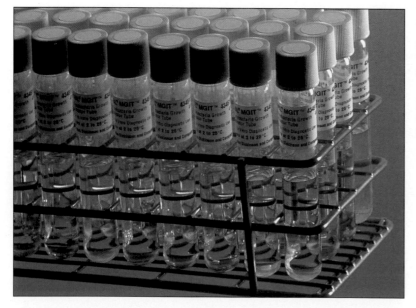

FIGURE 4-18 Rapid detection of mycobacterial growth by the luciferase mycobacteria growth indicator tube. The mycobacteria growth indicator tube (Becton Dickinson) is a novel new diagnostic test that assays light production after infection of mycobacteria by a recombinant mycobacteriophage expressing firefly luciferase. Resistance can be detected within 48 hours by demonstrating light production despite treatment with antibiotics. Tubes with growth are seen to fluoresce brightly compared with tubes in which growth is inhibited [8]. (*Courtesy of* Becton Dickinson.)

Immunopathogenesis

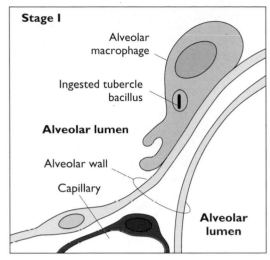

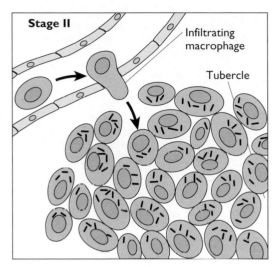

FIGURE 4-19 Pathogenesis of pulmonary tuberculosis (rabbit model), stage I. Tuberculosis in rabbits closely resembles the disease in humans, with the exception being that in humans the stages do not occur in an orderly progression. In the initial stage, after inhalation of a few tubercle bacilli into the terminal air spaces, bacilli are ingested by alveolar macrophages. Alveolar macrophages of rabbits and humans are usually in an activated state from nonspecific stimulation and probably destroy or inhibit more than 90% of bacilli. Within tissue macrophages, the remaining mycobacteria evade the host's microbicial killing. (*Illustration by* L. Duprey and S. Hung.) (*From* Dannenberg [9]; with permission.)

FIGURE 4-20 Pathogenesis of pulmonary tuberculosis, stage II. During stage II, the tubercle bacilli that are not destroyed by alveolar macrophages multiply intracellularly and are released on macrophage death. Released bacilli attract unactivated monocytes and macrophages from the bloodstream, and an early primary tubercle forms. The phagocytic vacuole in the cytoplasm of unactivated macrophages provides an ideal environment for bacilli, which multiply logarithmically. During this stage, a symbiosis exists between multiplying bacilli and accumulating macrophages, with neither being destroyed. (*Illustration by* L. Duprey and S. Hung.) (*From* Dannenberg [9]; with permission.)

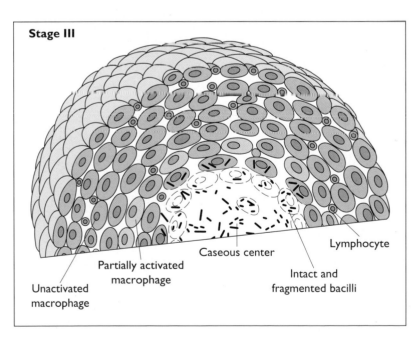

FIGURE 4-21 Pathogenesis of pulmonary tuberculosis, stage III. At 2 to 3 weeks into infection, delayed hypersensitivity and cellular immunity develop. Only delayed hypersensitivity can halt the logarithmic growth by killing bacilli-laden macrophages. This results in the formation of a caseous necrotic center in the tubercle, which consists of dead and live bacilli and cellular debris surrounded by granulation tissue containing lymphocytes and macrophages. Bacilli are unable to multiply within caseous tissue due to anoxia, low pH, and toxic fatty acids. (*Illustration by* L. Duprey and S. Hung.) (*From* Dannenberg [9]; with permission.)

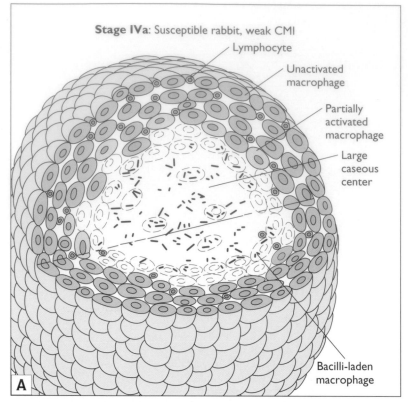

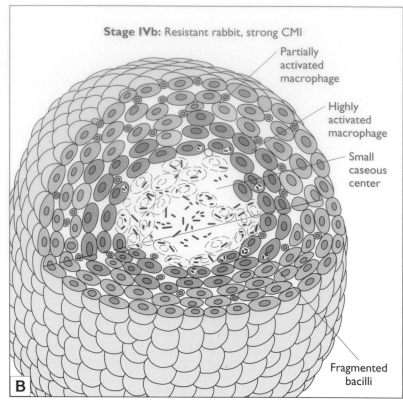

FIGURE 4-22 Pathogenesis of pulmonary tuberculosis, stage IV. After 3 weeks, multiplication of bacilli is controlled. **A**, In rabbits with weak cell-mediated immunity (CMI), the caseous center enlarges, and lung tissue is destroyed as released bacilli are ingested by relatively unactivated macrophages, resulting in the pathologic features of tuberculosis. **B**, In animals with strong CMI, bacilli released from the caseous center are ingested by highly activated macrophages that accumulate around the caseous center with little tissue destruction. The latter scenario takes place in more than 90% of healthy humans, who develop positive tuberculin reactions without clinical evidence of disease, although viable bacilli may remain. In immunocompromised patients, as in animals with weak immunity, infection is not contained, and both rapid progression of recent infection and a high rate of reactivation occur. (*Illustrations by* L. Duprey and S. Hung.) (*From* Dannenberg [9]; with permission.)

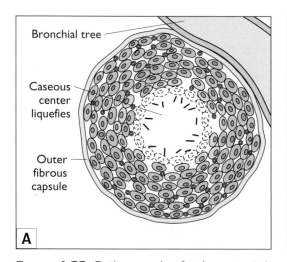

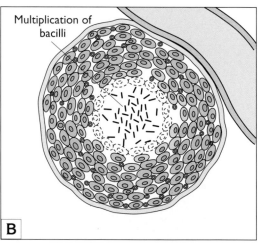

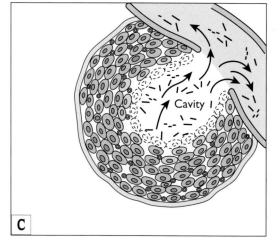

FIGURE 4-23 Pathogenesis of pulmonary tuberculosis, stage V. **A**, In the final stage of infection, liquefaction of the solid caseous focus occurs. **B**, In this favorable environment, bacilli multiply extracellularly. The large dose of bacillary antigens causes extensive tissue damage secondary to delayed hypersensitivity. **C**, Erosion of nearby bronchi occurs, followed by cavity formation when digestion of caseous tissue occurs by host hydrolytic enzymes. Spread of bacilli via the bronchial tree to other parts of the lung extends disease and may result in tuberculous pneumonia. (*Illustrations by* L. Duprey and S. Hung.) (*From* Dannenberg [9]; with permission.)

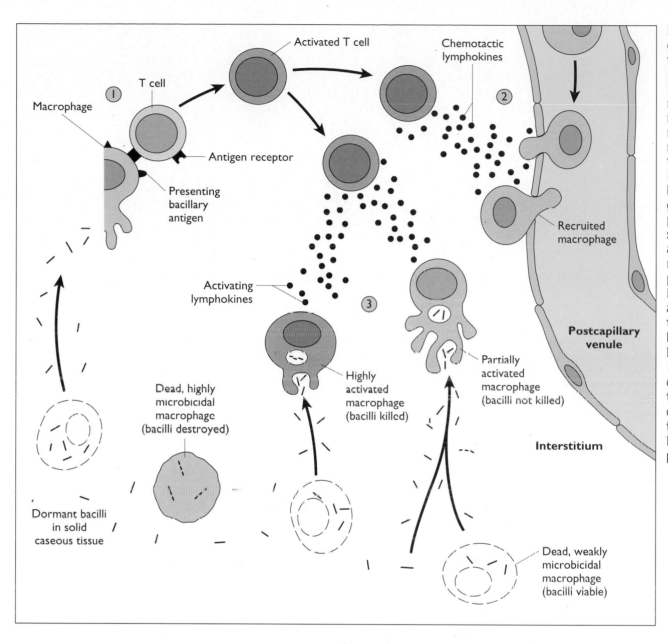

FIGURE 4-24 Activation of cell-mediated immunity after *Mycobacterium tuberculosis* infection. Initial activation of cell-mediated immunity results in production of many highly activated macrophages in the tuberculous lesion. Macrophages ingest bacilli and present antigens to specific T lymphocytes (*1*), which secrete lymphokines that attract and activate monocytes and macrophages (*2*) to enhance intracellular killing (*3*) and increase cellular infiltration to the site. It has been suggested that the host response to *M. tuberculosis* has a significant autoimmune effect that contributes to the caseation and liquefaction process. (*From* Dannenberg [9]; with permission.)

Clinical Manifestations

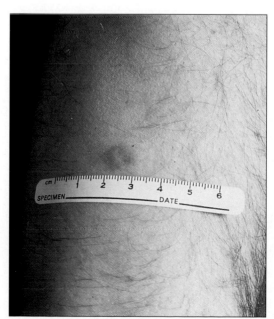

FIGURE 4-25 Mantoux test (tuberculin skin test). The Mantoux test is performed by intradermal injection of 5 tuberculin units of purified protein derivative into the volar aspect of the forearm. The reaction is read at 48 to 72 hours, with a positive test usually defined as > 10 mm of induration (5 mm in HIV-infected and other high-risk individuals). False-positive reactions are usually secondary to infection with other nontuberculous species of mycobacteria or recent vaccination with bacille Calmette-Guérin. False-negative reactions may be seen in conditions of cellular immune hyporesponsiveness and, occasionally, during acute tuberculous infection. The larger the area of induration, the greater the probability of infection. Reactivity can be accentuated by repeated testing, referred to as the booster effect [10].

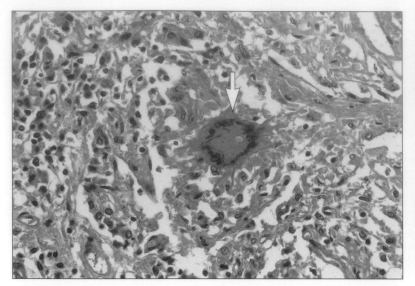

FIGURE 4-26 Epithelioid cell granuloma containing Langhans' giant cells. Epithelioid cells are highly stimulated macrophages. The Langhans' giant cell (*arrow*) represents fused macrophages oriented around tuberculous antigen, with the multiple nuclei in a peripheral position. Activated macrophages secrete a fibroblast-stimulating substance that leads to collagen production and eventual fibrosis. This hard tubercle is able to contain infection and heals with fibrosis, encapsulation, and scar formation (*see* Fig. 4-21). (*Courtesy of* G. Sidhu, MD.)

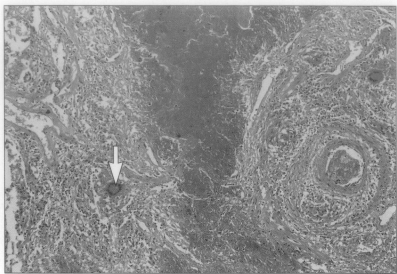

FIGURE 4-27 Tubercle with a large area of caseation in the center. The *arrow* points to the granuloma seen under higher power in Fig. 4-26. (Hematoxylin-eosin stain; original magnification, × 25.) (*Courtesy of* G. Sidhu, MD.)

Clinical presentations of pulmonary tuberculosis
Primary tuberculosis: asymptomatic, primary "Ghon" complex, chronic infection
Postprimary tuberculosis: apical caseation, cavity formation, fibrosis
Lower-lobe tuberculosis: elderly, HIV
Endobronchial tuberculosis
Tuberculomas

FIGURE 4-28 Clinical presentation of pulmonary tuberculosis. In most instances, following tuberculin positivity and development of cellular immunity, bacteria are destroyed and the only remaining evidence of infection is a positive skin test. In a smaller number of cases, infection progresses to the primary complex stage, and in an even smaller number, infection progresses to chronic pulmonary tuberculosis.

Classification of pulmonary tuberculosis		
0	No exposure, PPD–	
I	Exposure, no infection, PPD–	
II	Infection without disease, PPD+	
III	Infection with disease	
	1) Location	
	2) Bacteriologic status	
	3) Chemotherapy	
PPD—purified protein derivative.		

FIGURE 4-29 Classification of pulmonary tuberculosis. The present classification of pulmonary tuberculosis defines disease by exposure, as indicated by a positive tuberculin test, and by evidence of infection according to location of disease (pulmonary and/or extrapulmonary), microscopy with culture information, and specific treatment.

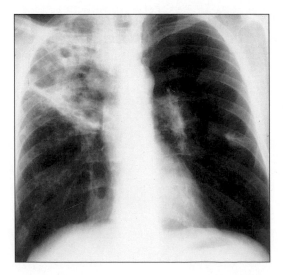

FIGURE 4-30 Chest radiograph of a 39-year-old man with acute upper lobe tuberculosis demonstrating typical cavitary infiltrates. Apical localization of pulmonary tuberculosis is characteristic of adult infection. This localization has been attributed to the hyperoxic environment of the apices, but another theory proposes that lymph production is deficient at the apices, favoring retention of antigens at this location [11]. (*Courtesy of* N. Ettinger, MD.)

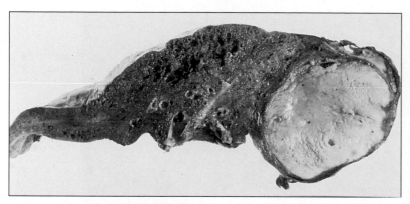

FIGURE 4-31 Gross pathology of chronic pulmonary tuberculosis with marked emphysema and a large caseous nodule. Necrosis in tuberculosis tends to be incomplete, resulting in solid or semisolid, acellular, and amorphous material referred to as caseous because of its cheesy consistency. The chemical environment and oxygen tension in this material is not favorable to bacillary multiplication, but caseous necrosis is unstable and may liquefy and discharge through the bronchial tree. The resulting tuberculosis cavity promotes explosive multiplication of mycobacteria with subsequent spread of bacilli-rich material through the bronchial tree. (*Courtesy of* J. Jagirdar, MD.)

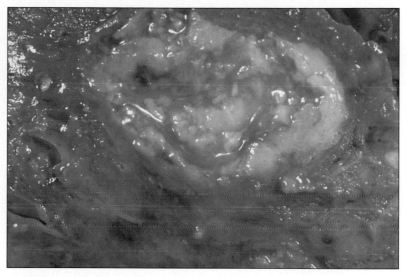

FIGURE 4-32 Gross photograph of a tuberculous cavity with caseous content. An active, freshly opened cavity exemplifies the many pathologic reactions that occur with tuberculous infection. Microscopically, the cavity contains a central core of many bacilli lined by a layer of caseous material with fewer organisms; a more peripheral layer of macrophages and lymphocytes with still fewer organisms; a layer of epithelioid cells and Langhans' giant cells; and finally a layer of encapsulating fibrosis. (*Courtesy of* G. Sidhu, MD.)

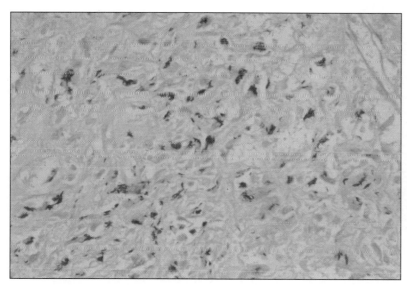

FIGURE 4-33 Lung biopsy specimen showing a granulomatous area with numerous acid-fast bacilli. Diagnostic fiberoptic bronchoscopy with transbronchial biopsy and bronchial washings is an effective way to obtain diagnostic materials when sputum examination is unrevealing, in the early diagnosis of miliary disease, and in lower lobe tuberculosis when the number of bacilli may be small. (Kinyoun stain.)

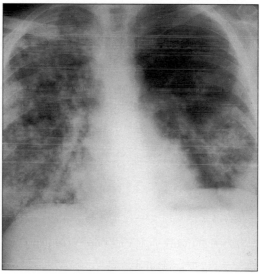

FIGURE 4-34 Chest radiograph of a 48-year-old alcoholic man showing diffuse infiltrates secondary to tuberculous pneumonia. Bronchogenic spread caused by recent spillage of the infectious contents of a tuberculous cavity or breakdown of endobronchial disease leads to multiple, fluffy, or confluent infiltrates. (*Courtesy of* N. Ettinger, MD.)

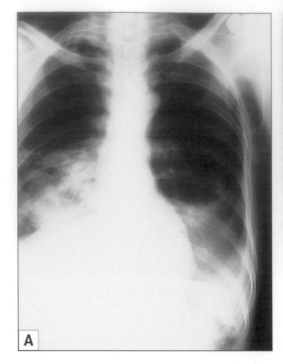

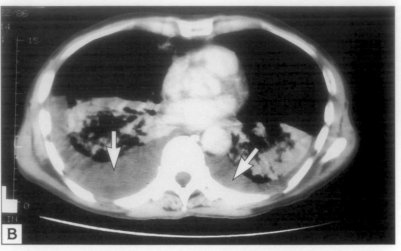

FIGURE 4-35 Lower lobe tuberculosis and pleural effusion. **A** and **B**, A chest radiograph and computed tomography scan of a 68-year-old man show a right lower lobe infiltrate and bilateral pleural effusions (panel 35B, *arrows*) secondary to tuberculosis. When new tuberculosis occurs in an older, previously tuberculin-negative individual, the picture may be of a nonspecific, nonresolving pneumonitis in the lower or middle lobes. Lower lobe tuberculosis is radiographically nonspecific and may appear as nonresolving pneumonia, atelectasis, mass lesions, or cavities. (*Courtesy of* N. Ettinger, MD.)

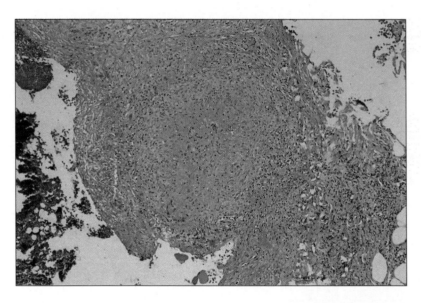

FIGURE 4-36 Low-power photomicrograph of a pleural biopsy specimen in tuberculous pleuritis. Serofibrinous pleurisy with effusion is seen in early postprimary infection but can also occur in patients with chronic infection. It results from necrosis and rupture into the pleural cavity of a subpleural caseous focus and subsequent exudation of fluid and cells from pleural surfaces. Tuberculous pleurisy usually resolves spontaneously, but patients often progress to chronic tuberculosis within 5 years if not treated [12]. (*Courtesy of* J. Jagirdar, MD.)

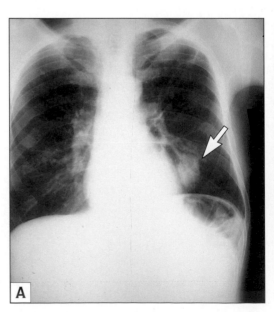

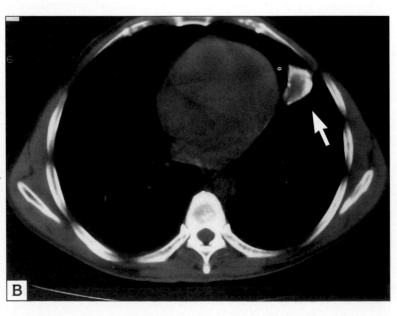

FIGURE 4-37 Tuberculoma. **A** and **B**, A chest radiograph and computed tomography scan from a 45-year-old man show a 3.5-cm × 2-cm tuberculoma in the lingula (*arrows*). The diagnosis was made at surgery. Asymptomatic round lesions may develop around the parenchymal residua of the initial infection or as a result of fibrous encapsulation of a caseous lesion. Tuberculomas may be confused with malignancy. (*Courtesy of* N. Ettinger, MD.)

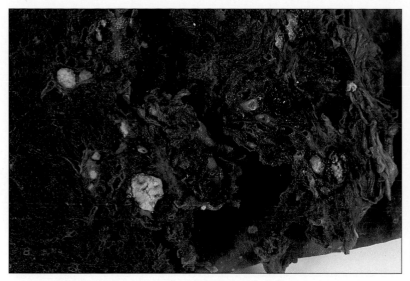

FIGURE 4-38 Gross lung with marked emphysema, extensive parenchymal fibrosis, and many tuberculous nodules containing caseous material. In chronic pulmonary tuberculosis, disease spreads by drainage into the bronchial tree, where the bacillary contents are aerosolized and spread widely throughout the lung by coughing. New foci of infection develop in susceptible areas followed by caseation, fibrosis, and new cavity formation. (*Courtesy of* G. Sidhu, MD.)

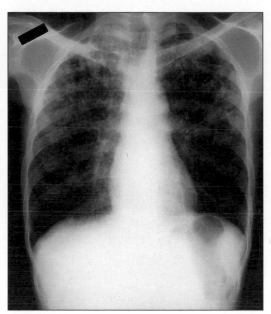

Figure 4-39 Chest radiograph of miliary tuberculosis showing widespread, small, discrete densities. Hematogenous dissemination of infection occurs before development of hypersensitivity. In the vast majority of people, dissemination stops when hypersensitivity develops, but in some individuals, it progresses to the clinical syndrome of acute miliary disease. (*Courtesy of* N. Ettinger, MD.)

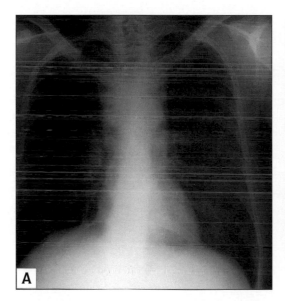

Figure 4-40 Miliary tuberculosis. A 38-year-old man on chronic prednisone therapy for asthma was admitted with fever and cough of 3 weeks' duration. **A** and **B**, A chest radiograph and computed tomography scan show mediastinal lymphadenopathy and a fine miliary pattern. The diagnosis of miliary tuberculosis was made by the finding of acid-fast bacilli on bronchoscopic washings. Chronic hematogenous, or late generalized tuberculosis, occurs when immune mechanisms are compromised and hematogenous spread occurs after primary infection, often from chronic extrapulmonary foci. (*Courtesy of* N. Ettinger, MD.)

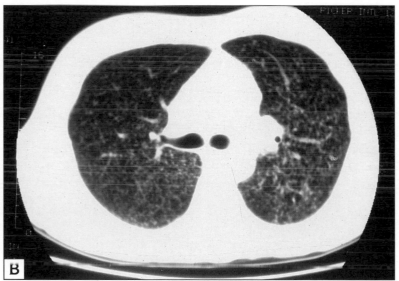

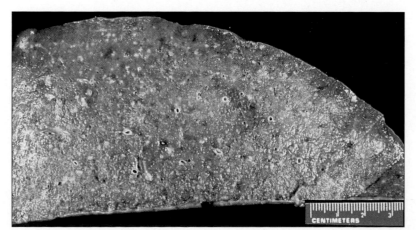

FIGURE 4-41 Gross specimen of lung parenchyma showing numerous 1- to 2-mm yellow-white nodules typical of miliary tuberculosis. Fulminant miliary tuberculosis may be associated with the adult respiratory distress syndrome and disseminated intravascular coagulation. Treatment, including adjuvant therapy with steroids, should be initiated promptly because the mortality rate remains significant. (*Courtesy of* J. Jagirdar, MD.)

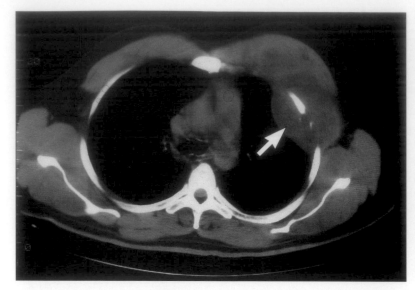

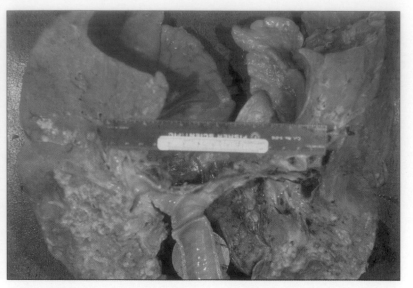

FIGURE 4-42 Chest computed tomography scan showing a left-sided tuberculous chest wall abscess with associated rib destruction. It is rare for tuberculosis to present as single or multiple cold abscesses of the chest wall (*arrow*). Some, as in this case, are associated with tuberculous osteomyelitis of ribs. Others may arise from dissection of pus from underlying caseous intercostal lymph nodes [13]. (*Courtesy of* N. Ettinger, MD.)

FIGURE 4-43 Bilateral fibrocaseous tuberculosis at autopsy. The segment of lung containing the initial cavity is typically involved with patchy disease. Spread via the bronchi often leads to secondary involvement of the contralateral apex and bilateral disease. (*Courtesy of* G. Sidhu, MD.)

Multidrug-Resistant Tuberculosis

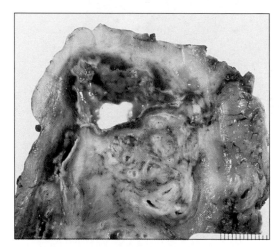

FIGURE 4-44 Lung at autopsy from a patient who died of multidrug-resistant tuberculosis. The lung is shrunken with massive pleural fibrosis and extensive cavitary fibrocaseous tuberculosis. Multidrug-resistant strains of *Mycobacterium tuberculosis* are increasing in prevalence and have been responsible for outbreaks of infection in hospitals and prisons. In a study of drug-resistant isolates in New York City, there was an association with previous therapy, HIV infection, and intravenous drug use. Patients with AIDS were more likely to die of tuberculosis if infected with a resistant strain [14]. (*Courtesy of* J. Jagirdar, MD.)

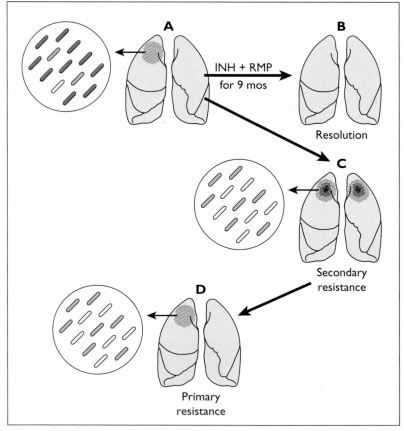

FIGURE 4-45 Mechanism of drug resistance in tuberculosis. In a patient presenting with apical tuberculosis, the lesions contain drug-sensitive organisms (*red*) but also small numbers of resistant organisms (*blue*, isoniazid [INH] resistance; *yellow*, rifampin [RMP] resistance) (*A*). Compliance with the full course of therapy leads to resolution of infection (*B*). If therapy is interrupted, infection progresses to cavitation, with large numbers of organisms that are now resistant to multiple drugs (secondary resistance) (*C*). When this patient transmits infection to a previously tuberculin-negative person, multidrug-resistant disease develops (primary resistance) (*D*).

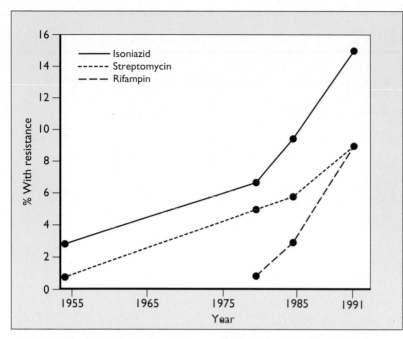

FIGURE 4-46 Incidence of multidrug-resistant tuberculosis in New York City in 1991. During the 1970s, primary resistance in *Mycobacterium tuberculosis* to at least one drug was observed in less than 3% of cases in the United States. Over the past decade, however, the incidence of primary resistance has risen dramatically, as illustrated in statistics from New York City. (*From* Frieden *et al.* [14]; with permission.)

Factors favoring acquisition and infection with MDR TB
Previous treatment with antituberculous medications
Contact with drug-resistant case
Foreign-born persons from areas of high prevalence
(Asia, Africa, Latin America)
Homelessness
Illicit drug use
HIV infection
Institutionalization
MDR TB—multidrug-resistant tuberculosis.

FIGURE 4-47 Factors favoring acquisition and infection with multidrug-resistant tuberculosis. The factors predisposing to infection with a multidrug-resistant strain of *Mycobacterium tuberculosis* are outlined. Inadequate therapy remains the most common mechanism by which resistance develops.

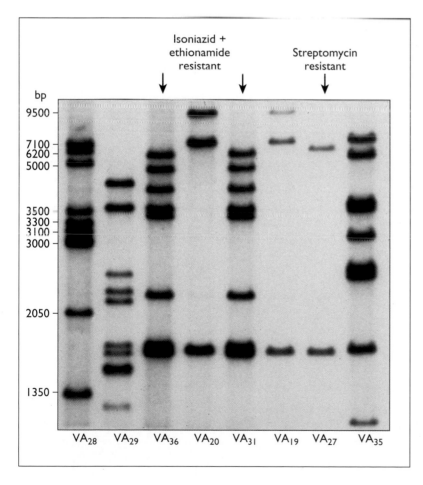

FIGURE 4-48 DNA restriction fragment length polymorphism (RFLP) analysis of a multidrug-resistant strain of *Mycobacterium tuberculosis*. DNA "fingerprinting" uses a repetitive DNA element specific to the *M. tuberculosis* complex that is carried on a transposon present at multiple sites on the chromosome. Variability in the number and size of probed fragments allows definition of unique strains. The technique has been used to trace transmission of particular strains of *M. tuberculosis* during outbreaks and has the potential for early recognition of resistant strains, prior to availability of standard susceptibility data [15]. (*Courtesy of* M. Lutfey.)

TREATMENT

Drugs used in the treatment of tuberculosis

Drug	Daily adult dosage	Major toxicity
First-line agents		
Isoniazid	300 mg orally or im	Hepatitis, neuropathy
Rifampin	600 mg orally or iv	Hepatitis, flulike syndrome
Pyrazinamide	1.5–2.5 g orally	Hepatitis, hyperuricemia
Ethambutol	15–25 mg/kg orally	Optic neuritis
Streptomycin	0.5–1 g im	Vestibular dysfunction, deafness, renal (rare)
Second line agents		
Cycloserine	250–500 mg twice a day orally	Seizures, psychiatric symptoms, CNS dysfunction
Ethionamide	250–500 mg twice a day orally	Nausea, vomiting, hepatitis, psychiatric symptoms
Capreomycin	0.5–1 g im, then 1 g 2–3 times a day	Deafness, vestibular dysfunction, renal damage
Kanamycin	15 mg/kg im or iv	Deafness, renal damage
Amikacin	15 mg/kg im or iv	Auditory, renal
PAS	4–6 mg twice a day orally	GI, lupuslike syndrome
Ciprofloxacin	500–750 mg twice a day orally	Nausea, abdominal pain, rash, CNS symptoms
Ofloxacin	300–400 mg twice a day orally	Nausea, abdominal pain, rash, CNS symptoms
Clofazamine	100–200 mg orally	GI, hyperpigmentation

CNS—central nervous system; GI—gastrointestinal; im—intramuscularly; iv—intravenously; PAS—*para*-aminosalicyclic acid.

FIGURE 4-49 Drugs used in treatment of tuberculosis. The daily adult dosage and major toxicities of the drugs used to treat tuberculosis are outlined. Isoniazid combined with rifampin makes up the cornerstone of antituberculous therapy.

Treatment regimens for tuberculosis due to sensitive strains of *Mycobacterium tuberculosis*

INH 300 mg + RMP 600 mg daily for 9 mo

INH 900 mg + RMP 600 mg twice weekly for 9 mo

INH 300 mg + RMP 600 mg + PZA 25–35 mg/kg + EMB (15–25 mg/kg) or STM (1 g) for 2 months, followed by INH + RMP daily for 4 mo

INH 300 mg + EMB 15 mg/kg for 18–24 mo

EMB—ethambutol; INH—isoniazid; PZA—pyrazinamide; RMP—rifampin; STM—streptomycin.

FIGURE 4-50 Treatment regimens for tuberculosis due to sensitive strains of *Mycobacterium tuberculosis*. Selection of a drug regimen for infection by sensitive strains of *M. tuberculosis* depends on patient compliance and drug toxicity. Directly observed therapy eliminates the problem of compliance and the likelihood of resistance emerging. For both standard 9-month regimens of insoniazid and rifampin, addition of pyrazinamide and either ethambutol or streptomycin is recommended initially pending susceptibility results. The isoniazid–ethambutol regimen is recommended for less extensive disease or severe liver disease.

Treatment of multidrug-resistant tuberculosis

Resistance	Suggested regimen	Duration of therapy	Comments
Isoniazid, streptomycin, + pyrazinamide	Rifampin Pyrazinamide Ethambutol Amikacin	6–9 mo	Anticipate 100% response rate and < 5% relapse rate
Isoniazid + ethambutol (± streptomycin)	Rifampin Pyrazinamide Ofloxacin or ciprofloxacin Amikacin	6–12 mo	Efficacy should be comparable to above regimen
Isoniazid + rifampin (± streptomycin)	Pyrazinamide Ethambutol Ofloxacin or ciprofloxacin Amikacin	18–24 mo	Consider surgery
Isoniazid, rifampin, + ethambutol (± streptomycin)	Pyrazinamide Ofloxacin or ciprofloxacin Amikacin Plus 2 (ethionamide, cycloserine, or PAS)	24 mo after conversion	Consider surgery
Isoniazid, rifampin, + pyrazinamide (± streptomycin)	Ethambutol Ofloxacin or ciprofloxacin Amikacin Plus 2 (ethionamide, cycloserine, or PAS)	24 mo after conversion	Consider surgery
Isoniazid, rifampin, pyrazinamide, + ethambutol (+ streptomycin)	Ofloxacin or ciprofloxacin Amikacin Plus 3 (ethionamide, cycloserine, or PAS)	24 mo after conversion	Surgery, if possible

PAS—*para*-aminosalicylic acid.

FIGURE 4-51 Treatment of multidrug-resistant tuberculosis. Initiation of antituberculous therapy in patients with proven multidrug-resistant strains requires assessment of prior drug therapy and data from *in vitro* susceptibility testing. If there is resistance to amikacin, kanamycin, and streptomycin, an alternative agent is capreomycin. Injectable agents are usually continued for 4 to 6 months if toxicity does not develop. All injectable drugs are given daily (two or three times weekly) by either intravenous or intramuscular routes. (*From* Iseman [16]; with permission.)

Criteria for prescribing isoniazid chemoprophylaxis in persons exposed to tuberculosis

	Age group	
Category	**< 35 yrs**	**≥ 35 yrs**
With risk factor	Treat all ages if reaction to 5 TU (PPD) ≥ 10 mm (or ≥ 5 mm and patient is recent contact, HIV infected, or has radiographic evidence of old TB)	
No risk factor, high incidence group	Treat if PPD ≥ 10 mm	Do not treat
No risk factor, low-incidence group	Treat if PPD ≥ 15 mm	Do not treat

PPD—purified protein derivative; TB—tuberculosis; TU—tuberculin unit.

FIGURE 4-52 Criteria for prescribing isoniazid chemoprophylaxis in persons exposed to tuberculosis. The most current recommendations from the Centers for Disease Control and Prevention regarding isoniazid chemoprophylaxis of persons exposed to *Mycobacterium tuberculosis* without evidence of active infection (positive tuberculin test only) are listed. Risk factors include HIV infection, known recent exposure, recent skin-test conversion, abnormal chest radiograph, intravenous drug abuse, and certain medical risk factors (*see* Fig. 4-6). For no-risk, low-incidence groups, a cutoff lower or higher than purified protein derivative ≥ 15 mm may be used, depending on the prevalance of *M. tuberculosis* infection and nonspecific cross-reactivity in the population. (*Adapted from* Centers for Disease Control and Prevention [6]; with permission.)

MYCOBACTERIUM KANSASII

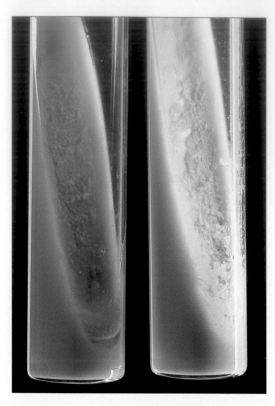

FIGURE 4-53 *Mycobacterium kansasii* colonies on Löwenstein-Jensen media. The distinctive feature of this photochromogenic species is dependence on light exposure for production of yellow pigment. Both tubes are shielded from light during incubation; the tube on the right was exposed to light for several hours and developed pigmented colonies. Typical strains grow at about the same rate or slightly faster than *Mycobacterium tuberculosis*. Colonies are intermediate between fully rough and fully smooth.

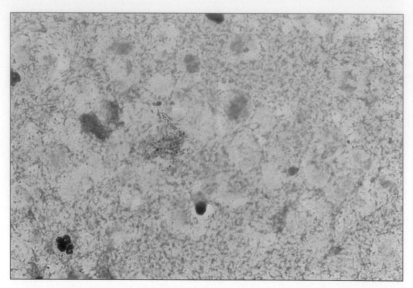

FIGURE 4-54 Acid-fast smear of *Mycobacterium kansasii*. This organism appears long, thick, and cross-barred on acid-fast staining. This distinctive morphology may provide a clue to identification. *M. kansasii* strains have a uniform antigenic structure that most closely resembles that of *Mycobacterium tuberculosis*. Among the nontuberculous mycobacteria, *M. kansasii* is the least likely to be recovered from nonhuman sources.

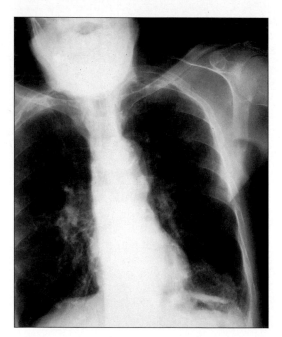

FIGURE 4-55 Chest radiograph of *Mycobacterium kansasii* infection demonstrating a left lower lobe infiltrate, calcified nodes in the right hilum, and linear stranding in the right apex. Underlying lung disease, particularly emphysema and pneumoconioses, predisposes patients to infection. Disseminated infection has been reported in immunocompromised patients. *M. kansasii* produces a chronic lung infection similar to but milder than classic tuberculosis, usually involving the upper lobes. Multiple thin-walled cavities, scarring, and endobronchial spread are seen radiographically. The combination of isoniazid, rifampin, and ethambutol has been the traditional treatment for infection, but sulfamethoxazole and quinolones hold promise as future therapeutic options [17].

MYCOBACTERIUM AVIUM-INTRACELLULARE COMPLEX

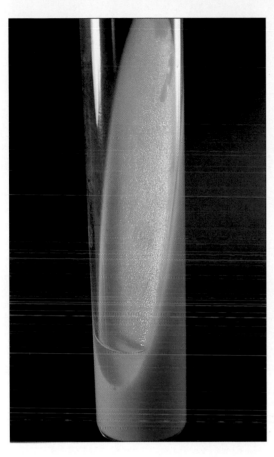

FIGURE 4-56 *Mycobacterium avium-intracellulare* complex on Löwenstein-Jensen media. Colonies can be thin, translucent, and cream-colored or domed, opaque, and yellow-colored. These two species are so similar biochemically and antigenically that they are considered as one group, but they may be distinguished serologically. The organisms are ubiquitous and found in many environmental sites, including water, soil, dust, and air. The lungs are the most frequent site of infection in immunocompetent hosts, with preexisting pulmonary disease an important risk factor. Pulmonary infection may occur in the absence of recognized risk factors [18].

Clinical signs and symptoms of pulmonary *Mycobacterium avium* complex disease		
	Patients, %	Range
Symptom		
Cough	84	78–89
Sputum production	79	49–97
Weight loss	39	14–58
Fever	24	14–51
Hemoptysis	21	8–35
Radiographic findings		
Localized disease	26	23–28
Diffuse disease	74	72–76
Cavitation	5	24–87

FIGURE 4-57 Clinical signs and symptoms of pulmonary *Mycobacterium avium* complex (MAC) disease. Symptoms of pulmonary disease due to MAC are nonspecific and often have an insidious onset, delaying diagnosis. (*From* Havlir and Ellner [19]; with permission.)

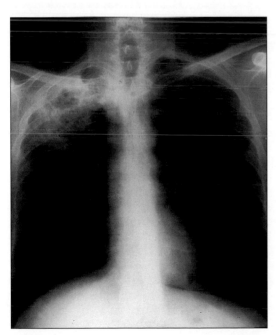

FIGURE 4-58 Chest radiograph from a 50-year-old man with chronic *Mycobacterium avium-intracellulare* pulmonary infection. This radiograph, taken after 2 years of therapy with a five-drug antibiotic regimen, shows persistence of a right upper lobe infiltrate with areas of cavitation. In most immunocompetent patients, infection follows an indolent course and is similar to tuberculosis radiographically. Treatment is complicated by the wide resistance of strains to the first-line agents. Treatment regimens include ethambutol, a macrolide antibiotic (clarithromycin or azithromycin), ciprofloxacin, rifabutin, clofazamine, and amikacin. In non-AIDS patients, resectional surgery may be used in conjunction with chemotherapy [20]. (*Courtesy of* N. Ettinger, MD.)

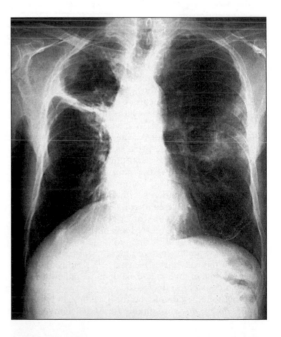

FIGURE 4-59 Chest radiograph of a middle-aged man with pulmonary infection due to *Mycobacterium avium* complex. Right upper lobe cavitation, peritracheal adenopathy, and a left midlung infiltrate are present. (*From* Havlir and Ellner [19]; with permission.)

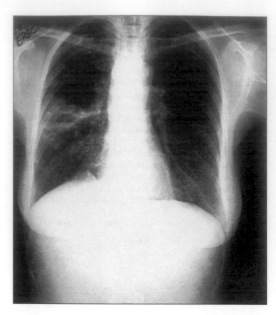

FIGURE 4-60 Chest radiograph of a middle-aged woman with bronchiectasis and pulmonary infection due to *Mycobacterium avium* complex. There is a cavity in the right midlung field with an air-fluid level and right upper and left lower lobe infiltrates. The patient improved after 2 years of therapy. (*From* Havlir and Ellner [19]; with permission.)

Treatment of *Mycobacterium avium* complex infections

Clinical syndrome	Treatment
Cervical adenitis	Surgical resection
Pulmonary disease	
Nodule	Surgical resection
Infiltrates	Rifampin (600 mg daily), ethambutol (25 mg/kg/day × 2 mo, then 15 mg/kg/day), and streptomycin (1 g 5 day/wk × 6–12 wks, then 1 g 3 times a wk). Clarithromycin (500 mg orally twice a week) may be beneficial.
Localized infiltrate	Surgery may be considered as adjunctive therapy to above antibiotics for localized disease.
Disseminated disease	Clarithromycin (500 mg twice a week) or azithromycin (500 mg daily) and ethambutol (15 mg/kg/day), plus at least one of the following: clofazimine (100 mg daily), rifampin (600 mg daily), rifabutin (300–450 mg daily), ciprofloxacin (500–750 mg twice a week), or amikacin (500–750 mg intravenously daily).

FIGURE 4-61 Treatment of *Mycobacterium avium* complex infections. The treatment of pulmonary infection due to *M. avium* complex depends on the extent of disease. Combined medical and surgical therapy is often employed in localized disease. Optimal dosages for clarithromycin and rifabutin in disseminated disease are not yet determined. (*From* Havlir and Ellner [19]; with permission.)

MYCOBACTERIUM FORTUITUM-CHELONAE COMPLEX

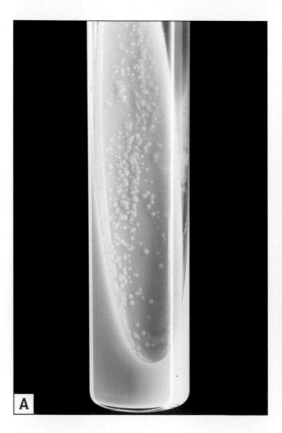
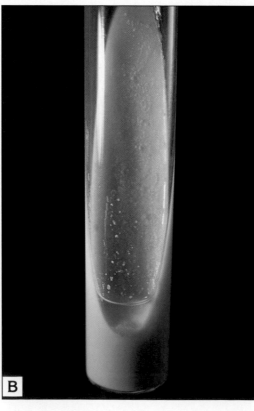

FIGURE 4-62 *Mycobacterium fortuitum* and *Mycobacterium chelonae* on Löwenstein-Jensen agar. These two rapid-growing mycobacterial species are often referred to as the *M. fortuitum-chelonae* complex but can be distinguished by biochemical tests. These organisms are often pleomorphic on acid-fast staining, and unlike the other mycobacteria, they do not stain with auramine or rhodamine. Colonies are nonpigmented, convex, and smooth in consistency, and they usually grow within 3 to 5 days on both routine and specialized mycobacterial media. **A**, *M. fortuitum*. **B**, *M. chelonae*.

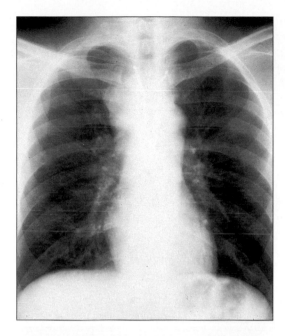

FIGURE 4-63 Chest radiograph showing areas of scarring and cavitation bilaterally, mainly in the midlung fields, secondary to *Mycobacterium chelonae* infection. In many cases, chronic pulmonary disease due to *M. chelonae* resembles *Mycobacterium kansasii* or *Mycobacterium avium-intracellulare* infection. Histologically, polymorphonuclear leukocytes are seen together with granulomatous inflammation. Necrosis is present, but caseation is minimal. *M. chelonae* organisms are characterized by a high degree of resistance *in vitro* to antituberculous drugs [21]. (*Courtesy of* G. McGuinness, MD.)

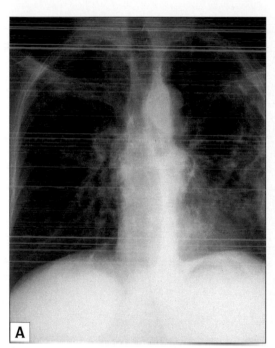

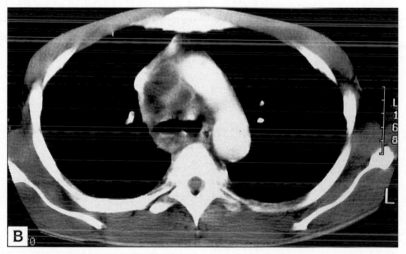

infiltrates that spare the upper lobes without cavity formation. Infection is seen in patients with underlying pulmonary diseases, such as cystic fibrosis and chronic obstructive pulmonary disease, and in immunocompromised hosts, as in this 45-year-old man. Infection has also been documented in nonsmokers without lung disease. (*Courtesy of* T. Harkin, MD.)

FIGURE 4-64 Interstitial infiltrates due to *Mycobacterium fortuitum*. **A** and **B**, Chest radiograph and computed tomography scan demonstrating enlarged paratracheal nodes and interstitial infiltrates secondary to *M. fortuitum* infection. Typically, *M. fortuitum* infection presents as reticulonodular

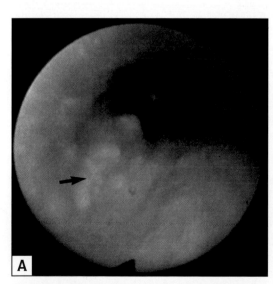

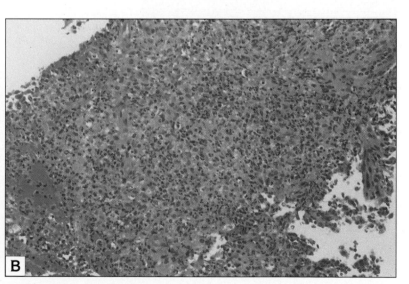

FIGURE 4-65 Paratracheal lymphadenitis due to *Mycobacterium fortuitum*. **A**, Bronchoscopy in the patient seen in Fig. 4-64 shows enlarged lymph nodes indenting the trachea (*arrow*). **B**, Transbronchial biopsy revealed suppurative inflammation with hemorrhage. Infection with *M. fortuitum* can resemble pyogenic abscesses with an acute inflammatory reaction or can cause chronic inflammation. (*Courtesy of* T. Harkin, MD.)

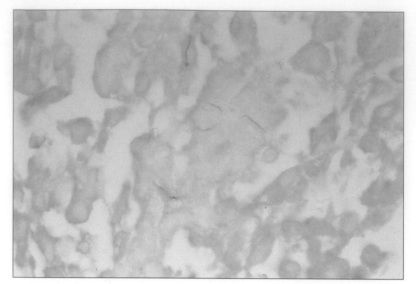

FIGURE 4-66 Acid-fast smear of *Mycobacterium fortuitum*. An acid-fast smear of purulent material obtained from the aspirate in the patient seen in Fig. 4-64 shows long nonbeaded bacilli that were subsequently identified as *M. fortuitum*. *M. fortuitum* may show filamentous extensions on acid-fast staining. In general, this organism is resistant to standard antituberculous drugs and is susceptible to cefoxitin, amikacin, clarithromycin, imipenem, and sulfamethoxazole. (*Courtesy of* T. Harkin, MD.)

MYCOBACTERIUM XENOPI

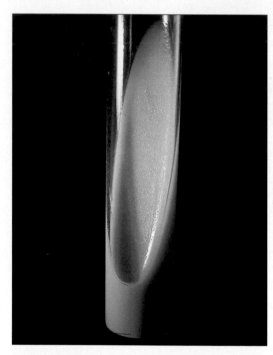

FIGURE 4-67 *Mycobacterium xenopi* colonies on Löwenstein-Jensen agar. Colonies are slow growing, tiny, and dome shaped and produce yellow pigment. On smear, organisms appear as long, filamentous rods with tapered ends, often arranged in palisades. Birds are the natural reservoir, and the organism has been isolated from tap water.

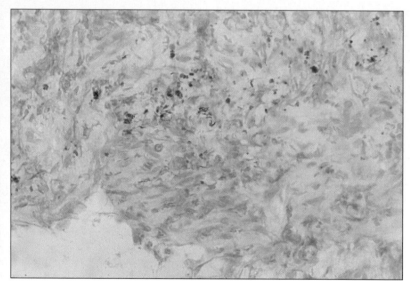

FIGURE 4-68 Lung biopsy specimen of *Mycobacterium xenopi* pulmonary infection showing numerous acid-fast bacilli. *M. xenopi* was previously considered nonpathogenic, but recent reviews confirm its increasing prevalence and tendency to relapse. Most patients have either preexisting lung disease or another condition such as malignancy, alcoholism, or diabetes. Most pulmonary infection resembles tuberculosis, but disseminated disease has been reported in patients with severe underlying immunodeficiency states. Radiographic appearance is variable, ranging from consolidation to mass lesions. Treatment is unpredictable because of variable resistance to many antibiotics [22].

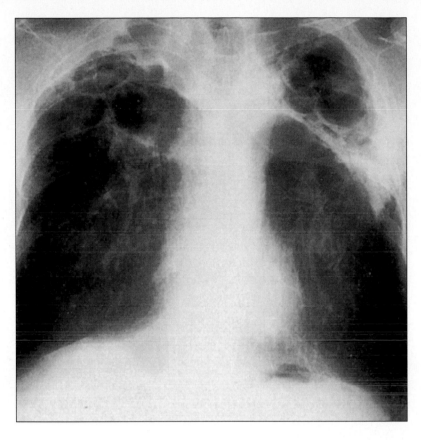

Figure 4-69 Chest radiograph of a 75-year-old man with severe obstructive lung disease and bilateral apical cavitary disease due to *Mycobacterium xenopi. M. xenopi* lung disease usually presents with chronic productive cough, hemoptysis, and few constitutional symptoms. (*From* Griffith and Wallace [23]; with permission.)

ACKNOWLEDGMENTS

The author thanks Howard Radzyner, Herbert Koch, and Anthony Morales for their photographic support, and Richard Ziegenfuss for his assistance in the Mycobacteriology Laboratory.

REFERENCES

1. Salo WL, Aufderheide AC, Buikstra J, Holcomb TA: Identification of *Mycobacterium tuberculosis* DNA in a pre-Colombian Peruvian mummy. *Proc Natl Acad Sci U S A* 1994, 91:2091–2094.

2. Morell V, Mummy settles antiquity debate. *Science* 1994, 263.1606–1607.

3. American Thoracic Society: Control of tuberculosis in the United States. *Am Rev Respir Dis* 1992. 146:1623–1633.

4. Jereb JA, Kelly GD, Dooley SW, *et al.*: Tuberculosis mortality in the United States, final data, 1990. *MMWR* 1991, 40(SS-3):23–27.

5. Sudre P, ten Dam G, Kochi A: Tuberculosis: A global overview of the situation today. *Bull WHO* 1992, 70:149–159.

6. Centers for Disease Control and Prevention: Screening for tuberculosis infections in high-risk populations, and the use of preventive therapy for tuberculosis infection in the United States: Recommendations of the Advisory Council for the Elimination of Tuberculosis. *MMWR* 1990, 39(RR-8):1–12.

7. Eisenach KD, Sifford MD, Cave D, *et al.*: Detection of *Mycobacterium tuberculosis* in sputum samples using a polymerase chain reaction. *Am Rev Respir Dis* 1991, 144:1160–1163.

8. Jacobs WR, Barletta RG, Udani R, *et al.*: Rapid assessment of drug susceptibilities of *Mycobacterium tuberculosis* using luciferase reporter phage. *Science* 1993, 260:819–822.

9. Dannenberg AM: Immunopathogenesis of pulmonary tuberculosis. *Hosp Pract* 1993, 28:51–58.

10. Huebner RE, Schein MF, Bass JB: The tuberculin skin test. *Clin Infect Dis* 1993, 17:968–975.

11. Goodwin RA, des Prez RM: Apical localization of pulmonary tuberculosis, chronic pulmonary histoplasmosis, and progressive massive fibrosis of the lung. *Chest* 1983, 83:801–805.

12. Berger HW, Mejia E. Tuberculous pleurisy. *Chest* 1973, 63.88–92.

13. Brown TS: Tuberculosis of the ribs. *Clin Radiol* 1980, 31:681–684.

14. Frieden TR, Sterling T, Pablos-Mendez A, *et al.*: The emergence of drug-resistant tuberculosis in New York City. *N Engl J Med* 1993, 328:521–526.

15. Alland D, Kalkut GE, Moss AR, *et al.*: Transmission of tuberculosis in New York City: An analysis by DNA fingerprinting and conventional epidemiologic methods. *N Engl J Med* 1994, 330:1710–1716.

16. Iseman MD: Treatment of multidrug-resistant tuberculosis. *N Engl J Med* 1993, 329:784–791.

17. Lillo M, Orengo S, Cernoch P, Harris RL: Pulmonary and disseminated infection due to *Mycobacterium kansasii*: A decade of experience. *Rev Infect Dis* 1990, 12:760–767.

18. Prince DS, Peterson DD, Steiner RM, *et al.*: Infection with *Mycobacterium avium* complex in patients without predisposing conditions. *N Engl J Med* 1989, 321:963–968.

19. Havlir DV, Ellner JJ: *Mycobacterium avium* complex. *In* Mandell GL, Bennett JE, Dolin R (eds.): *Principles and Practice of Infectious Diseases*, 4th ed. New York: Churchill Livingstone; 1995:2250–2264.

20. Iseman MD, Corpe RF, O'Brien RJ, *et al.*: Diseases due to *Mycobacterium avium-intracellulare. Chest* 1985, 87(suppl):139S–149S.

21. Singh N, Yu VL: Successful treatment of pulmonary infection due to *Mycobacterium chelonae*: Case report and review. *Clin Infect Dis* 1992, 14:156–161.

22. Weber J, Mettang T, Staerz E, *et al.*: Pulmonary disease due to *Mycobacterium xenopi* in a renal allograft recipient: Report of a case and review. *Rev Infect Dis* 1989, 11:964–969.

23. Griffith DE, Wallace RJ: Lung disease caused by nontuberculous mycobacteria. *In* Pennington JE (ed.): *Respiratory Infections: Diagnosis and Management*, 3rd ed. New York: Raven Press; 1994:672.

SELECTED BIBLIOGRAPHY

Barnes PF, Barrows SA: Tuberculosis in the 1990s. *Ann Intern Med* 1993, 119:400–410.

Dannenberg AM: Immunopathogenesis of pulmonary tuberculosis. *Hosp Pract* 1993, 28:51–58.

Haas DW, Des Prez RM: *Mycobacterium tuberculosis*. *In* Mandell GL, Bennett JE, Dolin R (eds.): *Principles and Practice of Infectious Diseases*, 4th ed. New York: Churchill Livingstone; 1995:2213–2243.

Horowitz EA, Sanders WE Jr.: Other *Mycobacterium* species. *In* Mandell GL, Bennett JE, Dolin R (eds.): *Principles and Practice of Infectious Diseases*, 4th ed. New York: Churchill Livingstone; 1995:2264–2273.

Woods GL, Washington JA: Mycobacteria other than *Mycobacterium tuberculosis*: Review of microbiologic and clinical aspects. *Rev Infect Dis* 1987, 9:275–294.

CHAPTER 5

Fungal Infections

Scott F. Davies
George A. Sarosi

Classification of fungal infections

T-cell opportunists
  Endemic mycoses
    Histoplasmosis
    Blastomycosis
    Coccidioidomycosis
    Paracoccidioidomycosis
  Cryptococcosis (worldwide)
Phagocyte opportunists
  Aspergillosis
  Mucormycosis
  Pseudoallescheria boydii and other aspergillus-like soil organisms (rare)
Overlap disease (T-cell opportunist on mucosal surfaces but phagocyte opportunist for deep invasion)
  Candidiasis

FIGURE 5-1 Classification of fungal infections (by predispositions to infection).

HISTOPLASMOSIS

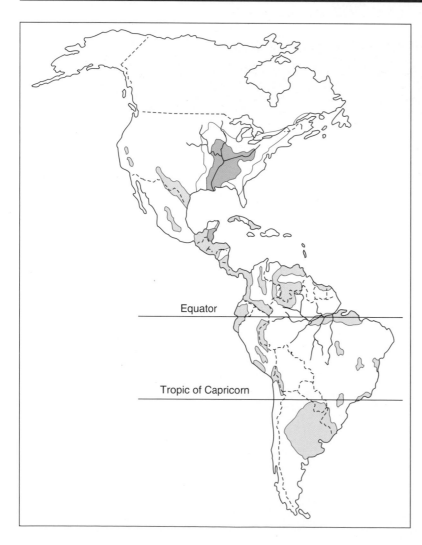

FIGURE 5-2 Map of areas endemic for histoplasmosis. Histoplasmosis, like the other endemic mycoses, is predominantly an infection of the western hemisphere. The area of highest disease activity is the central United States, encompassing the Mississippi and Ohio River valleys. Other endemic areas include the Caribbean islands and Central America. The fungus is also widely distributed throughout the world with some disease activity in many river valleys, especially in temperate climates. However, in no place on earth does the density of the infection approach that of the central United States. In Tennessee and Kentucky, for example, there are counties where 90% of residents have become skin test positive by age 18 years. In contrast, virtually no disease activity is seen in Europe or Australia. (*Darker shaded areas* denote higher disease activity.) (*Adapted from* Rippon [1]; with permission.)

Equator

Tropic of Capricorn

Clinical manifestations of histoplasmosis	
Habitat	Soil enriched by organic nitrogen in the form of bird or animal feces
Portal of entry	Lung
Primary infection	Mild, usually self-limited Occasional ARDS
Tissue response	Granulomatous
Extrapulmonary spread	Always (benign fungemia) Progressive in T-cell–immunocompromised hosts Reticuloendothelial organs
Complications in HIV infection	Common

ARDS—acute respiratory distress syndrome.

FIGURE 5-3 Clinical manifestations of histoplasmosis. Histoplasmosis is always acquired by inhalation, and the primary infection is in the lungs. The organism is dimorphic. In nature, it grows as a mycelium in nitrogen-enriched soil (especially soil contaminated with bird droppings or bat droppings). Once inhaled, it converts to a yeast form that grows intracellularly in macrophages. In disseminated infections, there is spread to the reticuloendothelial system, including liver, spleen, bone marrow, and lymph nodes. The centers of the granulomas may undergo necrosis and eventually become hyalinized or even calcified. The acute tissue response is totally granulomatous, unlike the other three endemic mycoses (blastomycosis, coccidioidomycosis, and paracoccidioidomycosis), which have a mixed pyogenic and granulomatous inflammatory response (*see* Fig. 5-32B).

FIGURE 5-4 Diagnosis of histoplasmosis.

Diagnosis of histoplasmosis	
Histopathology (special stains)	2–5 μm, single budding yeast (Silver or periodic acid–Schiff stain)
Culture	Time-consuming, up to 30 days Tuberculate macroconidia may be seen by 5–7 days Exoantigen testing quicker
Rapid diagnosis by examination of fresh specimen	Silver stain of sputum may show small yeasts, but unreliable and low sensitivity Organisms may be seen on peripheral blood smear, especially in AIDS patients
Serology	Immunodiffusion not sensitive Complement fixation is 75% sensitive Four-fold rise usually takes 3–6 weeks Histoplasma polysaccharide antigen is sensitive only in disseminated disease and is most helpful in AIDS patients

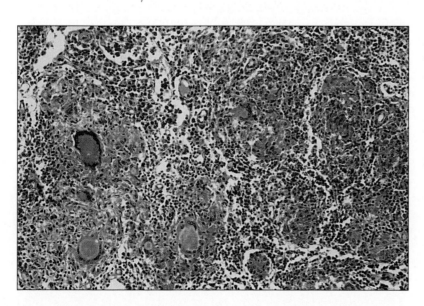

FIGURE 5-5 Histopathologic appearance of histoplasmosis in tissue. The tissue response in histoplasmosis is granulomatous with epithelioid histiocytes and giant cells surrounded by lymphocytes. Special stains (usually one of the silver stains, including methenamine silver and Grocott stains) might show rare or moderate yeast. In general, the better developed and tighter the granulomas (the more they look like sarcoidosis), the harder it is to find the organisms on routine or specially stained sections. (Hematoxylin-eosin stain; original magnification, × 400.) (*From* Salfelder *et al.* [2]; with permission.)

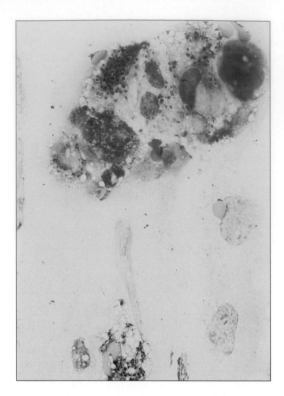

FIGURE 5-6 Wright stain of bone marrow aspirate in histoplasmosis. The photomicrograph shows collections of macrophages that have multiple small intracellular organisms characteristic of *Histoplasma capsulatum*. The small clearer area around the yeast resembles a capsule but is actually a drying artifact. The yeast are 1 to 2 μm in diameter. This morphologic appearance is highly typical for this fungus and is diagnostic of disseminated histoplasmosis. This patient was a renal transplant recipient on chronic therapy with prednisone and azathioprine who presented with high fever, no localizing symptoms, and a normal chest radiograph. (Original magnification, × 1000.)

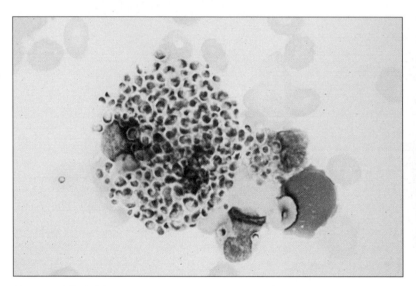

FIGURE 5-7 Wright-stained smear of peripheral blood buffy coat in a patient with AIDS and disseminated histoplasmosis. A macrophage is shown that is full of 1- to 2-μm yeast of *Histoplasma capsulatum*. Again, faint staining artifacts are seen around the individual yeast, suggesting capsules. This image is pathognomonic for disseminated histoplasmosis. Peripheral blood smears are positive in up to 50% of AIDS patients with disseminated histoplasmosis. (Original magnification, × 1000.)

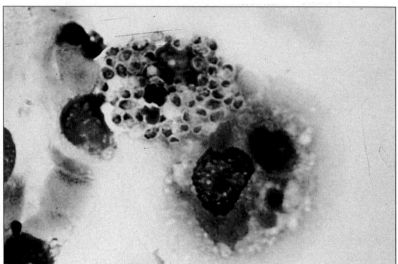

FIGURE 5-8 Bronchoalveolar lavage fluid stained with Wright stain showing typical histoplasma yeast in an alveolar macrophage. These organisms (1–2 μm in diameter) are pathognomonic for histoplasmosis. They are seen in high numbers in HIV-infected patients who have disseminated histoplasmosis but are unusual in immunocompetent patients with pulmonary or systemic forms of histoplasmosis. When present, they are diagnostic of infection. (*From* Stanley *et al.* [3]; with permission.)

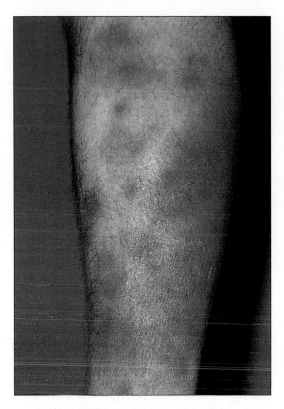

FIGURE 5-9
Erythema nodosum on the lower extremity. Erythema nodosum occurs in a small percentage of patients with primary pulmonary histoplasmosis. It is usually bilateral and symmetric, and the lesions are often very painful. Lesions are nodular but usually lack discrete borders and can be confluent. The differential diagnosis includes tuberculosis and sarcoidosis. (*From* Fitzpatrick *et al.* [4]; with permission.)

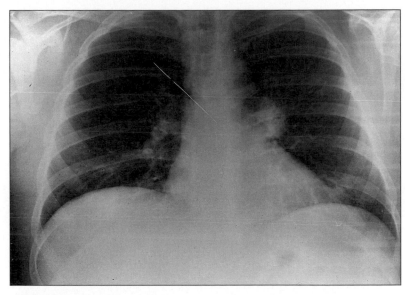

FIGURE 5-10 Chest radiograph showing patchy infiltrate and hilar lymphadenopathy in acute pulmonary histoplasmosis. A posteroanterior chest radiograph from a 30-year-old man shows a patchy infiltrate in the lower lobe and a very large left hilar lymph node. The diagnosis was confirmed by a serologic testing. The complement fixation titer was 1:128 to the yeast antigen of *Histoplasma capsulatum*. The patient recovered without antifungal therapy. (*From* Bone *et al.* [5]; with permission.)

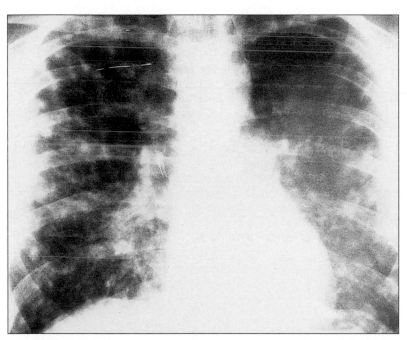

FIGURE 5-11 Chest radiograph showing diffuse, bilateral micronodular infiltrates in inhalational histoplasmosis. A 32-year-old man was exposed to large concentrations of *Histoplasma capsulatum* spores in a closed space while cleaning an attic contaminated by large amounts of bat droppings. Exactly 2 weeks later, he presented with headache, cough, and fever. His chest radiograph showed diffuse micronodular infiltrates throughout both lung fields. Serologic tests were positive. An immunodiffusion test was positive for H and M bands, and the competent fixation test was positive at a titer of 1:64. The patient was febrile for almost 2 weeks but eventually made a complete recovery without any specific antifungal therapy.

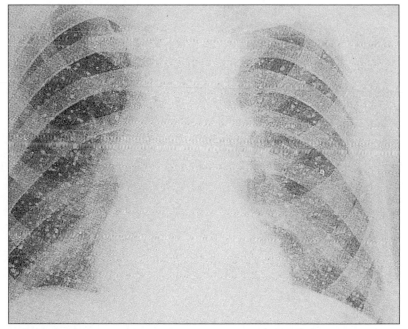

FIGURE 5-12 Posteroanterior chest radiograph showing "buckshot" calcifications (calcified granulomas) of healed histoplasmosis. This film was from an asymptomatic patient who grew up in the midwestern United States but had no past history of pneumonia. It shows small calcifications (so-called buckshot calcifications) scattered throughout both lung fields, which are the residua of acute inhalational histoplasmosis (*see also* Fig. 5-11). This appearance of buckshot calcifications on a chest radiograph is almost pathognomonic of remote histoplasmosis. The only possible alternative diagnosis is remote varicella pneumonia, which almost certainly would have been symptomatic. Many patients who have a chest radiograph with this finding cannot recall any discrete episode of pneumonia in their past life. (*From* Salfelder *et al.* [2]; with permission.)

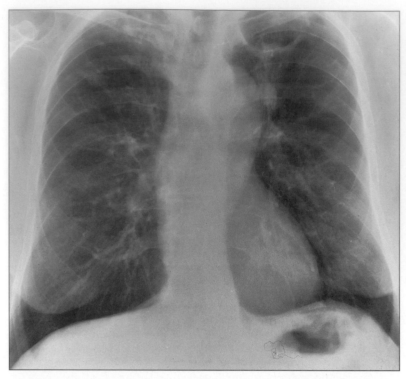

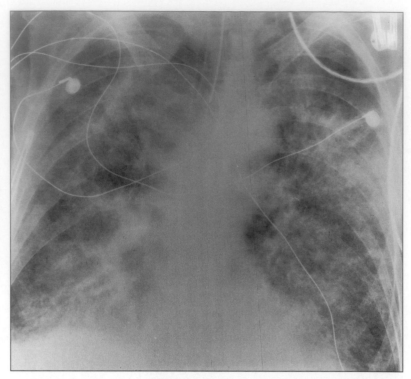

FIGURE 5-13 Chest radiograph showing fibronodular disease with chronic cavitary infiltrate in histoplasmosis. A posteroanterior chest radiograph shows bilateral, upper lobe, fibronodular disease, including a large cavity in the left upper lobe. The patient was a 58-year-old man with chronic productive cough, fever, night sweats, and weight loss. Sputum cultures were repeatedly positive for *Histoplasma capsulatum*. He was treated with oral imidazole therapy with good results. The patient had a negative tuberculin skin test and negative sputum cultures for tuberculosis. He had been a chronic smoker and had moderately severe chronic obstructive pulmonary disease. (*From* Bone *et al.* [5]; with permission.)

FIGURE 5-14 Chest radiograph showing diffuse bilateral infiltrates in histoplasmosis. The patient, a 62-year-old man, has an endotracheal tube in place because of severe hypoxemic respiratory failure. He had received a renal transplant 8 years earlier and was on therapy with prednisone and azathioprine. He presented with a febrile illness. Infiltrates were mild initially but progressed rapidly to respiratory failure over 5 days. This type of illness is most common in patients with underlying AIDS but also can be seen in other patients with deficient T-cell immunity. The best treatment is intravenous amphotericin B, but the mortality is high, even with appropriate therapy. (*From* Bone *et al.* [5]; with permission.)

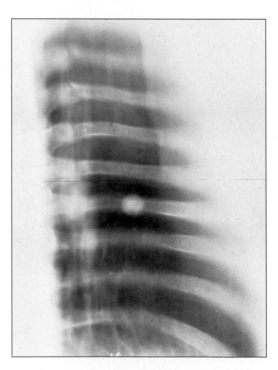

FIGURE 5-15 Computed tomography scan of a densely calcified histoplasmoma in the left lower lobe. The nodule is located posteriorly, near the ribs and shows dense uniform calcification of the entire lesion. Small nodules that are totally calcified or that have a round, perfectly central mass of calcium (a "target" lesion) are almost certainly histoplasmomas if the tuberculin skin test is negative and the patient is a resident of an area highly endemic for histoplasmosis. Residual lesions from remote tuberculosis, coccidioidomycosis, or other granulomatous infections may appear the same.

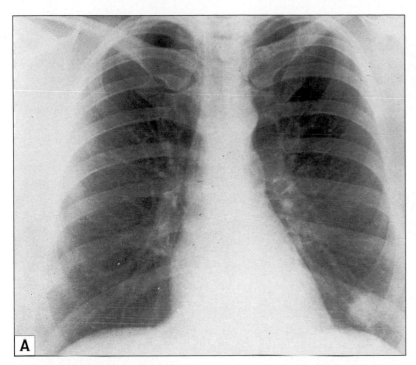

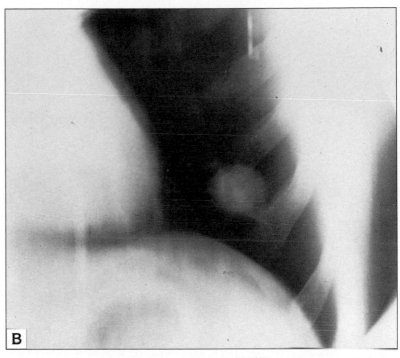

FIGURE 5-16 Histoplasmoma. **A,** A chest radiograph shows a round nodule in the left lower lobe. Older chest radiographs from this patient proved that the lesion was present for at least 5 years. Stable nodules like this one are almost certainly histoplasmomas if the tuberculin skin test is negative and the patient is a resident of an area highly endemic for histoplasmosis. Residual lesions from remote tuberculosis, coccidioidomycosis, or other granulomatous infections, as well as benign tumors, may also present in this way. **B,** Computed tomography scan of the nodule shows partial concentric rings of calcium, which are formed as the nodule very slowly enlarges. Sequential episodes of local inflammation followed by necrosis and eventual calcification cause the circumferential rings.

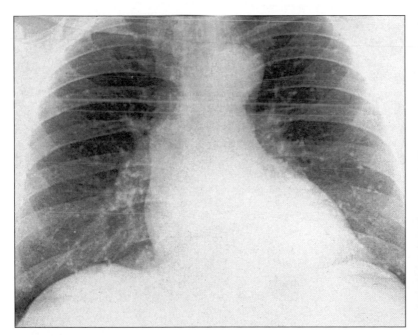

FIGURE 5-17 Chest radiograph showing multiple calcified granulomas typical of remote (healed) histoplasmosis. (*From* Bullock [6]; with permission.)

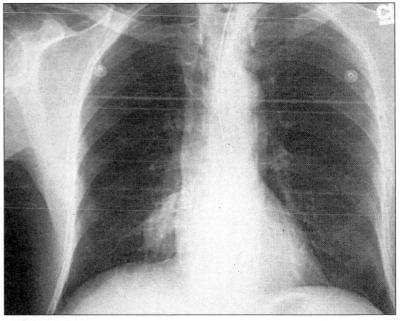

FIGURE 5-18 Chest radiograph showing a histoplasmoma. These lesions are very common in persons who live or have lived in endemic areas. (*From* Bullock [6]; with permission.)

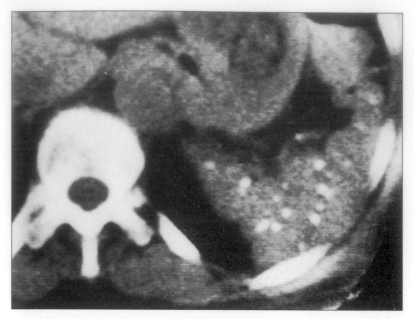

FIGURE 5-19 Abdominal computed tomography (CT) scan showing calcified granulomas in the spleen. The spleen has multiple, marble-sized, densely calcified nodules. Such splenic calcifications are very common in highly endemic areas and are diagnostic of remote histoplasmosis. They are seen on flat plates of the abdomen as well as on CT scans. Similar lesions are seen in the liver. Many patients give no history of symptomatic pneumonia. These nodules are evidence that many patients with primary pulmonary histoplasmosis have a benign fungemia at the time of their initial infection, even when it is quite mild. With advent of cell-mediated immunity, granulomas in the lung and distant sites heal uneventfully, leaving footprints in the form of these marble-sized calcifications. (*From* Lee *et al.* [7]; with permission.)

Usual therapy for histoplasmosis

		Immunosuppressed host	
	Immunocompetent host	**Without AIDS**	**With AIDS**
Acute	Observe	AMB (500–1000 mg) *then* ITRA (400 mg/day × 6 mo)	AMB (500–1000 mg) *then* ITRA (400 mg/day for life)
Acute, with ventilatory failure	AMB (500–1000 mg until improvement noted)	AMB (1000 mg) *then* ITRA (400 mg/day × 6 mo) *or* AMB (40 mg/kg, total dose)	Same as above
Cavitary	ITRA (400 mg/day × 6 mo) *or* KETO (400–800 mg/day × 6 mo) *or* AMB (35 mg/kg, total dose)	No specific information available; probably same as in immunocompetent host	No information; probably same as above
Progressive disseminated	AMB (500–1000 mg until stable) *then* ITRA (400 mg/day × 6 mo) *or* AMB (40 mg/kg, total dose)	AMB (1000 mg) *then* ITRA (400 mg/kg/day × 6 mo) *or* AMB (40 mg/kg, total dose)	AMB (1000 mg) *then* ITRA (400 mg/day for life)

AMB—amphotericin B; ITRA—itraconazole; KETO—ketoconazole.

FIGURE 5-20 Usual therapy for histoplasmosis.

BLASTOMYCOSIS

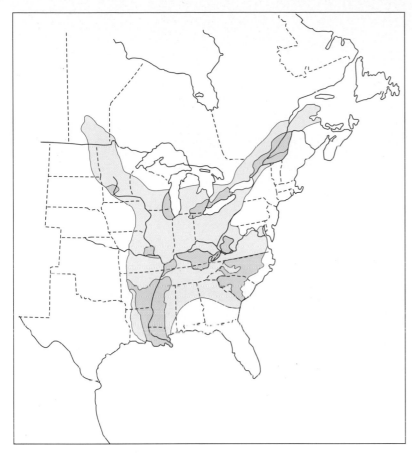

FIGURE 5-21 Map of areas endemic for blastomycosis. Blastomycosis, like the other endemic mycoses, is predominantly an infection of the western hemisphere. Some disease activity is seen in Africa, but the vast majority of cases come from the United States and Canada. Blastomycosis is coendemic with histoplasmosis over much of the central United States east of the Mississippi River. Disease activity extends northward across northern Wisconsin and Minnesota and into south central Canada. (*Darker shaded areas* denote higher disease activity.) (*Adapted from* Rippon [1]; with permission.)

Clinical manifestations of blastomycosis

Habitat	Soil enriched by organic nitrogen in the form of bird or animal feces
Portal of entry	Lung
Primary infection	Moderately severe May be self-limited, usually subacute and progressive Can mimic bacterial pneumonia
Tissue response	Pyogenic–granulomatous
Extrapulmonary spread	Frequent Skin and bone Often no evident T-cell abnormality
Complications in HIV infection	Rare

FIGURE 5-22 Clinical manifestations of blastomycosis. Blastomycosis is a dimorphic fungus. In nature, it grows as a mycelium, with microconidia (small spores) from the mycelia as the infectious particles. The disease is acquired by inhalation, and once within the lung, the spores convert to the yeast form. The primary infection is always in the lung. With disseminated disease, spread is most common to the skin and bones, similar to the pattern of spread of coccidioidomycosis but with less tendency for meningeal spread.

FIGURE 5-23 Diagnosis of blastomycosis.

Diagnosis of blastomycosis

Histopathology (special stains)	8–20 µm, single budding yeast, with broad neck of attachment; multiple nuclei; thick, doubly refractive wall Silver or periodic acid–Schiff stain
Culture	Time-consuming, up to 30 days Lollipop-shaped conidia by 5–7 days
Rapid diagnosis by examination of fresh specimen	Potassium hydroxide digest reliable Papanicolaou stain frequently positive
Serology	Tests are not reliable Immunodiffusion has fair specificity but poor sensitivity When positive, should lead to renewed efforts to investigate further with cultures and tissue biopsies for histopathology

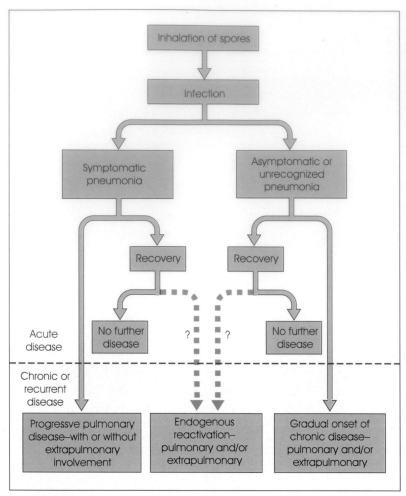

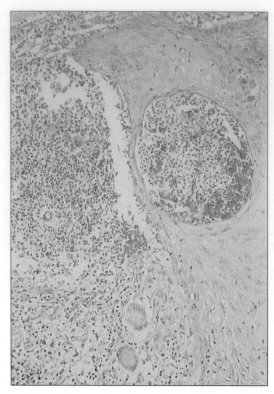

FIGURE 5-25 Histopathologic features of blastomycosis in skin biopsy. Blastomycosis causes a mixed pyogenic and granulomatous tissue response. This skin biopsy specimen shows giant cells but also small microabscesses containing neutrophils within both the epithelium and dermis. (Hematoxylin-eosin stain; original magnification, × 400.) (*From* Salfelder *et al.* [2]; with permission.)

FIGURE 5-24 Clinical classification of blastomycosis. (*Adapted from* Sarosi and Davies [8]; with permission.)

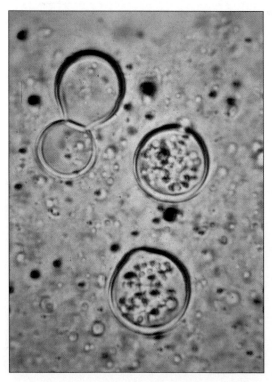

FIGURE 5-26 Sputum potassium hydroxide preparation showing the characteristic yeast form of *Blastomyces dermatitidis*. Because the infection is mixed with pyogenic and granulomatous components, many patients with pneumonia have secretions that are coughed up as purulent sputum. Direct smears of the sputum are often diagnostic, and the purulent material is usually also positive on culture. The yeast form is much larger than in histoplasmosis—about 8 to 20 μm in size. It has a highly characteristic morphology. The yeast has single buds. The daughter cell can be almost as large as the parent cell, and there is a broad base of attachment between the parent and the daughter cell. The cell wall is doubly refractile, and there are multiple nuclei within the cell. No other pathogenic yeast has similar broad-based single budding, so that the direct recognition of these forms is diagnostic of blastomycosis. Yeast may be seen in sputum or in material expressed from skin ulcers. (*From* Sarosi and Davies [8]; with permission.)

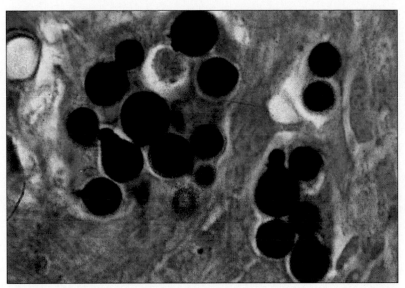

FIGURE 5-27 Silver staining of *Blastomyces dermatitidis* in histopathologic section. In histopathologic sections, the yeast is hard to see unless stained with a special stain. Silver stain colors the yeast a dark black and makes them very easy to see, but much valuable detail is lost. The periodic acid–Schiff stain also highlights the yeast in tissue sections but preserves morphologic detail better. In standard hematoxylin-eosin–stained tissue sections, the organisms are often difficult to see, and all tissue biopsy specimens showing a mixture of granulomatous and pyogenic inflammation should be stained with special stains to detect characteristic organisms. (*From* Salfelder *et al.* [2]; with permission.)

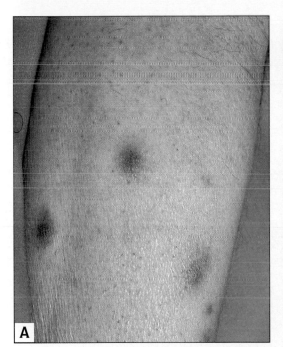
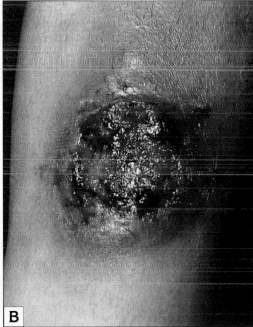

FIGURE 5-28 Skin lesions of blastomycosis. **A**, Inflammatory nodule beneath the epidermis. **B**, A large ulcer on an extremity. The skin is a preferred site for spread of blastomycosis. Often, the lesion begins as a small subcutaneous nodule and then erodes to the surface. The center of the area then undergoes ulceration. The edges may be heaped up, resembling that seen with a skin cancer. Biopsy of the edges reveals mixed granulomatous and pyogenic inflammation with characteristic yeast visible on special stains. Biopsy of the subcutaneous nodule also will show the characteristic organisms. Patients may have one or several skin lesions, sometimes at different stages. (Panel 28B *from* Fitzpatrick *et al.* [4]; with permission.)

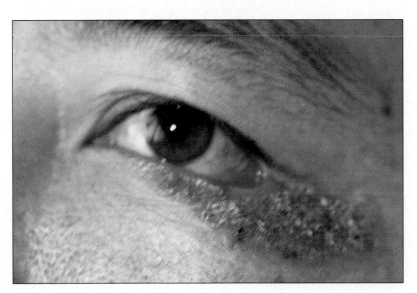

FIGURE 5-29 Solitary blastomycotic skin lesion on the lateral aspect of the lower eyelid and adjacent face. Many skin lesions of blastomycosis have a characteristic crusty surface. This patient was a 40-year-old Southeast Asian man who presented with no symptoms other than this lesion. Therapy with ketoconazole was not successful, but the lesion eventually was cured with oral fluconazole therapy.

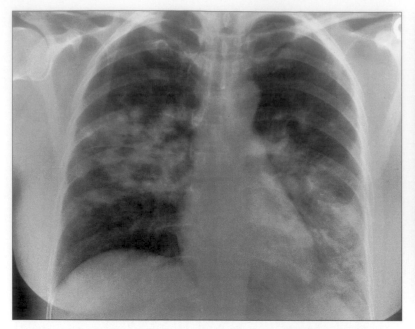

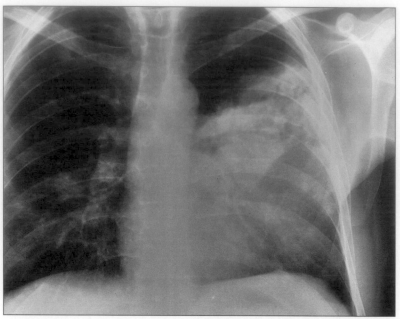

FIGURE 5-30 Chest radiograph showing multiple large nodular infiltrates in blastomycosis. A chest radiograph shows a dense infiltrate in the right upper lobe and multiple nodular lesions bilaterally. This was a 49-year-old woman presented with a subacute history of fever and chronic cough over several weeks. Direct smears of the sputum showed characteristic *Blastomyces* organisms on potassium hydroxide examination and on cultures. The patient responded well to therapy with oral ketoconazole. Large nodular infiltrates are very unusual in routine bacterial pneumonia. (*From* Bone *et al.* [5]; with permission.)

FIGURE 5-31 Chest radiograph showing dense alveolar infiltrate in blastomycosis. A posteroanterior chest radiograph shows a large, dense alveolar infiltrate involving the left midlung in a 33-year-old intravenous drug user. Direct smears of sputum after potassium hydroxide digestion were positive for *Blastomyces dermatitidis*. Sputum cultures were also positive. The dense alveolar infiltrates can resemble infiltrates of pneumococcal or other bacterial pneumonia. This patient was initially started on oral ketoconazole therapy, but while receiving that therapy, he developed multiple skin lesions and blastomycotic meningitis. Therapy was switched to intravenous amphotericin B, and he fully recovered. (*From* Bone *et al.* [5]; with permission.)

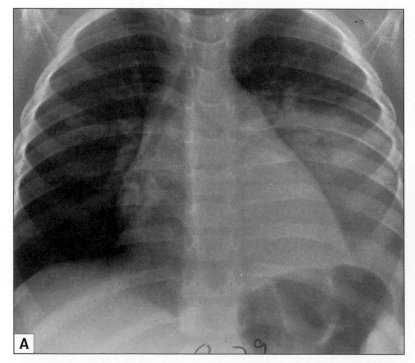

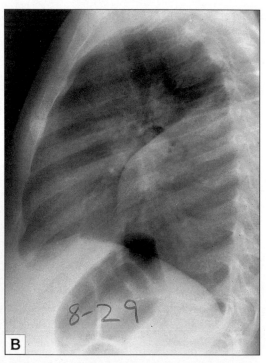

FIGURE 5-32 Chest radiographs showing lobar blastomycosis. **A,** A posteroanterior chest radiograph shows a dense lobar infiltrate in the left lower lobe of an infant less than 6 months of age. The patient had presented with fever and failed to respond to several courses of oral antibacterial therapy. She had briefly visited her grandmother who lived along a branch of the Arkansas River that had experienced recent flooding. **B,** A lateral chest radiograph shows the left lower lobe lobar infiltrate. Of note is a prominent bulging fissure, which suggests an edematous lobar pneumonia similar to that sometimes seen with *Klebsiella* pneumonia. Lobar blastomycosis with a bulging fissure is one clue to a high-risk infection with a high likelihood of rapid dissemination and fatal outcome. This patient developed progressive acute respiratory distress syndrome with diffuse alveolar infiltrates within a week of this film and ultimately died despite therapy with amphotericin B.

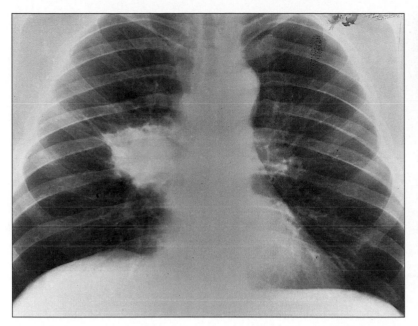

FIGURE 5-33 Chest radiograph showing a large right hilar mass in blastomycosis. The patient was relatively asymptomatic and had no fever, although he did have a mild chronic cough. He was a 68-year-old smoker, and the suspicion was bronchogenic carcinoma. Bronchoscopy showed no endobronchial lesion, and brushings obtained at bronchoscopy were positive for *Blastomycoses* yeast on direct smear and culture. The patient was treated with intravenous amphotericin B with good outcome. (*From* Bone *et al.* [5]; with permission.)

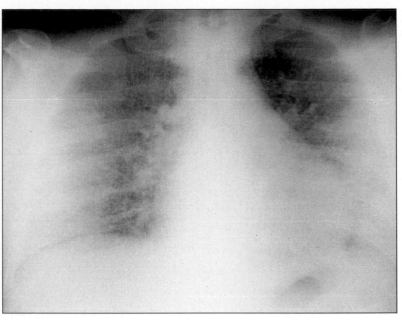

FIGURE 5-34 Chest radiograph showing diffuse interstitial-type infiltrates in blastomycosis. A 57-year-old forester, who had presented with hip pain of many months' duration, developed shortness of breath and increasing fever over a few days. Aspiration of his hip revealed *Blastomyces* organisms, and bronchoalveolar lavage was positive for *B. dermatitidis* on culture. The patient was treated with intravenous amphotericin B and recovered.

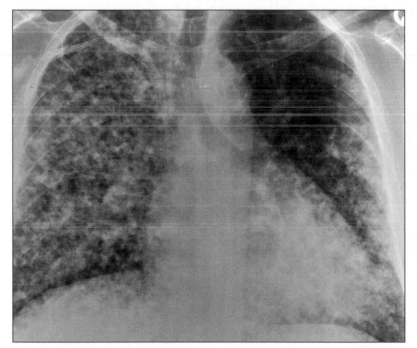

FIGURE 5-35 Chest radiograph showing diffuse nodular infiltrates in blastomycosis. A 50-year-old dialysis patient presented with fever and chills and progressive respiratory failure. The initial suspicion was tuberculosis, but an open-lung biopsy showed *Blastomyces dermatitidis* on histopathologic sections and on cultures. The patient recovered after treatment with intravenous amphotericin B. Diffuse infiltrates in blastomycosis can range from fine interstitial infiltrates (*see* Fig. 5-34) to diffuse nodular infiltrates or even to diffuse alveolar infiltrates with prominent air bronchograms typical for noncardiac pulmonary edema. (*From* Bone *et al.* [5]; with permission.)

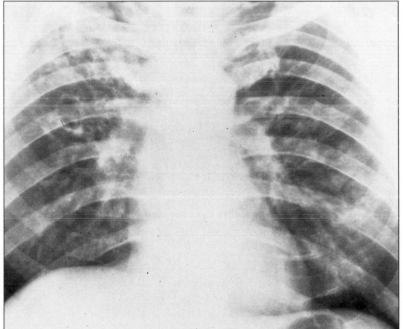

FIGURE 5-36 Chest radiograph showing a fibrocavitary infiltrate of blastomycosis. The infiltrate is most marked in the right upper lobe. The patient, a 22-year-old man, presented with chronic cough, low-grade fever, and night sweats, and the initial suspicion was tuberculosis. His sputum cultures were negative for mycobacteria, but direct potassium hydroxide–treated smear of sputum showed characteristic *Blastomyces* yeast with single broad-based buds. Sputum cultures were also positive.

Usual therapy for blastomycosis

| | Immunocompetent host | Immunosuppressed host | |
		Without AIDS	With AIDS
Acute	Observe only if clinically improving at diagnosis, otherwise—ITRA (400 mg/day × 6 mo) *or* KETO (400–800 mg/day)	AMB (1000 mg) *then* ITRA (400 mg/day × 6 mo) *or* AMB (2000–3000 mg, total dose)	AMB (500–1000 mg) *then* ITRA (400 mg/day for life)
Acute, with ventilatory failure	AMB (500–1000 mg until stable) *then* ITRA (400 mg/day) *or* KETO (400–800 mg/day)	Same as above	Same as above
Chronic pulmonary or extrapulmonary nonmeningeal	ITRA (400 mg/day × 6 mo) *or* KETO (400–800 mg/day × 6 mo) *or* AMB (2000 mg, total dose)	AMB (500–1000 mg until improvement noted) *then* ITRA (400 mg/day × 6–12 mo) *or* AMB (2000–3000 mg)	Same as above

AMB—amphotericin B; ITRA—itraconazole; KETO–ketoconazole.

FIGURE 5-37 Usual therapy for blastomycosis.

COCCIDIOIDOMYCOSIS

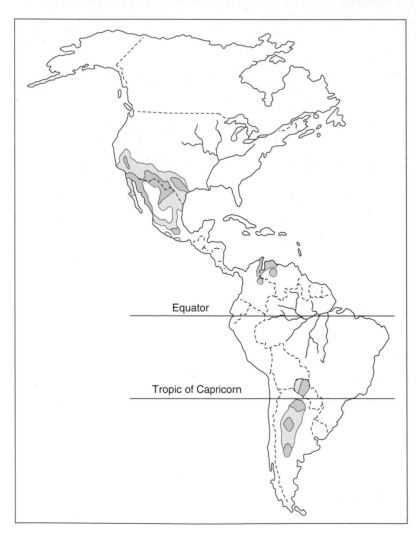

FIGURE 5-38 Map of areas endemic for coccidioidomycosis. Coccidioidomycosis, like the other endemic mycoses, is predominantly an infection of the western hemisphere. Although the disease was first described in Argentina, the most highly endemic areas are in the United States—in the central Arizona desert including Phoenix and in the San Joaquin Valley of southern California including Bakersfield—as well as adjacent areas of Mexico. There is virtually no overlap with the endemic area of histoplasmosis (*see* Fig. 5-2), except near San Antonio, Texas. (*Darker shaded areas* denote higher disease activity.) (*Adapted from* Rippon [1]; with permission.)

Clinical manifestations of coccidioidomycosis

Habitat	Soil enriched by organic nitrogen in the form of bird or animal feces
Portal of entry	Lung
Primary infection	Usually self-limited
	Progressive in a significant minority of patients
Tissue response	Pyogenic–granulomatous
Extrapulmonary spread	Skin, bone, prostate, meninges
	Unusual in normal hosts
	Men, blacks, T-cell–immmunocompromised hosts are at risk
Complications in HIV infection	Frequent

FIGURE 5-39 Clinical manifestations of coccidioidomycosis.

Diagnosis of coccidioidomycosis

Histopathology (special stains)	Huge, up to 100-μm giant spherule, with multiple endospores
	Hematoxylin-eosin and silver stains
Culture	Extreme biohazard; closed-system exoantigen testing avoids aerosol formation
	Barrel-shaped arthroconidia by 7 days
Rapid diagnosis by examination of fresh specimen	Papanicolaou stain positive in approximately 50%
	Potassium hydroxide digest less reliable
Serology	Immunodiffusion test is useful as initial screening test
	Complement fixation test is sensitive and provides prognostic information

FIGURE 5-40 Diagnosis of coccidioidomycosis.

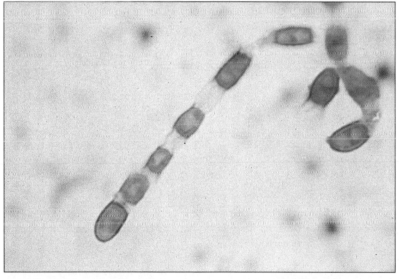

FIGURE 5-41 Arthrospores (mycelia) of *Coccidioides* in culture. *Coccidioides* is a dimorphic tissue fungus. This photomicrograph, stained with phenol cotton blue, shows the mycelial phase of the organism, as it grows in desert soil and in the laboratory at 22° C on fungal growth media. The fungal hyphae show the characteristic arthrospores, each alternating with an empty cell. These arthrospores are easily aerosolized and are the infectious particles. The disease is almost always acquired by inhalation—the only exceptions are rare cases of direct inoculation. Once in the mammalian host, the fungus transforms into an endospore, which then grows into a characteristic giant spherule. The spherule may eventually burst and release hundreds of endospores, each with potential to grow into a new spherule. (*From* Salfelder *et al.* [2]; with permission.)

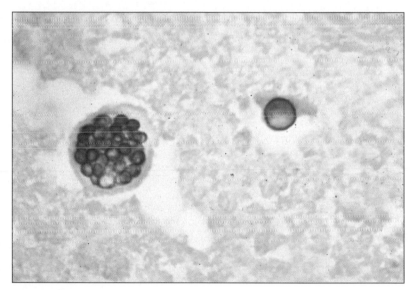

FIGURE 5-42 Giant spherule and endospores of *Coccidioides* in tissue sections on silver staining. This photomicrograph shows a single giant spherule packed with hundreds of endospores. Spherules can be 30 to 100 μm in diameter and are specific for coccidioidomycosis—there is nothing else that looks like these giant spherules. Also in the same field is a smaller endospore, which is not characteristic and could be confused with another yeast if the spherule was not in the same field. (Methenamine silver stain; original magnification, × 1000.)

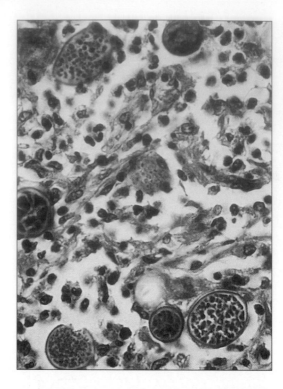

FIGURE 5-43 Giant spherules of *Coccidioides* on tissue section stained with hematoxylin-eosin. Spherules are so big and distinctive that they often can be seen in tissue biopsy specimens, even when the sections are stained routinely with hematoxylin-eosin. This high-power photomicrograph shows multiple spherules in an area of chronic inflammation. Because of their large size, the spherules stand out visually, even without a silver stain. Tissue biopsies usually show a mixed inflammatory response with pyogenic and granulomatous components, similar to that of blastomycosis. In individual biopsy specimens, one or the other component may predominate. The presence of spherules in tissue or on direct smears of secretions (such as sputum) is diagnostic of coccidioidomycosis. (*From* Salfelder *et al.* [2]; with permission.)

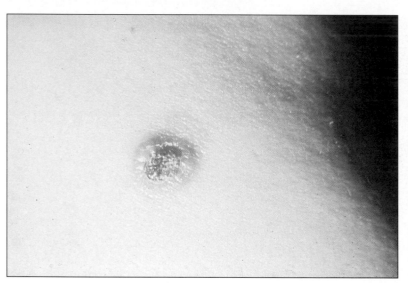

FIGURE 5-44 Skin ulcer of coccidioidomycosis. A small skin ulcer is seen on the wrist of an otherwise asymptomatic 50-year-old man, who had previously lived in the desert of the southwestern United States. The ulcer had a heaped-up border suggesting a skin cancer. Biopsy showed mixed granulomatous and pyogenic inflammation with multiple spherules. Skin lesions of coccidioidomycosis can be extensive and may be disfiguring when they occur on the face. Other skin ulcers may have less active borders. They are sometimes fixed to the deeper tissues and represent draining fistulas originating in infected bones deep to the ulcer. Biopsy of the fistulous opening usually shows characteristic spherules, and pus expressed from the area can be stained directly and cultured, also with high diagnostic yield. Dissemination in coccidioidomycosis (unlike in histoplasmosis) tends to involve the skin, bones, and meninges.

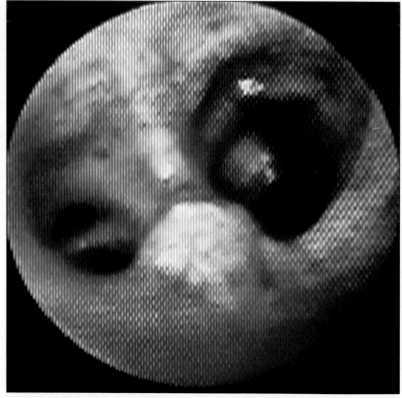

FIGURE 5-45 Endobronchial ulcer in coccidioidal pneumonia. A dime-sized endobronchial ulcer is seen in a patient with AIDS who underwent diagnostic bronchoscopy for pneumonia. Coccidioidal pneumonia is common in patients with AIDS who live in highly endemic areas. Endobronchial involvement is common and is often a diagnostic clue because it would not be expected with *Pneumocystis carinii* pneumonia or other opportunistic pulmonary infections complicating AIDS. Endobronchial biopsies of the edges of the ulcers usually show abundant spherules. (*Courtesy of* A. Thomas, MD.)

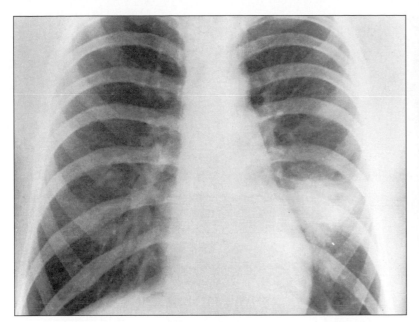

FIGURE 5-46 Chest radiograph showing acute focal infiltration in the left lower lobe in coccidioidomycosis. Focal infiltrates are the most common radiographic finding in acute pulmonary coccidioidomycosis. Many patients are not specifically diagnosed but rather are treated as having a community-acquired pneumonia, and they get better coincidentally as they receive antibacterial therapy. Serodiagnostic tests are sometimes obtained for an episode of nonspecific pneumonitis if the patient lives in a highly endemic area and are usually obtained if the initial febrile illness is accompanied by arthralgias (desert rheumatism), erythema nodosum ("the bumps"), or erythema multiforme. (*From* Hudson *et al.* [9]; with permission.)

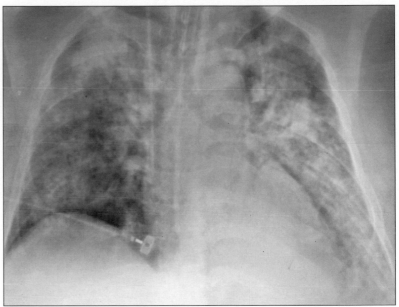

FIGURE 5-47 Chest radiograph showing diffuse pulmonary infiltrates in acute pulmonary coccidioidomycosis. Diffuse bilateral infiltrates occur in < 1% of immunocompetent patients with pulmonary coccidioidomycosis. In contrast, at least 20% of patients with AIDS who develop coccidioidomycosis have diffuse, often nodular infiltrates (*see* Fig. 5-48). This patient was not immunosuppressed and presumably inhaled a large number of organisms. Infection was proven by serologic tests and culture. (*Courtesy of* J. Smilack, MD.)

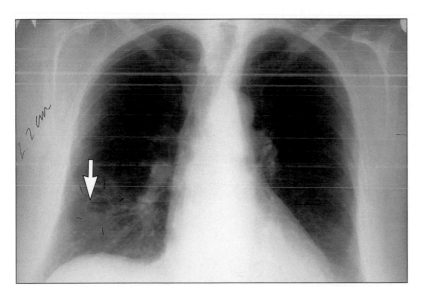

FIGURE 5-48 Chest radiograph showing a thin-walled cavity characteristic of pulmonary coccidioidomycosis. Cavities, seen here in the right lower lobe (*arrow*), are formed when small nodular infiltrates round up and become necrotic. The contents of the nodule are expectorated, leaving a thin-walled cavity. Most such cavities behave in a benign fashion and eventually close. Complications do occur, including hemoptysis, rupture into the pleural space (causing pyopneumothorax), and secondary bacterial infections.

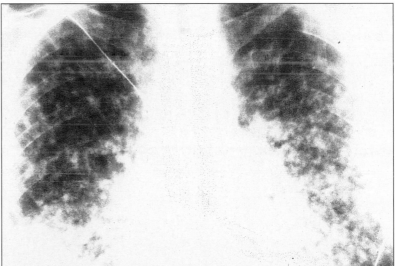

FIGURE 5-49 Chest radiograph showing diffuse macronodular pulmonary infiltrates in coccidioidomycosis. The individual nodules are larger than miliary nodules, even up to 1 to 2 cm in size. The patient was a 28-year-man with AIDS who lived half of each year in Phoenix, Arizona. He presented with fever and progressive dyspnea. At bronchoscopy, large endobronchial ulcers were seen at the right upper lobe and right middle lobe takeoffs. Endobronchial biopsy specimens showed spherules. Bronchoalveolar lavage was also positive for spherules and was negative for *Pneumocystis carinii* and other pathogens.

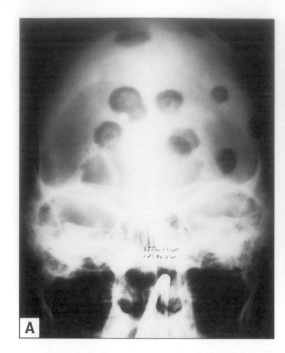

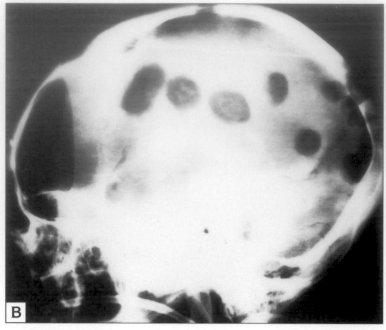

FIGURE 5-50 Coccidioidal osteomyelitis of the skull. **A** and **B**, Multiple lytic lesions are seen in the skull of a 30-year-old man with AIDS who was a resident of Texas. Coccidioidomycosis was confirmed by bone biopsy. The intracranial air visible in the lateral view was the result of a pneumoencephalogram, which is an unusual finding because this test had largely disappeared before the AIDS era. (*Courtesy of* J.T. Mader, MD.)

Usual therapy for coccidioidomycosis

	Immunocompetent host	Immunosuppressed host	
		Without AIDS	**With AIDS**
Acute	Observe, except for high-risk patients Rapid disease—AMB (1500–2000 mg, total dose) Slow disease—FLU (400–800 mg × 12 mo)	Rapid disease—AMB (1500–2000 mg, total dose) Slow disease—FLU (400 mg/day × 6–12 mo)	High-risk patients: Rapid disease—AMB (1500—2000 mg) *then* FLU (400–800 mg for life) Slow disease—FLU (400–800 mg for life)
Thin-walled cavity	Observe if stable Symptomatic, enlarging—FLU (400 mg/day × 6 mo) *or* resect High-risk, even without symptoms—same as above	FLU (400–800 mg/day × 6–12 mo)	FLU (400–800 mg for life)
Ruptured cavity with empyema, pneumothorax	AMB (1500–2500 mg, total dose)	AMB (1500–2500 mg, total dose) *then* FLU (400–800 mg/day × 12 mo)	AMB (2000–3000 mg) *then* FLU (for life)
Rapidly progressive miliary	AMB (2000–3000 mg, total dose)	AMB (2000–3000 mg, total dose)	AMB (2000–3000 mg) *then* FLU (400–800 mg for life)
Meningeal Patient awake	FLU (400–800 mg/day × 12 mo or longer, depending on symptoms)	FLU (400–800 mg/day, probably for life)	FLU (400–800 mg for life) or AMB (2000–3000 mg systemically + intracisternally 3 × wk); once awake and cultures negative, FLU (400–800 mg for life)
Patient confused	AMB (2000–3000 mg systemically + intracisternally 3×/wk until cultures negative, *then* decrease frequency); with improvement, FLU (400–800 mg/day × at least 12 mo)	Same as in immunocompetent host, but continue FLU (400–800 mg/day) for life (?)	Same as above

AMB—amphotericin B; FLU—fluconazole.

FIGURE 5-51 Usual therapy for coccidioidomycosis. High-risk patients include blacks and those with immunosuppression but without AIDS.

PARACOCCIDIOIDOMYCOSIS

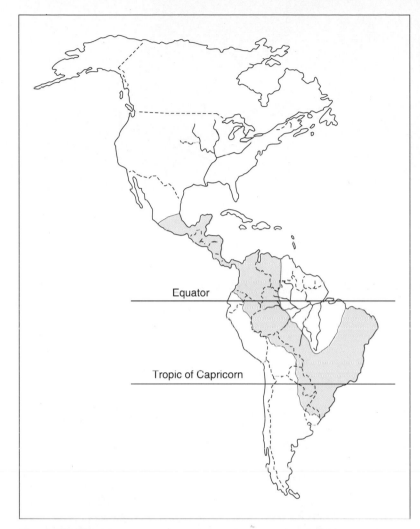

FIGURE 5-52 Map of areas endemic for paracoccidioidomycosis. Paracoccidioidomycosis, like the other endemic mycoses, is predominantly an infection of the western hemisphere. It is largely limited to Central and South America, with most disease activity centered in Columbia, Venezuela, and Brazil. (*Adapted from* Rippon [1]; with permission.)

Clinical manifestations of paracoccidioidomycosis

Habitat	Soil enriched by organic nitrogen in the form of bird or animal feces
Portal of entry	Lung
Primary infection	Often subacute and progressive
	Can mimic bacterial pneumonia
Tissue response	Pyogenic–granulomatous
Extrapulmonary spread	Oral mucosa
	Cervical and mediastinal lymph nodes
Complications in HIV infection	Uncommon

FIGURE 5-53 Clinical manifestations of paracoccidioidomycosis. *Paracoccidioidomycosis brasiliensis* is a dimorphic fungus. The mycelial form grows in the soil and has small spores that are aerosolized and then inhaled. Once in mammalian tissue at 37° C, the fungus converts to the parasitic yeast form. The tissue response is mixed granulomatous and pyogenic, and many patients have purulent secretions that are coughed up. The primary infection is in the lung. A direct smear of potassium hydroxide–digested sputum showing multiple, peripheral, thin-neck buds is diagnostic paracoccidioidomycosis.

Diagnosis of paracoccidioidomycosis

Histopathology (special stains)	5–10-µm yeast; multiple small peripheral buds with thin neck of attachment—resembles pilot's wheel
	Silver stain
Culture	Time-consuming, up to 30 days
Rapid diagnosis by examination of fresh specimen	Potassium hydroxide digest often helpful
Serology	Complement fixation test is useful clinically

FIGURE 5-54 Diagnosis of paracoccidioidomycosis.

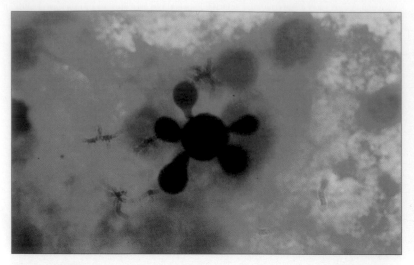

FIGURE 5-55 Characteristic "pilot-wheel" yeast form of *Paracoccidioides brasiliensis*. *P. brasiliensis* is a large yeast, often 8 to 15 µm in diameter. It has characteristic thin-necked buds that are smaller than the parent cell and distributed around the periphery of the organism, giving the budding yeast the appearance of a pilot wheel on a ship. If a yeast has only two small buds, it is sometimes referred to as a "Mickey Mouse" form. (Grocott silver stain; original magnification, × 1000.) (*From* Salfelder *et al.* [2]; with permission.)

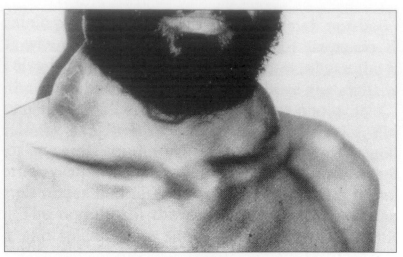

FIGURE 5-56 Bulky cervical lymphadenopathy in paracoccidioidomycosis. The large bulky cervical nodes in this patient clinically suggested malignant lymphoma but were proven to be due to paracoccidioidomycosis. Bulky cervical nodes are seen in paracoccidioidomycosis but not in other endemic mycoses. (*From* Franco *et al.* [10]; with permission.)

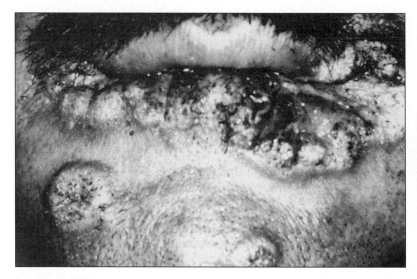

FIGURE 5-57 Indurated perioral ulcers in paracoccidioidomycosis. Another clinical feature that is unique to paracoccidioidomycosis among the endemic mycoses is the frequent presentation with pharyngeal, oral, and perioral ulcers. Crusty lesions and ulcerations on the face can be seen in patients with blastomycosis and coccidioidomycosis, but oral and pharyngeal ulcers are much more common with paracoccidioidomycosis than with these other mycoses. (*From* Franco *et al.* [10]; with permission.)

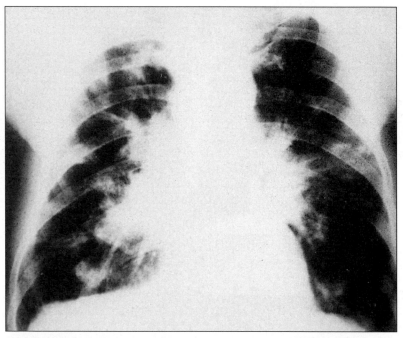

FIGURE 5-58 Chest radiograph showing bilateral perihilar infiltrates with bulky enlarged central mediastinal nodes in paracoccidioidomycosis. Patients with paracoccidioidomycosis may have focal, dense, infiltrates suggesting bacterial pneumonia. Mediastinal adenopathy is quite common. Bilateral central perihilar infiltrates are another recognized radiographic pattern. (*From* Franco *et al.* [10]; with permission.)

CRYPTOCOCCOSIS

Clinical manifestations of cryptococcosis	
Habitat	Soil enriched by organic nitrogen in the form of bird or animal feces
Portal of entry	Lung
Primary infection	Asymptomatic to mild
Tissue response	Usually little or no inflammatory response
	Occasional granuloma
Extrapulmonary spread	Rare in normals
	Extremely common in T-cell–immuno-compromised hosts
	Meninges, bones, prostate, kidney, skin
Complications in HIV infection	Very common

FIGURE 5-59 Clinical manifestations of cryptococcosis. The infection is acquired by inhalation, and the primary infection occurs in the lung. The pulmonary infection is often asymptomatic or minimally symptomatic, and there is an unusual tropism for the central nervous system. In fact, chronic meningitis is the most common clinical presentation of cryptococcal infection.

Diagnosis of cryptococcosis	
Histopathology (special stains)	Encapsulated single budding yeast; capsule size variable
	Silver or mucicarmine stain on tissue
	India ink preparation for CSF and other fluids
Culture	Rapid, 3–5 days
	Capsule formation variable
Rapid diagnosis by examination of fresh specimen	India ink preparation of CSF or prostatic secretions is highly specific and 70% sensitive
Serology	Antigen determination is highly sensitive in CSF
	Serum antigen usually positive in AIDS patients but negative in others

CSF cerebrospinal fluid.

FIGURE 5-60 Diagnosis of cryptococcosis. *Cryptococcus* is the only encapsulated fungal organism that infects humans. It exists both in nature and in the mammalian host as a small budding yeast. The size of the yeast varies from 2 to 10 μm, and the yeast has a carbohydrate capsule.

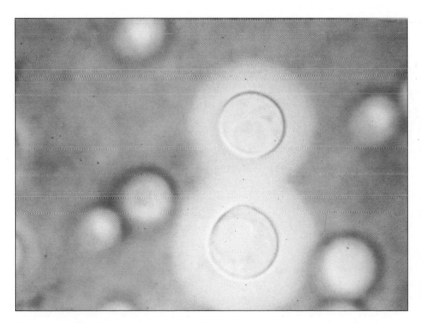

FIGURE 5-61 *Cryptococcus neoformans* in cerebrospinal fluid (CSF) on a direct India ink preparation. Because the yeast has a large carbohydrate capsule, there is often a clear "halo-like" space around the individual yeast organisms. An India ink preparation of CSF can dramatically illustrate the clear space. A similar effect can be seen with direct stains, including Gram stain of sputum, and with histopathologic stains (including routine hematoxylin-eosin) on tissue sections. (Original magnification, × 1000.)

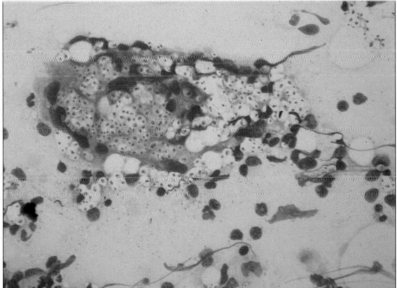

FIGURE 5-62 Wright stain of bronchoalveolar lavage fluid showing capsular *Cryptococcus neoformans*. Small yeast are obvious within the macrophages and are about the same size as *Histoplasma capsulatum* organisms. However, there is a larger clear space around the organisms that suggests an actual capsule rather than the staining artifact that is sometime seen around *Histoplasma* organisms. If capsular material is suspected, a mucicarmine stain will demonstrate it (*see* Fig. 5-63). (Original magnification, × 1000.)

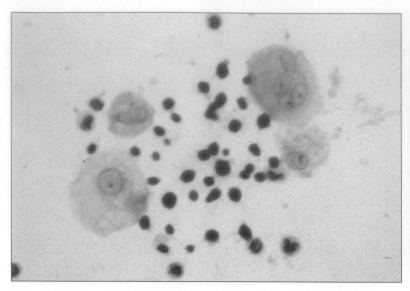

FIGURE 5-63 Mucicarmine stain of bronchoalveolar lavage fluid showing capsule around *Cryptococcus neoformans*. Mucicarmine stain colors that carbohydrate capsule of *C. neoformans* a bright crimson. In a sample of body fluid or a histopathologic section of tissue, the presence of yeast staining bright red with a mucicarmine stain is diagnostic of cryptococcal infection, because *Cryptococcus* is the only pathogenic fungus that has a carbohydrate capsule. (Original magnification, × 1000.) (*From* Stanley *et al.* [3]; with permission.)

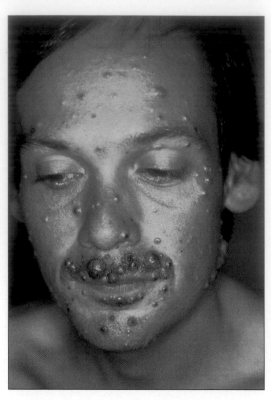

FIGURE 5-64 Multiple nodular cryptococcal skin lesions on the face of a patient with AIDS. These lesions are not very inflammatory and actually resemble molluscum contagiosum. A biopsy specimen, however, showed abundant cryptococcal yeast. In patients with AIDS, similar subcutaneous nodules can be seen in disseminated histoplasmosis and coccidioidomycosis. Sometimes, these cutaneous cryptococcal nodules are redder and more inflammatory in appearance. Cryptococcosis can also present on the skin as a spreading cellulitis. (*From* Vaillant [11]; with permission.)

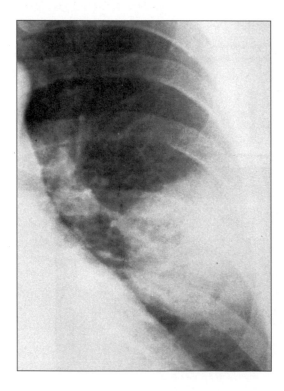

FIGURE 5-65 Chest radiograph showing a large focal mass in cryptococcosis. The patient, who had very few symptoms and was immunocompetent, showed a relatively large focal mass in the left lower lobe on chest radiography. Other patients with pulmonary cryptococcosis may present with nodules or focal infiltrates. (*From* Fraser and Paré [12]; with permission.)

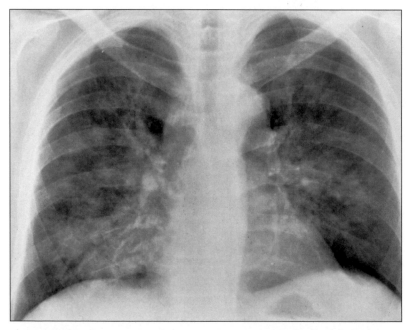

FIGURE 5-66 Chest radiograph showing diffuse bilateral infiltrates in cryptococcosis. The patient, who was receiving high-dose prednisone for collagen vascular disease, presented with fever and then progressive shortness of breath. Blood cultures were positive for *Cryptococcus neoformans*. Diffuse pulmonary infiltrates from cryptococcal infection are most common in patients with AIDS. AIDS patients with cryptococcal infection, unlike immunocompetent patients, usually have positive cryptococcal antigen in the serum at a titer higher than that in cerebrospinal fluid.

Usual therapy for cryptococcosis

	Immunocompetent host	Immunosuppressed host	
		Without AIDS	With AIDS
Pulmonary	Observe if LP negative; alternatively, FLU* (200–400 mg/day)	AMB (0.7 mg/kg/day) with or without 5-FC (150 mg/kg/day) × 6 wk or until stable, *then* FLU* (200–400 mg/day × 12 mo)	AMB (0.7 mg/kg/day) + 5-FC (100 mg/kg/day) until stable, *then* FLU (200–400 mg for life)
Extrapulmonary nonmeningeal	If stable—FLU (400 mg/day × 6 mo) If sick—AMB (0.4 mg/kg/day) + 5-FC (150 mg/kg/day) × 4 wk	Same as above	Same as above
Meningeal	AMB (0.4 mg/kg/day) + 5-FC (150 mg/kg/day) × 4 wk If awake and stable—FLU* (400 mg/day × 6–12 mo)	AMB (0.7 mg/kg/day) + 5-FC (150 mg/kg/day) × 6 wk If awake and stable—FLU* (400 mg/day × 6–12 mo)	Same as above

*Role of this drug untested for this condition.
AMB—amphotericin B; 5-FC—5-fluorocytosine (flucytosine); FLU—fluconazole; LP—lumbar puncture.

FIGURE 5-67 Usual therapy for cryptococcosis.

ASPERGILLOSIS

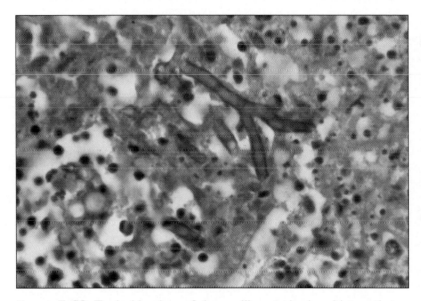

FIGURE 5-68 Typical hyphae of *Aspergillus* species in a histopathologic section. The hyphae of *Aspergillus* spp are 5 to 10 μm in diameter, have dichotomous acute-angle branching, and are septate. The hyphae often lie in the same tissue plane so that parallel strands of fungus are visible across the whole field. *Aspergillus* is not a dimorphic fungus and exists only as a mycelium with hyphae, both in nature and in infected mammalian tissue. Similar hyphae are seen with rare opportunistic fungi, including *Pseudoallescheria boydii* and *Fusarium* spp. Differentiation must be made by culture.

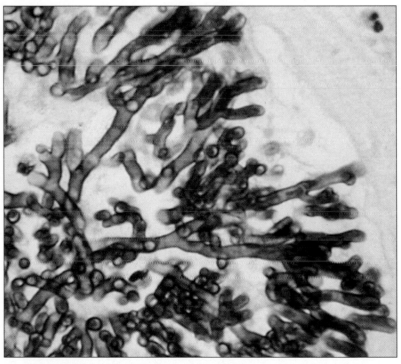

FIGURE 5-69 Typical hyphae of *Aspergillus* growing within a blood vessel. The organisms show parallel hyphae in the same tissue plane, exhibiting cross-striations or septae and also dichotomous acute-angle branching. *Aspergillus* tends to be angioinvasive, growing in blood vessels and causing distal hemorrhage and infarction of tissue. *Aspergillus fumigatus* is the most common pathogenic species, with *A. flavus* and *A. niger* also being important pathogens. (*From* Hudson *et al.* [9]; with permission.)

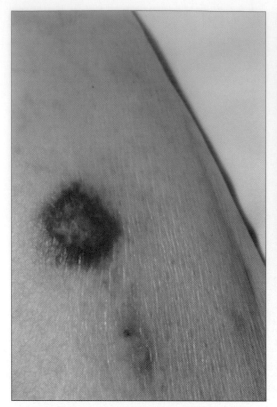

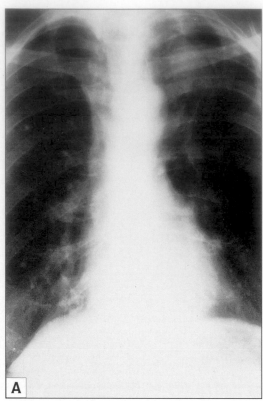

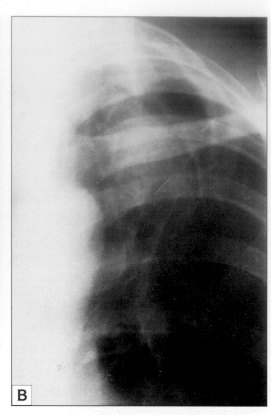

A

B

FIGURE 5-70 Chronic skin lesion of aspergillosis. A chronic skin lesion is seen on the extremity of a 74-year-old man with prolonged neutropenia from myelofibrosis. Biopsy of the skin lesion showed typical *Aspergillus* organisms growing within blood vessels and also more widely within the tissue. Invasive pulmonary aspergillosis is acquired by inhalation and usually complicates profound neutropenia or other neutrophil dysfunction. The fungus invades blood vessels, causes local infarction, and can spread through the bloodstream to distant sites including the skin, brain, and viscera.

FIGURE 5-71 Pulmonary aspergilloma. **A**, A chest radiograph shows a rounded mass in the left upper lobe with a faintly visible crescent of air around the mass. There is no infiltrate in the surrounding lung tissue. The patient was asymptomatic, and the rounded mass was an aspergilloma colonizing a preexisting space in the lung. The crescent of air around the fungus ball is called *Monod's sign*. **B**, A computed tomography scan clearly shows the crescent of air surrounding the large fungus ball within the cavity.

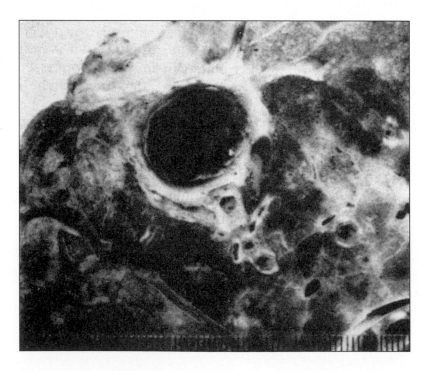

FIGURE 5-72 Gross pathology of an aspergilloma in the lung apex. Contiguous pleura is thickened. (*From* Bennett [13]; with permission.)

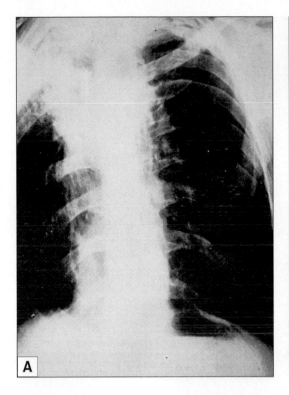

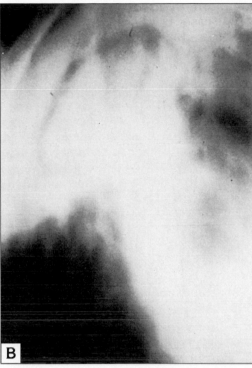

FIGURE 5-73 Chronic necrotizing aspergillosis. **A**, A chest radiograph shows a dense right upper lobe infiltrate extending to the pleural surface with overlying pleural thickening. Cultures of the sputum were positive for *Aspergillus*, and biopsies of the tissue showed *Aspergillus* organisms. This radiographic pattern is not seen with a simple aspergilloma but rather represents chronic necrotizing aspergillosis with local infection of the surrounding lung and overlying pleural space. **B**, A computed tomography scan clearly shows a fungus ball in the central cavity with a crescent of air around it. However, the active infection in the surrounding lung tissue and in the overlying pleural space suggest more than an uncomplicated aspergilloma. Patients with necrotizing aspergillosis have chronic symptoms including productive cough, night sweats, and weight loss and may have chronic anemia and elevated sedimentation rate. There is little tendency for distant spread through the bloodstream. (*From* Rippon [1]; with permission.)

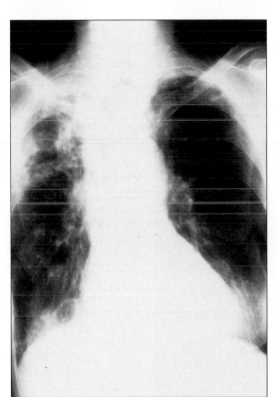

FIGURE 5-74 Chest radiograph showing chronic cavitary aspergillosis involving the right upper lobe. In this case, there was no aspergilloma, and the initial diagnostic impression was probable tuberculosis. Sputum cultures were negative for mycobacteria but were positive on repeated occasions for *Aspergillus fumigatus*. There is a fibrocavitary infiltrate with extensive pleural thickening. Transbronchial biopsy showed *Aspergillus* organisms growing in the lung tissue.

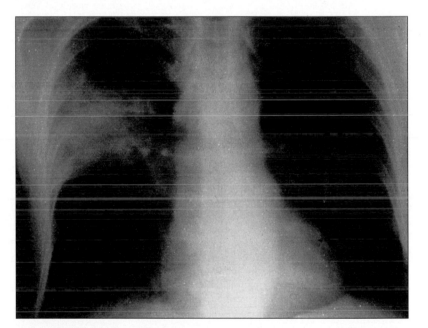

FIGURE 5-75 Chest radiograph in invasive aspergillosis showing a dense wedge-shaped infiltrate in the right upper lobe. The patient was a 74-year-old man with prolonged neutropenia (*see* Fig. 5-70). Invasive aspergillosis complicates prolonged neutropenia or severe neutrophil dysfunction, including phagocyte dysfunction caused by prolonged therapy with high-dose prednisone. The disease is angioinvasive and can present with a wedge-shaped peripheral infiltrate. Patients can have hemoptysis and pleuritic pain and present with a syndrome resembling pulmonary infarction.

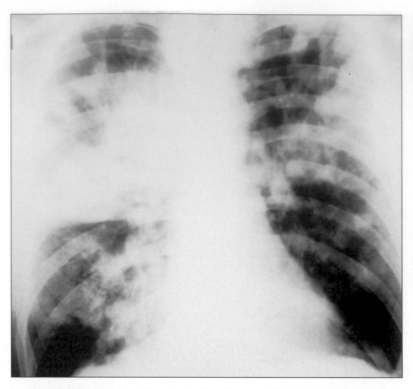

FIGURE 5-76 Chest radiograph showing multiple peripheral nodular infiltrates in invasive pulmonary aspergillosis. This is another radiographic pattern of invasive pulmonary aspergillosis associated with neutropenia. (*From* Hudson *et al.* [9]; with permission.)

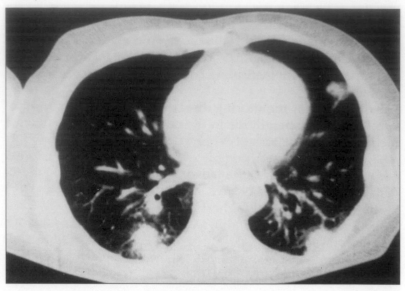

FIGURE 5-77 Computed tomography scan of the chest showing multiple peripheral nodules in invasive pulmonary aspergillosis. Invasive aspergillosis begins in the lung has a high tendency for pyemic spread to other organs, including brain, skin, and viscera. (*From* Zerhouni [14]; with permission.)

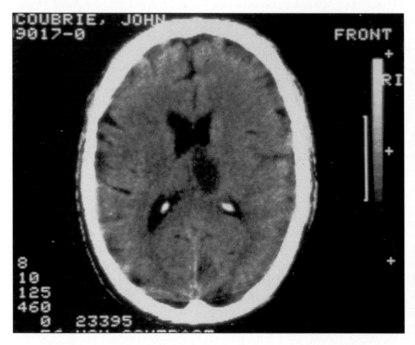

FIGURE 5-78 Cranial computed tomography (CT) scan showing metastatic foci of aspergillosis. A noncontrast-enhanced CT scan shows two large lucent areas, one just behind the ventricles and one in the occipital lobe. These abscesses were proven at autopsy to be metastatic foci of aspergillosis. (*From* Al-Doory and Wagner [15]; with permission.)

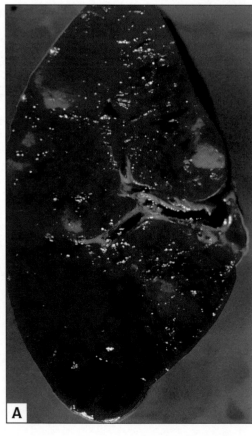

FIGURE 5-79 Multiple foci of aspergillosis in the spleen. **A,** Autopsy examination showed multiple white nodules on the surface of the spleen. On histopathologic section, these proved to be hematogenous foci of aspergillosis in a patient who died of invasive aspergillosis complicating prolonged neutropenia. (*continued*)

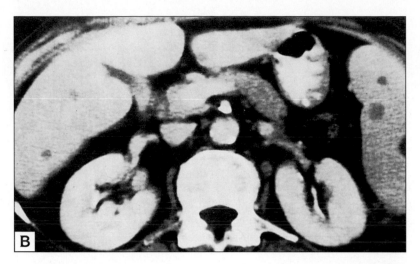

FIGURE 5-79 (*continued*) **B**, A non-contrast–enhanced computed tomography scan of the abdomen shows multiple low-density lesions in the spleen and liver. This is the typical radiographic presentation of hematogenous aspergillosis lesions. (Panel 79B *from* Lee *et al.* [7]; with permission.)

MUCORMYCOSIS

Pathogenic agents of mucormycosis

Absidia
  A. corymbifera
  A. ramosa
Mucor
  M. circinelloides
Rhizomucor
  R. pusillus
Rhizopus
  R. oryzae
  R. arrhizus
  R. rhizopodiformis

FIGURE 5-80 Pathogenic agents of mucormycosis.

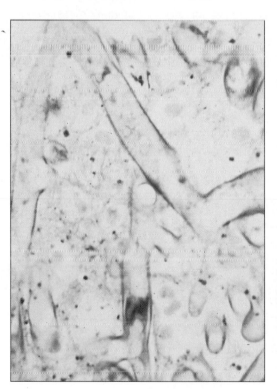

FIGURE 5-81 Typical hyphae of *Mucor* species. This fungus always occurs as a mycelium, both in nature and in infected tissue. Its hyphae are broader than those of *Aspergillus* spp, ranging in width from 10 to 20 μm. In general, the hyphae are not oriented in a parallel fashion, so only short stubby pieces are seen in any one tissue section. The side branches are also short and stubby and come off at right angles. There are no septae. The hyphae are often difficult to see in tissue sections and are sometimes better seen on routine hematoxylin-eosin–stained sections than on sections stained with special stains. Biopsy specimens of infected tissue often show a great deal of necrosis. The fungus is often difficult to culture.

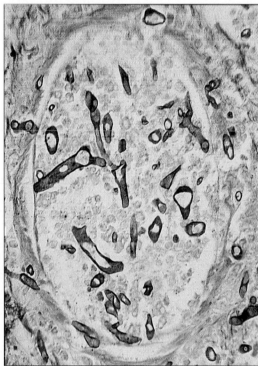

FIGURE 5-82 Typical hyphae of *Mucor* species within an occluded blood vessel. Like *Aspergillus* spp, *Mucor* tend to be angioinvasive and cause infarction and necrosis of tissue. Mucormycosis complicates prolonged neutropenia, uncontrolled diabetic ketoacidosis (because it tends to grow well in an acidic, high-glucose environment), and deferoxamine chelation therapy (used for iron-overload states). (*From* Salfelder *et al.* [2]; with permission.)

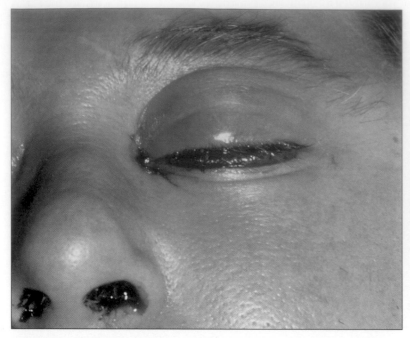

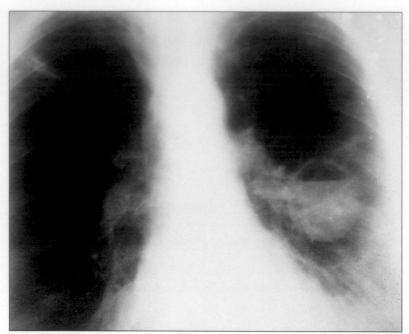

FIGURE 5-83 Rhinocerebral mucormycosis involving the left nose and orbit. The usual predisposition to rhinocerebral mucormycosis is uncontrolled diabetic ketoacidosis. Spores of *Mucor* spp impact on the nasal mucosa, and the hyphae invade the turbinates and paranasal sinuses, extending to the adjacent orbit. Eventually, they invade backward along the cavernous sinuses and cause infarction in the brain. This is the most lethal fungal infection of humans. Treatment involves control of the diabetic ketoacidosis, intravenous amphotericin B, and extensive debridement of infarcted necrotic tissue.

FIGURE 5-84 Chest radiograph in mucormycosis showing a large cavitary mass in the left lower lobe. The patient was a 60-year-old woman who had idiopathic thrombocytic purpura being treated with high-dose prednisone. She also had diabetes induced by the prednisone and was receiving insulin. She presented with fever and this radiographic mass on chest radiographs. Specimens drawn by transthoracic fine-needle aspiration showed typical hyphae of *Mucor*, and the cultures were also positive. The patient was treated by reducing the prednisone dose and with intravenous amphotericin B and recovered.

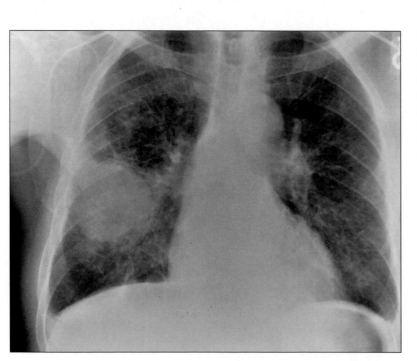

FIGURE 5-85 Chest radiograph in mucormycosis showing a large rounded mass in the right lower lobe. The patient was an elderly man with prolonged neutropenia from myelofibrosis. Biopsy of the mass showed typical hyphae of *Mucor* spp and cultures were also positive. Other radiographic presentations of mucormycosis include cavitary wedge-shaped peripheral infiltrates and single and multiple nodules. Mucormycosis, like invasive aspergillosis, also can spread to skin, brain, and internal viscera. (*From* Rubenstein and Federman [16]; with permission.)

CANDIDIASIS

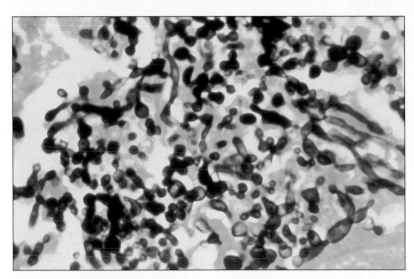

FIGURE 5-86 Typical *Candida* organisms in tissue biopsy. The key feature in identifying *Candida* is the mixture of yeast and hyphae together in the same tissue section. The hyphae are formed by serial budding of the yeast (sprout mycelia), causing an elongated structure. Because the pseudohyphae are formed by serial budding, the walls are not totally parallel, like the walls of *Aspergillus* and *Mucor* spp in tissue sections. Also, in the same field will be small yeast, some with thin-necked single buds. *Candida albicans* typically has pseudohyphae and yeast in tissue biopsy specimens, but some non-*albicans* spp have only yeast forms in the infected tissue.

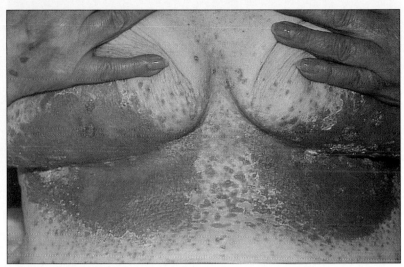

FIGURE 5-87 Cutaneous candidiasis involving the moist skinfolds under the breasts. The lesions are very red, and there are small red satellite lesions surrounding the main area of involvement. The typical location and the presence of satellite lesions make the gross image highly suggestive of cutaneous candidiasis. There is little tendency for deep tissue invasion with this type of lesion. (*From* Fitzpatrick *et al.* [4]; with permission.)

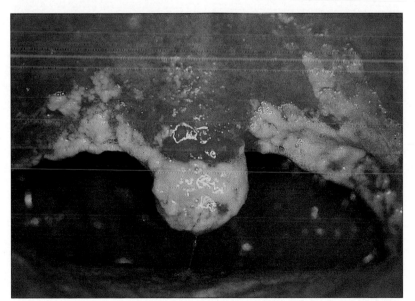

FIGURE 5-88 Extensive pharyngeal candidiasis involving the soft palette and uvula of a patient with AIDS. Oral pharyngeal candidiasis can be a marker of T-cell immunosuppression. T cells are required to control candida growth on the mucosal surfaces. However, adequate neutrophil number and function are enough to prevent deep invasion, and there is surprisingly little tendency to develop disseminated candidiasis in patients who are T-cell deficient. (*From* Fitzpatrick *et al.* [4]; with permission.)

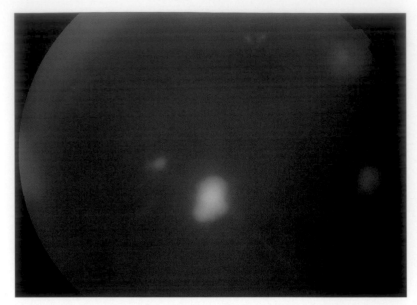

FIGURE 5-89 Cottonwool exudates on the retina due to disseminated candidiasis. Patients with disseminated candidiasis often have microabscesses in multiple organs. This disease generally complicates prolonged neutropenia or a neutrophil dysfunction, including that induced by high-dose prednisone, as well as multiple abdominal surgeries. Candida is the only fungus that is part of the normal flora of humans and is found on the skin, pharynx, and stool. Generally, the organism gains access to the circulation across the bowel wall and spreads through the bloodstream to multiple organs. It can also gain access to the body across the skin along intravascular catheters. It is not acquired by inhalation. The patient generally presents with a nonspecific febrile illness. Microabscesses can develop in deep viscera and subcutaneous tissue. The eyes can sometimes be involved, and cottonwool exudates, seen in the eye grounds here, are diagnostic of disseminated candidiasis. Positive blood cultures are suggestive of disseminated candidiasis but are not sensitive. Almost half of patients found at autopsy to have disseminated candidiasis never had a positive blood culture during life. (*Courtesy of* J.L. Davis, MD, and A.G. Palestine, MD.)

SPOROTRICHOSIS

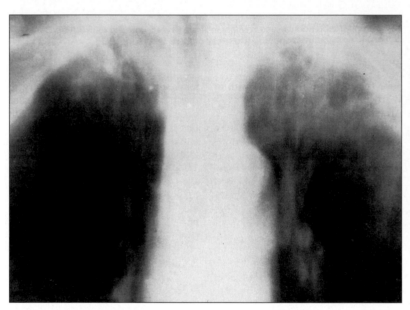

FIGURE 5-90 Computed tomography scan of the chest showing extensive fibronodular disease in both apices due to sporotrichosis. These infiltrates are most suggestive of tuberculosis, and in fact, this patient was initially treated for tuberculosis despite multiple negative cultures for mycobacteria. Eventually, the correct diagnosis was made and the appropriate treatment begun. Similar upper lobe fibronodular infiltrates can be seen in tuberculosis, chronic cavitary histoplasmosis, and chronic necrotizing aspergillosis. (*From* Rippon [1]; with permission.)

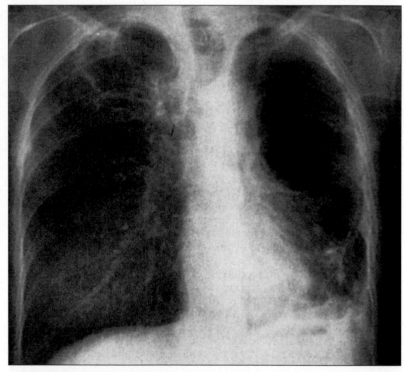

FIGURE 5-91 Chest radiograph showing extensive bilateral cavitation in pulmonary sporotrichosis. Pulmonary sporotrichosis is a very rare presentation (much less common than lymphocutaneous disease). (*From* Rex [17]; with permission.)

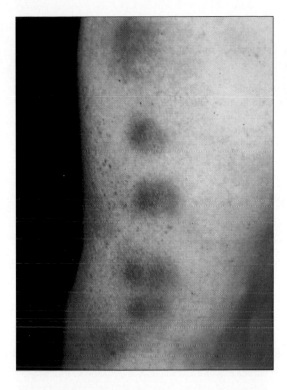

FIGURE 5-92 Lymphocutaneous nodules of sporotrichosis. These red and inflamed nodules are located along the lymphatics of the lower extremity. This presentation is highly characteristic for sporotrichosis and is the most common manifestation of sporotrichosis. This lymphocutaneous form is an inoculation disease and spreads proximally along draining lymphatics from the inoculation point, usually distal on an extremity. The mechanism of infection of pulmonary sporotrichosis may be inhalation of spores, similar to that with other pulmonary fungal infections. (*From* Fitzpatrick *et al.* [4]; with permission.)

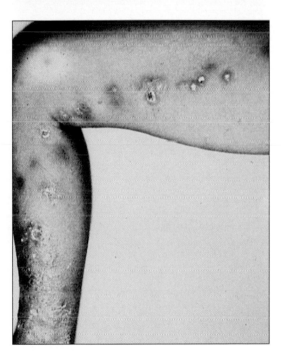

FIGURE 5-93 Stable chronic skin lesions of the lower extremity in sporotrichosis. This presentation of sporotrichosis is a more chronic fixed disease, with crusted lesions extending to the skin overlying the infected lymph nodes. (*From* Salfelder *et al.* [2]; with permission.)

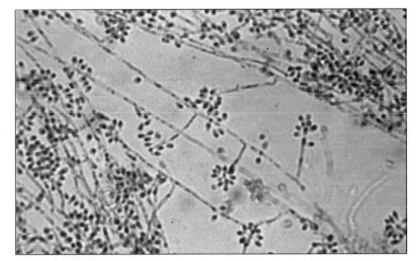

FIGURE 5-94 Culture of *Sporothrix schenckii*. *Sporothrix* is a dimorphic fungus. In tissue, it is a small yeast and not a specific finding. However, on culture at 26° C (as illustrated), the organism shows the characteristic morphology of small, petal-shaped spores. (*Courtesy of* G.J. Raugi, MD.)

REFERENCES

1. Rippon JW: *Medical Mycology: The Pathogenic Fungi and the Pathogenic Actinomycetes*, 3rd ed. Philadelphia: W.B. Saunders; 1988.

2. Salfelder K, deLiscano TR, Sauerteig E: *Atlas of Fungal Pathology*, vol 17. Boston: Kluwer Academic Publishers; 1990.

3. Stanley MW, Henry-Stanley MJ, Iber C: *Bronchoalveolar Lavage: Cytology and Clinical Applications.* New York: Igaku-Shoin; 1991:108.

4. Fitzpatrick TB, Johnson RA, Polano MK, *et al.* (eds.): *Color Atlas and Synopsis of Clinical Dermatology*, 2nd ed. New York: McGraw-Hill; 1992.

5. Bone RC, *et al.* (eds.): *Pulmonary and Critical Care Medicine, Care Volume*, vol. 2. St. Louis: Mosby; 1993.

6. Bullock WE: *Histoplasma capsulatum. In* Mandell GL, Bennett JE, Dolin R (eds.): *Principles and Practice of Infectious Diseases*, 4th ed. New York: Churchill Livingstone; 1995:2344.

7. Lee JK, Sagel SS, Stanley RJ (eds.): *Computed Body Tomography with MRI Correlation*, 2nd ed. New York: Raven Press; 1989.

8. Sarosi GA, Davies SF: Blastomycosis. *Am Rev Respir Dis* 1979, 120:911–938.

9. Hudson ME, Starke ID, Corrin B, *et al.*: *Atlas of Chest Infections.* New York: Gower Medical Publishing; 1992.

10. Franco M, da Silva Lacaz C, Restrepo-Moreno A, Del Negro G (eds.): *Paracoccidioidomycosis*. Boca Raton, FL: CRC Press; 1994.

11. Vaillant L: Disseminated cryptococcosis. *Acta Derm Venereol (Stockh)* 1989, 69:365–367.

12. Fraser RG, Paré JA: *Diagnosis of Diseases of the Chest*, vol IV, 2nd ed. Philadelphia: W.B. Saunders; 1979:2182.

13. Bennett JE: *Aspergillus* species. *In* Mandell GL, Bennett JE, Dolin R (eds.): *Principles and Practice of Infectious Diseases*, 4th ed. New York: Churchill Livingstone; 1995:2307.

14. Zerhouni EA (ed.): *CT and MRI of the Thorax*. New York: Churchill Livingstone; 1990:8.

15. Al-Doory Y, Wager GE (eds.): *Aspergillosis*. Springfield, IL: Charles C Thomas; 1985:104.

16. Rubenstein E, Federman DD (eds.): *Scientific American Medicine*, vol. 3. New York: Scientific American; 1993:15.

17. Rex JH: *Sporothrix schenckii. In* Mandell GL, Bennett JE, Dolin R (eds.): *Principles and Practice of Infectious Diseases*, 4th ed. New York: Churchill Livingstone; 1995:2322.

SELECTED BIBLIOGRAPHY

Davies SF: An overview of pulmonary fungal infections. *Respir Infect* 1987, 8:495–512.

Davies SF: Diagnosis of pulmonary fungal infections. *Semin Respir Infect* 1988, 3:162–171.

Davies SF: Fungal pneumonia. *Med Clin North Am* 1994 (in press).

Sarosi GA, Davies SF: Blastomycosis. *Am Rev Respir Dis* 1979, 120:911–938.

Sarosi GA, Davies SF (eds.): *Fungal Diseases of Lung*, 2nd ed. New York: Raven Press; 1993.

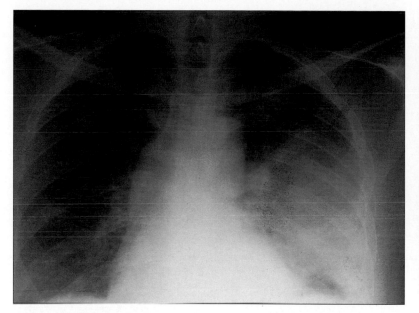

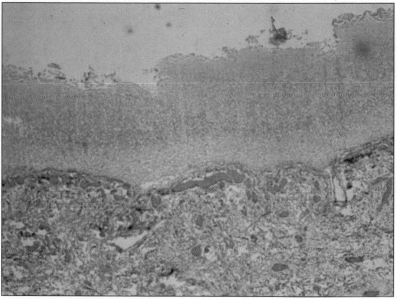

FIGURE 6-4 Chest radiograph showing anaerobic empyema. Anaerobes now account for 30% to 50% of empyemas. This suppurative complication of anaerobic pneumonitis, or lung abscess with bronchopleural fistula, requires adequate drainage of the pleural space as is indicated for any grossly purulent empyema. Pleural fluid is an easily accessible source for uncontaminated cultures, simplifying isolation of anaerobes.

FIGURE 6-5 Histologic examination of pleura in the exudative phase of empyema. The progression of pathologic changes in empyema is divided into three stages: an exudative phase with leukocyte migration and pus formation; a fibropurulent phase during which lung expansion begins to be limited by fibrosis; and an organizing phase in which the pleura becomes thickened and significant restrictive pulmonary dysfunction occurs. (Hematoxylin-eosin stain.) (*Courtesy of J. Jagirdar, MD.*)

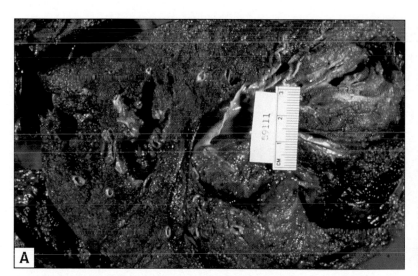

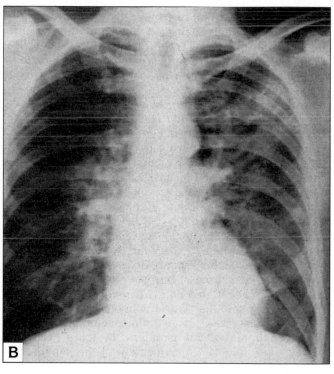

FIGURE 6-6 Confluent anaerobic necrotizing bronchopneumonia with lung abscess. **A,** Gross pathology. This acute process has been likened to "pulmonary gangrene" and is often associated with empyema. Patients are usually toxic appearing, with putrid sputum. **B,** Chest radiograph of a patient with such a process, showing left-sided cavitating infiltrates and blunting of the left costophrenic angle. (Panel 6B *from* Finegold [1]; with permission.)

Etiologic Agents

Anaerobes commonly encountered in pleuropulmonary infection

Gram-negative bacilli
 Pigmented *Prevotella* or *Porphyromonas*
 Prevotella oralis group
 P. oris
 P. buccae
 P. bivia
 Bacteroides ureolyticus group (especially *B. gracilis*)
 B. fragilis group
 Fusobacterium nucleatum
 F. necrophorum
 F. naviforme
 F. gonidiaformans

Gram-positive cocci
 Peptostreptococcus (especially *P. micros, P. anaerobus, P. magnus, P. asaccharolyticus, P. prevotii, P. intermedius**)
 Microaerophilic streptococci

Gram-positive spore-forming bacilli
 Clostridium perfringens
 C. ramosums

Gram-positive nonspore-forming bacilli
 Actinomyces spp
 Propionibacterium propionicum
 Bifidobacterium dentium

*This organism officially belongs in the genus *Streptococcus.*

FIGURE 6-7 Anaerobes commonly encountered in pleuropulmonary infections. The emergency of β-lactamase production among the anaerobic gram-negative bacilli has prompted reevaluation of recommendations for empiric antimicrobial therapy. In nosocomially acquired infections, other pathogens, such as *Staphylococcus aureus* and aerobic gram-negative rods, are often involved. (*From* Finegold [1]; with permission.)

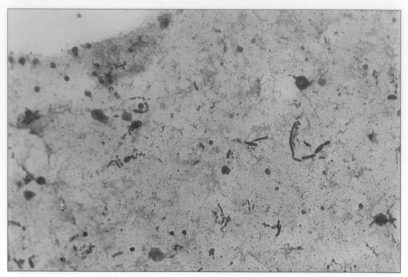

FIGURE 6-8 *Prevotella* or *Porphyromonas* species. Gram stain from a 72-hour colony on blood agar. These small coccobacillary forms contrast with the pleomorphism and variable staining of *Bacteroides* species (previously all classed as *Bacteroides fragilis* group) (*see* Fig. 6-13). These bacteria, most previously classed as *Bacteroides* species, are isolated in one half to three quarters of anaerobic bacterial infections of the lung. Increasing frequency of resistance of these isolates to penicillin has led most clinicians to abandon use of penicillin or ampicillin as single-agent therapy for lung abscesses.

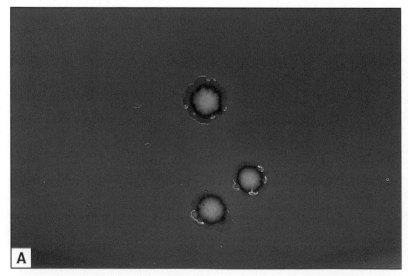

A

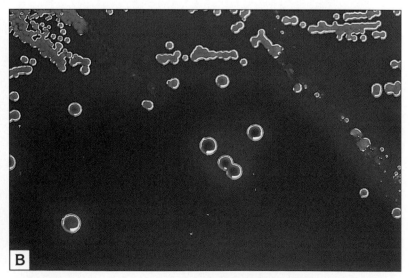

B

FIGURE 6-9 *Prevotella melaninogenica* colonies. **A,** After 7 days' incubation on blood agar, pigmentation is notable at the margins of colonies. It may be difficult to demonstrate pigmentation in some *Prevotella* strains. The use of laked blood agar (performed by freezing and thawing) is recommended for expression of pigment, which may develop only after 5 to 7 days. However, colonies may fluoresce brick-red under long-wave ultraviolet light (Woods' lamp) before pigment is produced. **B,** Further pigmentation developing after prolonged incubation.

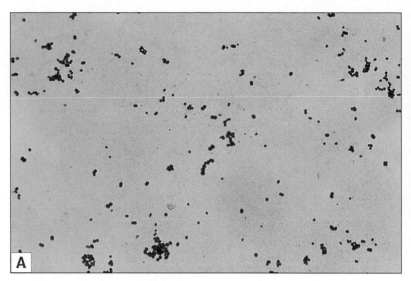

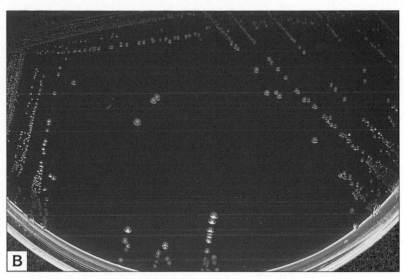

FIGURE 6-10 *Peptostreptococcus anaerobius.* **A,** Gram staining shows large gram-positive cocci in pairs, chains, and singles on specimens from a blood agar plate. The peptostreptococci are the second most frequent anaerobic isolates from pulmonary specimens, seen in 10% to 30% of cases. These differences in reported isolation rates probably reflect taxonomic changes between published surveys, such as the transfer of most *Peptococcus* species into the genus *Peptostreptococcus. P. micros, P. magnus,* and *P. anaerobius* are the most commonly isolated *Peptostreptococcus* species. **B,** *P. anaerobius* on blood agar. Colonies are gray to white and may be translucent or opaque. Colony size is < 0.5 to 2 mm in diameter.

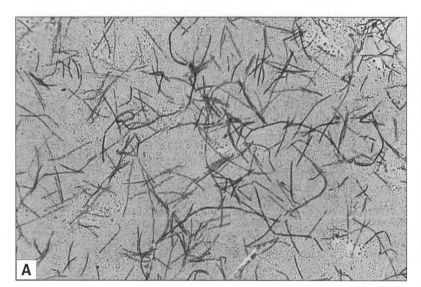

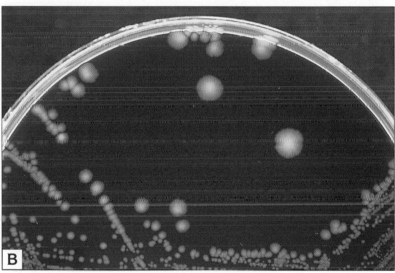

FIGURE 6-11 *Fusobacterium nucleatum.* **A,** Gram stain. The spindle-shaped cells appear as long filaments with tapered ends. This bacterium is regarded as one of the "big 3" pathogens of anaerobic pleuropulmonary infections. Fusobacteria also occur in brain abscesses, sinusitis, and various intra-abdominal infections. **B,** *F. nucleatum* colonies on blood agar. Colonies are 1 to 2 mm with so-called speckled opalescence, or internal flecking.

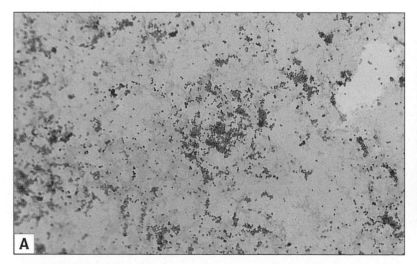

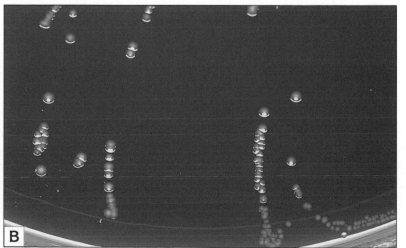

FIGURE 6-12 *Veillonella parvula.* **A,** Gram stain. Although a common isolate from saliva, *V. parvula* is thought to be a relatively infrequent pathogen. These small (< 0.5-µm-diameter) gram-negative cocci occur in masses or as diplococci. **B,** *Veillonella* colonies are blood agar. Colonies are small, convex, and translucent. They may fluoresce red under long-wave ultraviolet light.

A

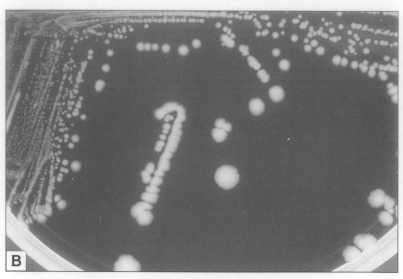

B

FIGURE 6-13 *Bacteroides fragilis*. **A**, Gram stain showing pale, pleomorphic, gram-negative bacilli with rounded ends. Although *B. fragilis*, which is generally resistant to penicillin G, has been isolated in as many as 15% of cases of lung abscesses, its pres-

ence per se in mixed infections of the lung is not believed to affect the efficacy of penicillin therapy. **B**, *B. fragilis* group colonies on blood agar are 1 to 3 mm in diameter, convex, gray to white, and glistening.

Susceptibility Testing

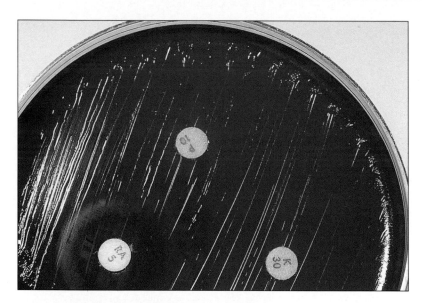

FIGURE 6-14 Antibiotic disk tests. A zone of inhibition around a 15-µg rifampin disk, but no inhibition around a 2-U penicillin disk or a 1000-µg kanamycin disk, is characteristic of the *Bacteroides fragilis* group. Although disk diffusion tests for certain antimicrobials may be useful qualitatively in identification of anaerobes, it is an unacceptable technique for susceptibility testing of anaerobes, particularly for slow-growing isolates.

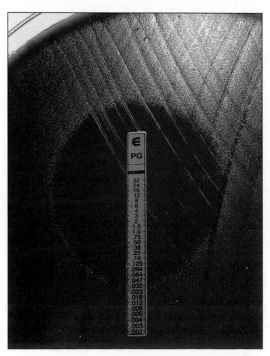

FIGURE 6-15 E-test for penicillin G susceptibility of an anaerobic isolate. Routine susceptibility testing of isolates from an individual patient is rarely indicated, given difficulties in correlating clinical success or failure of therapy with *in vitro* results. When susceptibility testing is performed in the clinical laboratory (as an alternative to the labor-intensive reference agar dilution method), sensitivities may be tested by broth microdilution or the E-test (AB-Biodisk). The E-test involves placement of a plastic strip impregnated with an antibiotic gradient on an agar plate. In the figure, a minimum inhibitory concentration of 0.032 µg/mL for penicillin G is observed. Wilkins-Chalgren agar is the medium recommended by the National Committee for Clinical Laboratory Standards (NCCLS). The broth disk elution system is no longer sanctioned by the NCCLS.

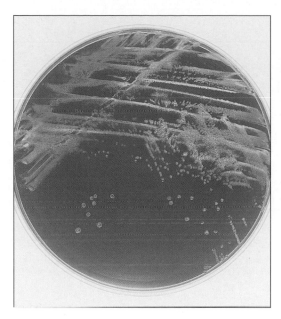

FIGURE 6-16
Esculin hydrolysis in a culture of *Bacteroides fragilis*. The blackening of media due to esculin hydrolysis is a useful characteristic in distinguishing the *B. fragilis* group from other anaerobic gram-negative bacilli.

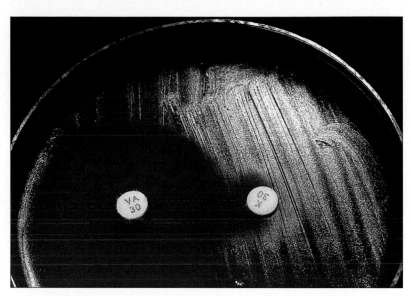

FIGURE 6-17 Kirby-Bauer testing of *Porphyromonas* to vancomycin and kanamycin. Sensitivity to vancomycin may be helpful in identifying the genus *Porphyromonas* among the pigmented anaerobic gram-negative bacilli.

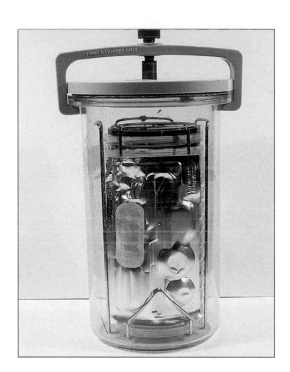

FIGURE 6-18 Gas-Pak system. Appropriate and expeditious transport of clinical specimens (in needle and syringe, where possible), plating, and incubation in an anaerobic system are essential to maximize the yield of anaerobes from empyema fluid, transtracheal or transthoracic aspirates, or protected-brush specimens. The Gas-Pak is the most commonly used anaerobic system in clinical laboratories in the United States. The catalyst of palladium-coated aluminum pellets removes oxygen from the chamber via reaction with H_2, provided by an H_2-CO_2 generator, to form water. Pellets should be replaced with each use of the jar.

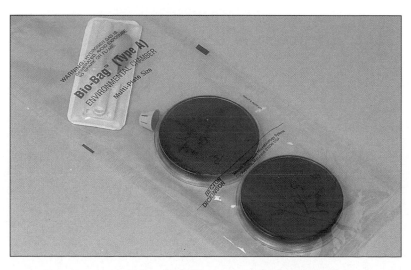

FIGURE 6-19 Bio-Bag system. The Bio-Bag is one of several anaerobic disposable bags available commercially. This system consists of a clear plastic bag, an H_2-CO_2 generator, cold palladium catalyst pellets, and a resazurin indicator. Following activation of the generator with water, the bag is heat sealed. The ability to inspect small numbers of plates for growth while maintaining anaerobic conditions is an advantage of these systems.

Pathogenesis

Predisposing conditions for pleuropulmonary anaerobic infections

Aspiration due to altered level of consciousness
  Alcohol use
  Cerebrovascular accident
  General anesthesia
  Drug overdose
  Seizure disorder
  Shock

Aspiration due to dysphagia
  Esophageal disease
  Neurologic disease
  Oral surgery
  Intestinal obstruction

Periodontal disease
Bronchiectasis
Septic embolization or bacteremia
"Postobstructive" pneumonia

FIGURE 6-20 Predisposing conditions for pleuropulmonary anaerobic infections.

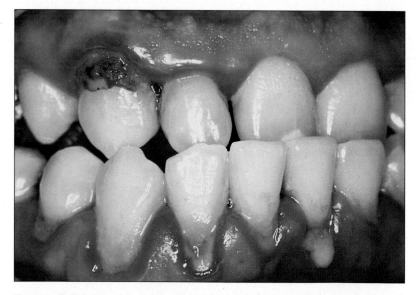

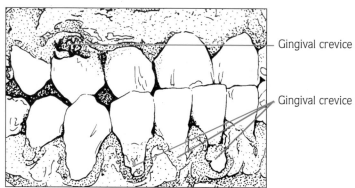

Gingival crevice

Gingival crevice

FIGURE 6-21 Severe periodontal disease. The presumed source of bacteria in anaerobic lung infections is the gingival crevice. In a patient with periodontitis, 200 mg of plaque may be present; bacteria may be found in concentrations of 10^{11} to 10^{12} bacteria per gram of plaque. This significant bacterial load is the inoculum in a patient with a predisposition to aspiration (*eg*, alcoholism, seizure disorder, general anesthesia). The presence of a lung abscess in an edentulous patient should prompt a search for an obstructing neoplasm in the lung. (*Courtesy of* G. Kazandjian, DDS.)

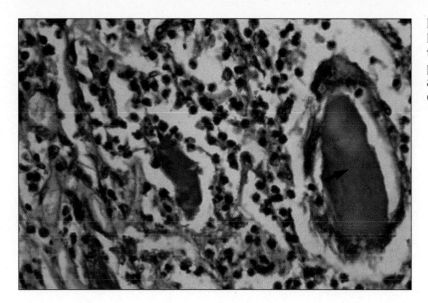

FIGURE 6-22 Histologic section showing meat fiber (*arrow*) in the lung of a patient following aspiration. Aspiration of saliva is thought to initiate anaerobic pneumonitis in most patients. However, larger particulate matter or foreign bodies may also be aspirated, providing a nidus for infection in other patients, in whom bronchial obstruction or atelectasis may also occur. (*Courtesy of* J. Jagirdar, MD.)

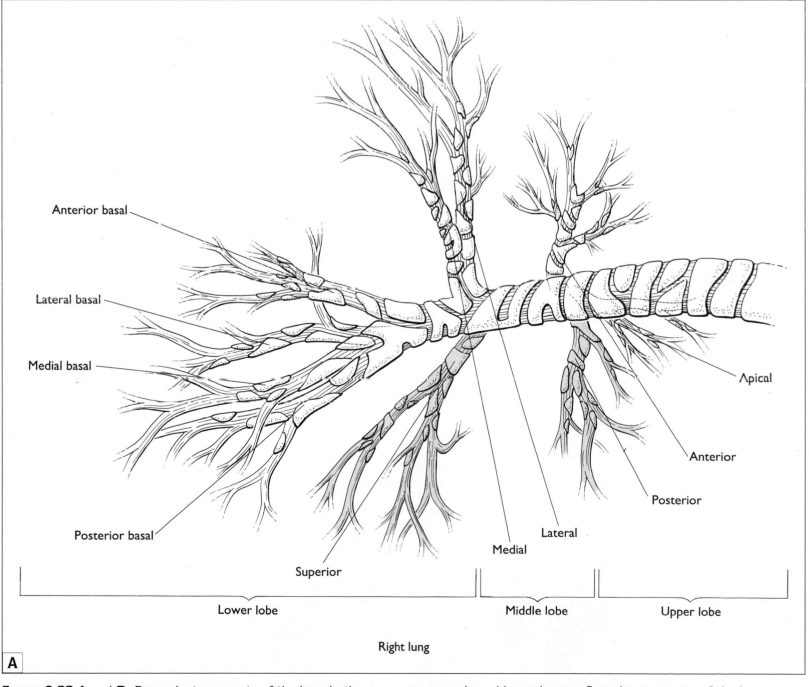

A

FIGURE 6-23 A and **B**, Dependent segments of the lung in the supine position. The posterior segment of the right upper lobe (*panel 23A*) is the most common segment involved in aspiration pneumonia and lung abscess. Superior segments of the lower lobes and posterior segments of *both* upper lobes are all frequently involved. (*continued*)

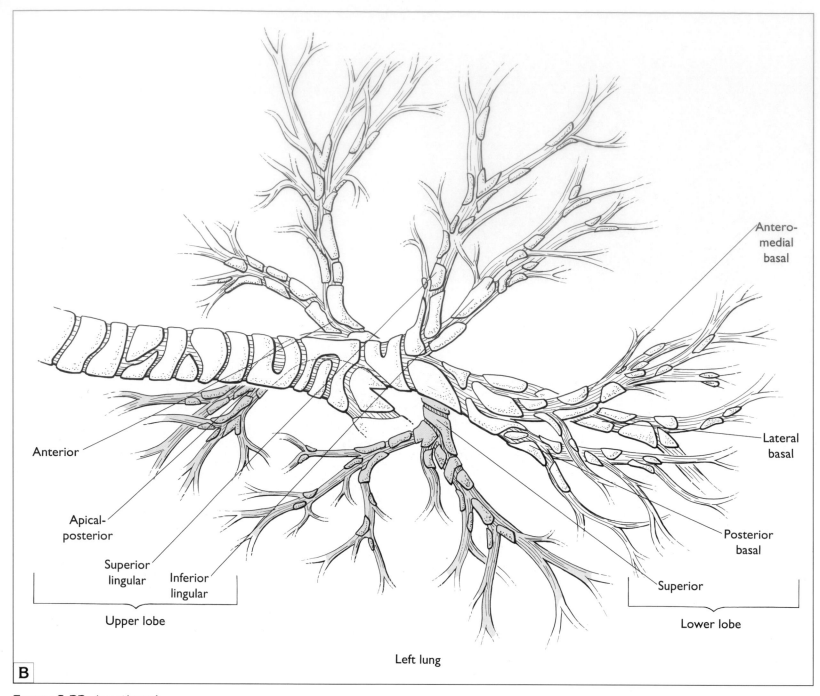

Antero-
medial
basal

Lateral
basal

Anterior

Apical-
posterior

Posterior
basal

Superior
lingular

Inferior
lingular

Superior

Upper lobe

Lower lobe

Left lung

B

FIGURE 6-23 (*continued*)

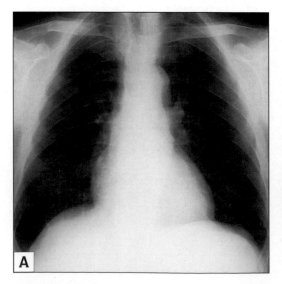

A

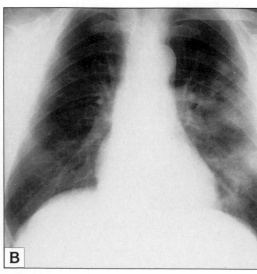

B

FIGURE 6-24 Aspiration pneumonia following esophagogastroduodenoscopy. **A**, Chest radiograph prior to the procedure. **B**, Chest radiograph taken 12 hours later shows left-sided infiltrates due to aspiration of gastric contents. These early inflammatory events are generally due to gastric acid and enzymes rather than established infection.

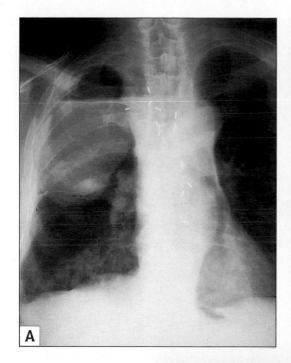

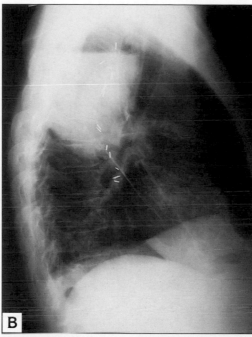

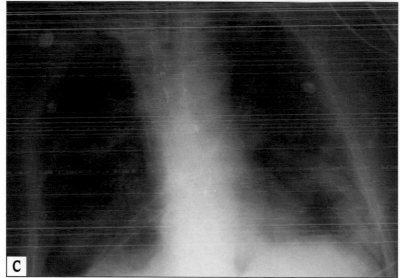

FIGURE 6-25 Drainage of lung abscess to contralateral lung with patient positioning. **A–C,** Chest radiographs of a 60-year-old man with a right-sided lung abscess show drainage of abscess contents into the contralateral lung following inadvertent placement of the patient in the left decubitus position. Although antimicrobials are the mainstay of therapy in lung abscess, *appropriate* postural drainage may expedite the safe expectoration of pus.

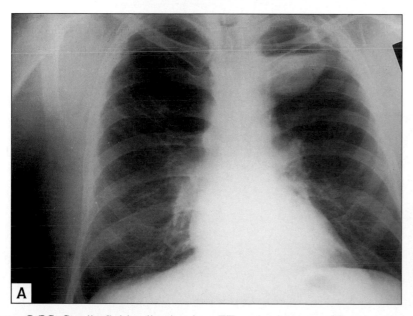

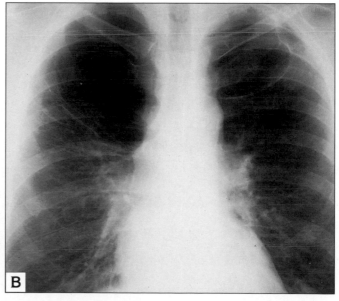

FIGURE 6-26 Sterile fluid collection in a 57-year-old man with a preexisting left upper lobe bulla. **A,** Chest radiograph revealed a fluid collection in a left upper lobe bulla. **B,** Prior chest film shows the bulla. Note the thin cyst wall and lack of surrounding pneumonitis. These collections, which may become infected with either oropharyngeal flora or community-acquired pathogens, are usually easily distinguishable from true lung abscesses by both radiographic and clinical features. Cyst walls are thinner, there may be no surrounding pneumonitis, and systemic symptoms are less common than in anaerobic lung abscess.

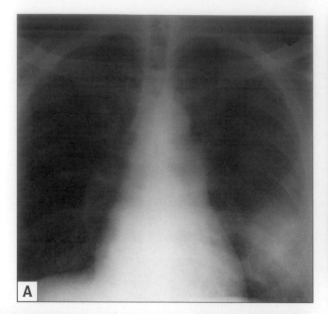

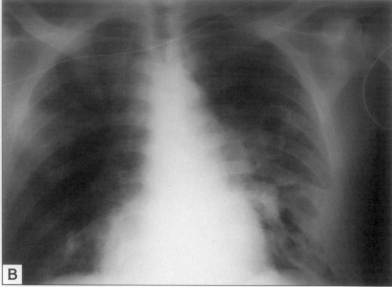

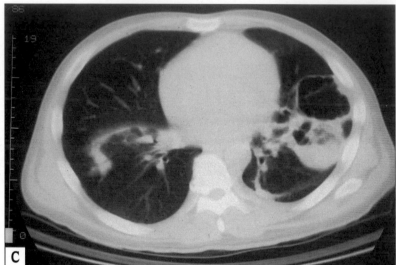

FIGURE 6-27 Femoral vein septic thrombophlebitis in a 49-year-old injecting drug user, showing evolution of multiple cavitating pulmonary lesions. **A** and **B**, Chest radiographs taken weeks apart. **C**, Chest computed tomography scan taken at the later date. *Bacteroides fragilis* and *Proteus vulgaris* were grown from blood cultures. Secondary lung abscesses may occur in various bacteremias, endocarditis, septic thrombophlebitis, subphrenic processes, and other processes. Septic emboli should be suspected when multiple cavities develop over an extended period.

Therapy

Empiric therapy for lung abscesses and aspiration pneumonia
Clindamycin *or* Cefoxitin *or* β-Lactam/β-lactamase-inhibitor combination (*ie*, ampicillin-sulbactam, ticarcillin-clavulanate, or piperacillin-tazobactam) *or* High-dose penicillin G *plus* metronidazole *or* Imipenem

FIGURE 6-28 Empiric therapy for lung abscesses and aspiration pneumonia. The use of penicillin G alone is no longer recommended, although the addition of metronidazole provides coverage for the penicillin-resistant gram-negative bacilli. Clindamycin may be ineffective against some strains of *Peptostreptococcus*, some *Bacteroides fragilis* groups, *Bacteroides gracilis*, *Fusobacterium varium*, and some non-*perfringens* clostridia. Cefoxitin is inactive against some non-*perfringens* clostridia as well, whereas the combination of β-lactam/β-lactamase inhibitors are active against essentially all clinically relevant anaerobes, as is imipenem. Should aerobic or facultative organisms warrant coverage, appropriate additional therapy may be necessary.

NOSOCOMIAL PNEUMONIAS

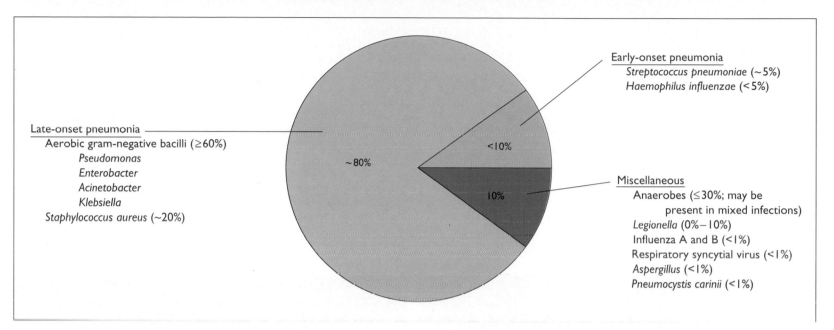

Late-onset pneumonia
  Aerobic gram-negative bacilli (≥60%)
    Pseudomonas
    Enterobacter
    Acinetobacter
    Klebsiella
  Staphylococcus aureus (~20%)

Early-onset pneumonia
  Streptococcus pneumoniae (~5%)
  Haemophilus influenzae (<5%)

Miscellaneous
  Anaerobes (≤30%; may be
    present in mixed infections)
  Legionella (0%–10%)
  Influenza A and B (<1%)
  Respiratory syncytial virus (<1%)
  Aspergillus (<1%)
  Pneumocystis carinii (<1%)

~80% <10% 10%

FIGURE 6-29 Causative organisms in nosocomial pneumonia. Nosocomial pneumonias may be divided into early-onset and late-onset disease. *Streptococcus pneumoniae*, *Haemophilus influenzae*, and *Moraxella catarrhalis* are among the early-onset pathogens, generally causing disease within 3 days of hospitalization. Late-onset disease is usually caused by aerobic gram-negative bacilli acquired in the hospital and accounts for most cases of nosocomial pneumonias, particularly in mechanically ventilated patients. Other pathogens occasionally reported include influenza A virus, *Legionella*, and *Aspergillus* [2].

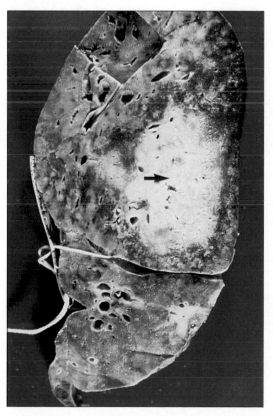

FIGURE 6-30 Autopsy specimen of lung showing necrotizing pneumonia (*arrow*) in a mechanically ventilated patient. Pneumonia causes the most deaths among the nosocomial infections. The mortality rate is estimated at 20% to 50% and is probably higher with some gram-negative isolates (such as *Pseudomonas aeruginosa*). Given the estimated rate of nosocomial pneumonia, as many as 100,000 patients may die annually in the United States from such infections.

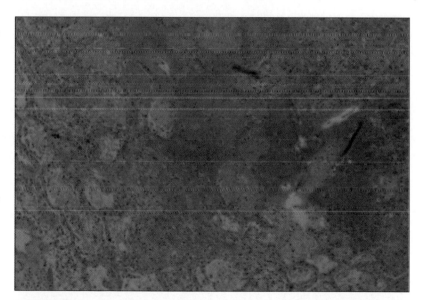

FIGURE 6-31 Histologic specimen showing bland necrosis due to *Pseudomonas aeruginosa* pneumonia. Aspiration of flora from a colonized oropharynx leads to infection. Factors favoring such colonization include exogenous sources, such as ventilators (*see* Fig. 6-35), and endogenous sources, such as the gastrointestinal tract. The loss of gastric acidity due to H_2-blocker or antacid therapy increase the rates of gastric colonization by gram-negative bacilli.

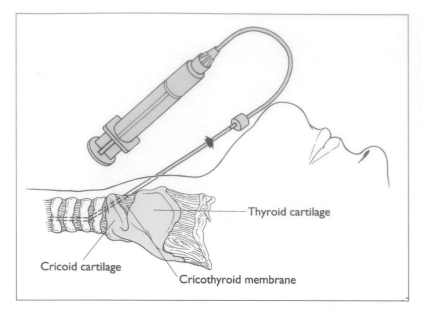

Thyroid cartilage

Cricoid cartilage

Cricothyroid membrane

FIGURE 6-32 Technique for transtracheal aspiration. Several approaches to obtaining uncontaminated sputum specimens for diagnosis of nosocomial pneumonias or for anaerobic culture have been investigated. In the early 1970s, transtracheal aspiration was extensively studied. Although adequate samples may be obtained through this method, the risks attendant to the procedure, including mediastinal emphysema, have led to its virtual abandonment in clinical practice.

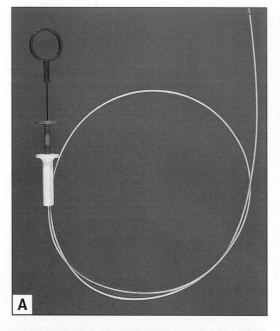

A

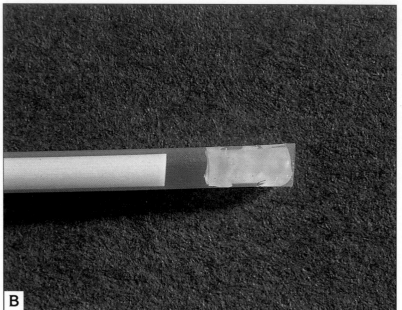

B

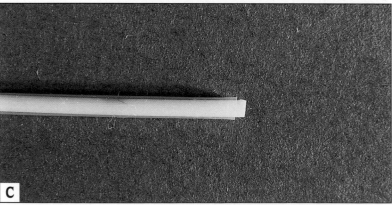

C

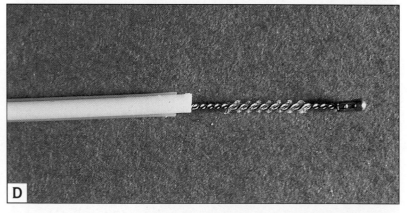

D

FIGURE 6-33 Protected-specimen brushing. The diagnosis of nosocomial pneumonia may be difficult, particularly in the intubated patient. Despite the promulgation of defined clinical, microbiologic, and radiographic criteria for epidemiologic surveys and therapeutic trials, correlation of clinical diagnosis and pathologic confirmation has been poor. Protected-specimen brushings with quantitative bacterial cultures have shown promising results in diagnosis, with both good sensitivity and specificity, especially in the seriously ill patient. **A**, The assembly of the protected-specimen brush (Microvasive, Boston Scientific, Watertown, MA) is advanced through the bronchoscope. **B**, A wax plug protects the brush tip from contamination. **C**, The plug is expelled near the target area. **D**, The brush is advanced to collect samples and is then retracted. Bronchoalveolar lavage, either with quantitative culture or observation of lavage cells with intracellular organisms, is another technique being actively investigated.

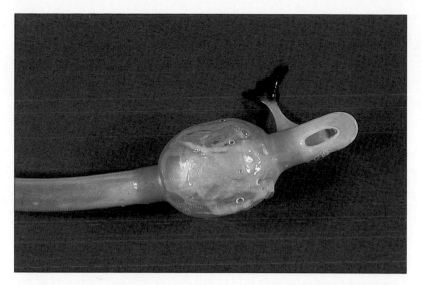

FIGURE 6-34 Endotracheal tube following extubation of a patient after 5 days of ventilatory support. Leakage of bacteria in secretions around the cuff of endotracheal tubes is believed to play a major role in nosocomial pneumonias in intubated patients, who have pneumonia rates 10 to 20 times those in other hospitalized patients. Nosocomial pneumonia more than doubles the case-fatality rate in mechanically ventilated patients and contributes significantly to the duration of hospitalization and intubation.

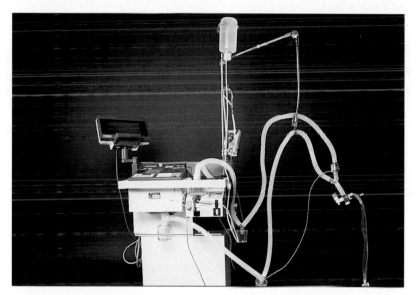

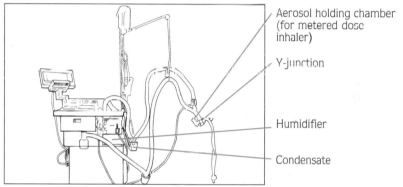

Aerosol holding chamber (for metered dose inhaler)

Y-junction

Humidifier

Condensate

FIGURE 6-35 Ventilator showing potential sources of bacterial contamination. Nebulization equipment has been implicated as a source of contamination, with small nebulized particles being able to reach terminal bronchioles and alveoli. Disinfection of nebulizers has been dramatically effective in reducing pneumonia rates. Humidifying cascades, which lead to condensate formation in the ventilator circuit, as well as in-line medication nebulizers may also pose risks. Devices apart from the ventilator, such as nasogastric tubes that may increase reflux and colonization of the oropharynx, may increase the incidence of nosocomial pneumonia. Enteral feedings may exacerbate that risk

Predisposing factors for nosocomial pneumonia

Mechanical ventilation with endotracheal intubation
Severe underlying disease
Postsurgical status
Advanced age

FIGURE 6-36 Predisposing factors for nosocomial pneumonia. Although other factors, such as chronic lung disease and antimicrobial use, have also been implicated as risks for the development of nosocomial pneumonia, the association of these factors with intubation and severity of disease makes assessment of their independent significance difficult.

REFERENCES

1. Finegold SM: Lung abscess. *In* Mandell GL, Bennett JE, Dolin R (eds.): *Principles and Practice of Infectious Diseases*, 4th ed. New York: Churchill Livingstone; 1995:643.

2. Horan T, Culver D, Jarvis W, *et al.*: Pathogens causing nosocomial infections. *Antimicrobic Newslett* 1988, 5:65–67.

SELECTED BIBLIOGRAPHY

Bartlett JG: Anaerobic bacterial infections of the lung and pleural space. *Clin Infect Dis* 1993, 16(suppl 4):S248–S255.

Bartlett JG, Finegold SM: Anaerobic infections of the lung and pleural space. *Am Rev Respir Dis* 1974, 110:56–77.

Craven DE, Steger KA, Duncan RA: Prevention and control of nosocomial pneumonia. *In* Wenzel RP (ed.): *Prevention and Control of Nosocomial Infections*. Baltimore: Williams & Wilkins; 1993:580–589.

Finegold SM, Jousimies-Somer HR, Wexler HM: Current perspectives on anaerobic infections: Diagnostic approaches. *Infect Dis Clin North Am* 1993, 7:257–275.

Scheld WM, Mandell GL: Nosocomial pneumonia: Pathogenesis and recent advances in diagnosis and therapy. *Rev Infect Dis* 1991, 13(suppl 9):S743–S751.

CHAPTER 7

Viral Pneumonias

Robert F. Betts
Ann R. Falsey
Caroline B. Hall
John J. Treanor

EPIDEMIOLOGY

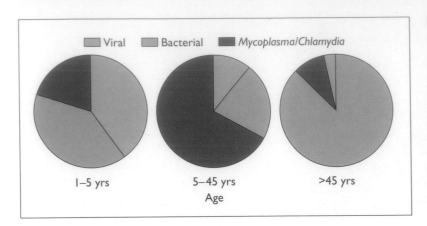

FIGURE 7-1 Prevalence of viral pneumonia by age group. Viral pneumonia is predominantly a disease of children, especially those < 5 years of age, and is very uncommon in adults in its pure form. What is often called viral pneumonia in adults is probably *Mycoplasma* or *Chlamydia* pneumonia. Both respiratory syncytial virus (RSV) and influenza can be isolated from elderly patients with segmental or lobar pneumonia on radiograph, but these patients have a nearly identical clinical course and respond in a similar fashion to antibiotics as do adults with segmental/lobar pneumonia occurring outside the influenza/RSV season. These charts show the relative proportion of different pneumonias that are of proven cause in patients according to age group. Community-derived *Legionella* pneumonia is included in the category of bacterial pneumonia in these charts, whereas nosocomial pneumonia is not.

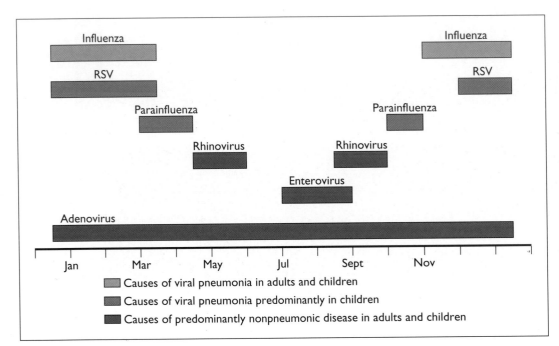

FIGURE 7-2 Seasonal variation in respiratory virus infections. Viral pneumonia is caused by relatively few virus types. Not included in this graph are the viruses that cause primarily rashes (*eg*, measles and varicella) and are occasionally complicated by pneumonia, especially in adults. Each of the viruses has its own season, and outside that season, these viruses are seldom isolated. A concentration of cases of viral pneumonia occurs in the winter, with fewer cases in the spring and fall. Although viral pneumonia in adults is uncommon, it is an important clinical problem, and the clinical course can be severe. During the viral season, when a patient presents severely ill with acute pneumonia that is "atypical" (because no bacterial cause can be identified), the physician often concludes that it must be due to *Legionella pneumophila*. However, cultures of respiratory secretions for virus often will yield virus, usually influenza A or B virus. Although influenza causes pneumonia in children, most cases occur in very young infants. Respiratory syncytial virus (RSV) is more common than influenza and also affects a greater age range. Parainfluenza is also an important pathogen, especially in the immunocompromised child. In the summer, the only virus that causes pulmonary infiltration is the hantavirus (not shown). In contrast to the winter, many of the "atypical" cases of pneumonia in the summer are caused by *Legionella*. In truth, *Legionella* pneumonia really resembles typical pneumonia, except that a bacterial pathogen is not readily identified.

INFLUENZA PNEUMONIA

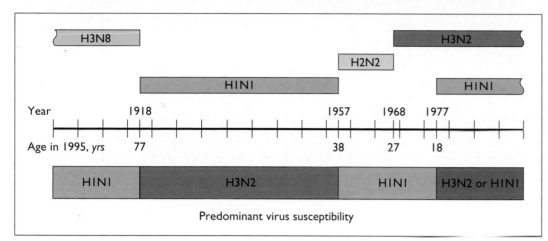

FIGURE 7-3 Age and susceptibility to influenza A virus subtypes. One incompletely understood aspect of influenza A infection is the "doctrine of original antigenic sin." This doctrine states that individuals develop prolonged immunity to the virus hemagglutinin (H) and neuraminidase (N) type that produces their first infection but not to the virus type that produces subsequent infections. Because almost everyone is infected in the first year or two of life, one can predict from the person's age which virus type will likely produce infection when he or she is older. Age provides the reference point to determine which virus was circulating when the person was an infant. As shown in this figure, in 1995, all persons over age 38 years, were originally infected with H1N1, which circulated between the early 1900s and 1957. Since 1977, when H1N1 reappeared on the scene, influenza H1N1 has rarely been isolated as a cause of infection from this age group. Persons between ages 18 and 37 (born between 1958 and 1977) form the age group whose first infection was with H2N2 or H3N2, and they were the ones afflicted by the epidemics of H1N1 beginning in 1977. Using similar logic, one can understand why between 1986 and 1990, on college campuses attended by 18- to 22-year-olds (born after 1968, the year of reappearance of H3N2), H3N2 outbreaks did not occur. In those persons born after 1977, it is very difficult to predict which will be the infective subtype because between 1977 and 1991, H1N1 circulated in some years, H3N2 in some years, and both in some years. The *bars* in the top part of this graph indicate the predominant circulating virus subtypes for periods since since 1900, the *bottom bar* then indicates the virus subtype to which persons born in those years remain susceptible.

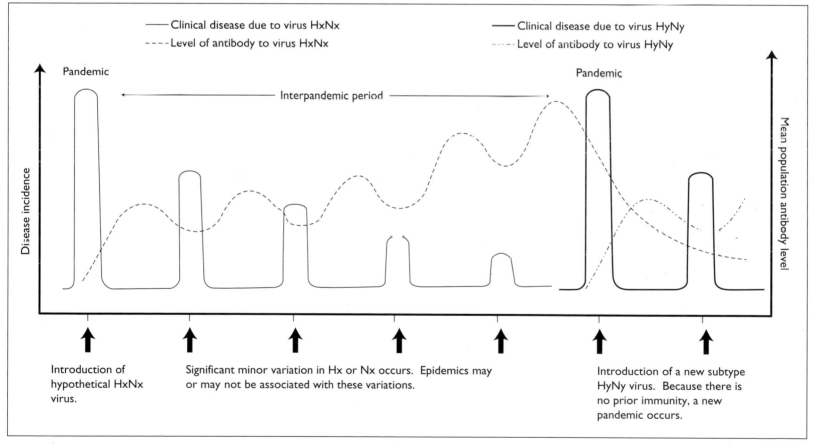

FIGURE 7-4 Occurrence of influenza pandemics and epidemics in relation to population antibody levels. A hypothetical virus bearing a novel hemagglutinin subtype (Hx) and neuraminidase subtype (Nx) is introduced into a population with little or no prior immunity. Worldwide severe illness occurs, referred to as a *pandemic*. As the population recovers from the pandemic, the level of immunity to Hx and Nx increases, so that the next year's epidemic is less severe. Over the next several seasons, antigenic variants are selected that generally differ from the preceding year's by a few amino acid changes in Hx or Nx and that cause epidemics of greater or lesser severity depending on the degree of antigenic change. This process generally is referred to as *antigenic drift*. At some unpredictable point in the future, a virus with an entirely new subtype of hemagglutinin (Hy) and/or neuraminidase (Ny) is introduced (*right*), and the pattern is repeated. The introduction of a new subtype is referred to as *antigenic shift*. Recent examples of antigenic shift include the introduction of H2N2 virus in 1957 and H3N2 virus in 1968. (*Modified from* Betts [1].)

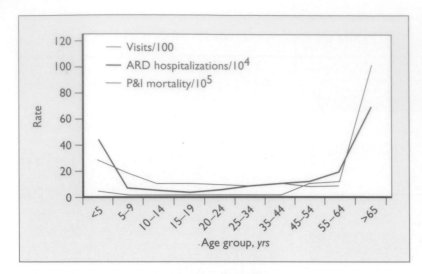

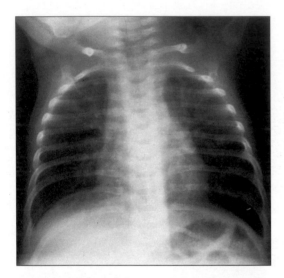

FIGURE 7-5 Age-specific attack rates, hospitalization rates, and mortality among patients with medically attended influenza. Studies conducted in Houston, Texas, indicate that the highest influenza attack rate and rate of hospitalizations occur at the extremes of life, but mortality occurs largely in those after age 65 years and rises with each year of age. Most deaths in older patients are due to either secondary bacterial pneumonia or cardiac complications. In other populations, experience on college campuses indicates that influenza causes outbreaks that afflict 25% of the population and force cancellation of classes or sports events; however, this age group does not come to the attention of the practicing physician and so is missed or undercounted when surveying only "medically attended" cases. Depending on the circulating virus in a given year (*see* Fig. 7-3), younger adults and middle-aged individuals can be included in the group developing influenza. (ARD—acute respiratory disease; P&I—pneumonia and influenza.) (*Adapted from* Glezen [2].)

FIGURE 7-6 Chest radiograph of bilateral interstitial pneumonia due to influenza A. This radiograph, from a 4-month-old infant, shows bilateral interstitial pneumonia, mainly in the upper lobes, which proved to be due to influenza A. Note the hyperaeration, which is presumably secondary to bronchial constriction provoked by virus infection, that accompanies the process. Because of the similarity to pneumonia caused by respiratory syncytial virus (RSV), the clinicians in this case had made that diagnosis until the culture results returned. Influenza A more commonly occurs in this very young population, which is a clue, but RSV also occurs at this age. Because influenza is transmitted by aerosols, bilateral distribution of infiltrates is characteristic. This contrasts to bacterial pneumonia or *Chlamydia/Mycoplasma* pneumonia, in which segmental localization is characteristic.

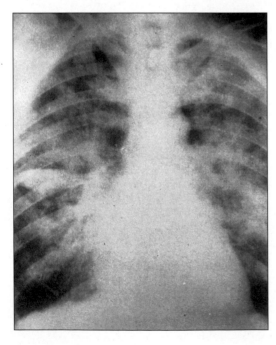

FIGURE 7-7 Admission chest radiograph of a 49-year-old man with primary influenza pneumonia superimposed on rheumatic heart disease with mitral stenosis and insufficiency. The density in the right midlung field represents a loculated interlobar effusion that was present prior to the acute illness. Diffuse interstitial infiltrates are seen bilaterally. This disease is typically associated with significant hypoxemia. (*From* Louria *et al.* [3]; with permission.)

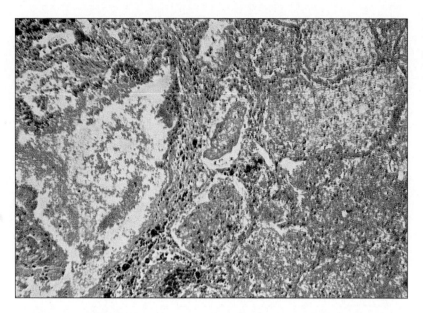

FIGURE 7-8 Hematoxylin-eosin–stained section of lung tissue from a fatal case of primary influenza pneumonia. The section shows ulceration of small bronchus in the right lower lobe. Note that adjacent alveoli are filled with erythrocytes mixed with fibrin. Neutrophilic leukocytes are present, but in small numbers. (*From* Louria *et al.* [3]; with permission.)

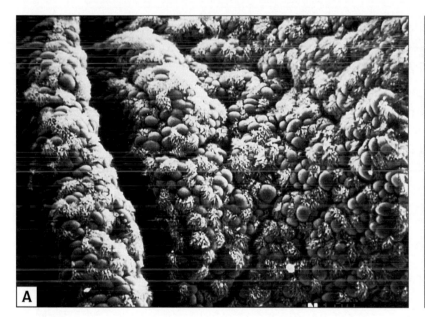

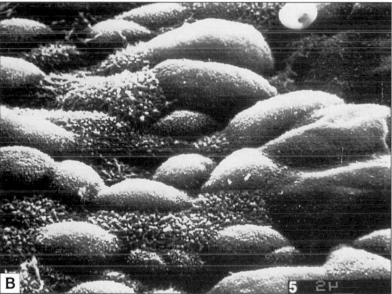

FIGURE 7-9 Scanning electron micrograph of mouse tracheal epithelium showing pathogenic changes induced by influenza. The mechanism by which influenza, and possibly other viruses, may predispose to bacterial superinfection can be visualized in this figure. **A**, Normal mouse trachea, seen by scanning electron microscopy, shows normal tracheal epithelial cells and cilia.

B, In mouse trachea seen 5 days after influenza virus infection, the epithelial cells have largely been sloughed, revealing the basement membrane. This wholesale destruction inactivates the normal ciliary clearing mechanisms and facilitates the adherence and invasion of bacteria, which can lead to bacterial pneumonia. (*From* Kilbourne [4]; with permission.)

A. Classic patterns of lower respiratory tract illness associated with influenza: Typical influenza with transient pulmonary signs	**B. Classic patterns of lower respiratory tract illness associated with influenza: Primary influenza virus pneumonia**
Symptoms: cough, pleuritic chest pain, dyspnea Physical findings: rales and wheezes Clinically diagnosed as bronchiolitis Complete recovery	All patients had underlying heart disease (predominantly mitral stenosis) Presentation with rapidly increasing severe dyspnea Productive cough, diffuse infiltrates Almost all died (mechanical ventilation was not available)

FIGURE 7-10 Four classic patterns of lower respiratory tract illness associated with influenza. These four patterns were first described during the H2N2 (Asian flu) pandemic of 1957. In practice, most patients with significant influenza causing lower respiratory tract disease present with mixtures of these syndromes [3]. **A**, Typical influenza with transient pulmonary signs. **B**, Primary influenza virus pneumonia. (*continued*)

C. Classic patterns of lower respiratory tract illness associated with influenza: Influenza followed by secondary bacterial pneumonia

One half of patients had preexisting diseases
Typical signs and symptoms of influenza, followed
  2–14 days later by recurrence of symptoms
Clinical course typical of community-acquired bacterial
  pneumonia
Streptococcus pneumoniae, Staphylococcus aureus, and
  Haemophilus influenzae commonly isolated

D. Classic patterns of lower respiratory tract illness associated with influenza: Concomitant viral and bacterial pneumonia

Most patients had underlying heart disease
Presented with typical influenza with gradual onset of lower
  respiratory tract symptoms
Streptococcus pneumoniae, Staphylococcus aureus, and mixed
  infections common
Mortality of ~ 33%, significantly higher than with secondary
  bacterial pneumonia

FIGURE 7-10 (*continued*) **C,** Influenza followed by secondary bacterial pneumonia.
D, Concomitant viral and bacterial pneumonia.

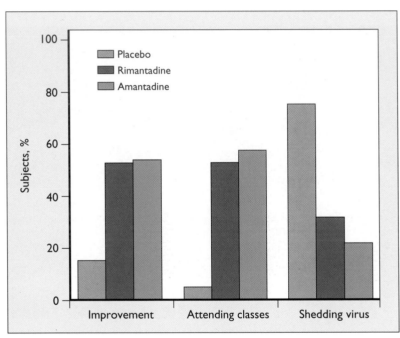

FIGURE 7-11 Treatment of H1N1 influenza with rimantadine versus amantadine in young adults. The first clinical evidence of effective antiviral treatment occurred in the treatment of influenza syndrome. Although outwardly the effect seems small, producing only a modest benefit in duration of fever and improvement in overall feeling of well-being, other evidence in fact suggests there is a greater impact. In a trial comparing rimantadine, amantadine, and placebo, the antiviral recipients not only improved more quickly than did placebo recipients, but also they returned to class more quickly following a bout of culture-proven influenza. Resuming classes (or work) has important economic ramifications, and because the individuals are clinically better, their performance may add to the difference. In addition, improvement was correlated with an antiviral effect. Conceivably, the shorter duration of viral shedding in the antiviral recipients could reduce transmission to susceptible persons, adding a second layer of benefit. (*Adapted from* Van Voris *et al.* [5].)

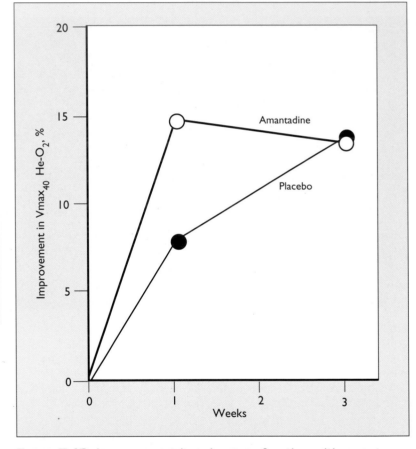

FIGURE 7-12 Improvement in pulmonary function with amantadine treatment of influenza. Small airways dysfunction shows improvement over time in patients with culture-proven H3N2 who received amantadine versus placebo. At 1 week, placebo recipients still have the abnormal test results that were present at the onset of disease, whereas in amantadine recipients, test results have returned to normal. These pulmonary function abnormalities at 1 week postinfection were detectable in individuals who were in the recovery phase of their illness. Perhaps the persistence of these abnormalities in the untreated individual may provide the groundwork for establishment of the late bacterial complications of influenza that are so characteristic, especially in the elderly. Although studies do not exist to prove that antiviral treatment for influenza prevents bacterial complications, this avenue for study is reasonable. (*Adapted from* Little *et al.* [6].)

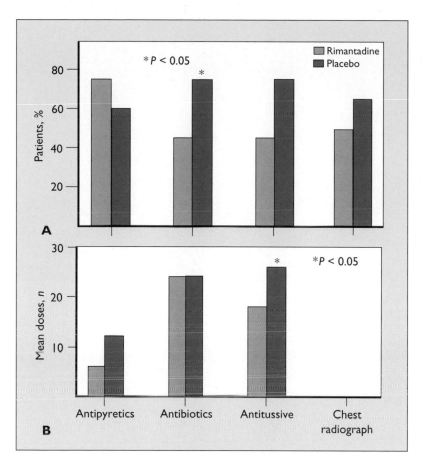

A

B

FIGURE 7-13 Clinical improvement of elderly patients with influenza A after rimantadine treatment. In a treatment trial of patients > 84 years of age with proven influenza A, rimantadine recipients defervesced faster and felt better sooner than placebo recipients. This figure depicts other measures that their blinded physicians took to provide these patients comfort or to evaluate their clinical course. **A,** This graph shows the percentage of patients in each group receiving additional medications. Antipyretics and antitussives were given at the onset of the illness, whereas chest radiographs were ordered and antibiotics administered when the patients did not seem to be responding. **B,** This graph illustrates the mean number of doses of additional medications administered, showing the more rapid improvement in patients receiving rimantadine.

RESPIRATORY SYNCYTIAL VIRUS PNEUMONIA

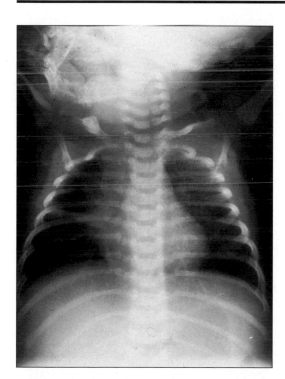

FIGURE 7-14 Right middle lobe consolidation seen in a chest radiograph of a 3-month-old infant with respiratory syncytial virus (RSV) pneumonia. One of the characteristic features of RSV pneumonia is right middle lobe consolidation. A left upper lobe process is also present. RSV produces striking bronchiolitis, which leads to air trapping and, as shown here, hyperinflation of the lungs on chest film. Wheezing is very characteristic of RSV infection at any age, and in the young infant, this manifests as bronchiolitis. In the asthmatic patient, exacerbation of asthma in the winter can often be ascribed to RSV reinfection. In the elderly, wheezing that has not previously been documented is a marker of RSV infection (*see* Fig. 7-20). Wheezing may be due in part to an IgE response to viral infection, and IgE plus antigen leads to histamine release.

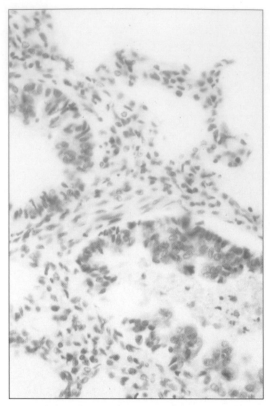

FIGURE 7-15 Histopathologic specimen obtained from the lung of a baby dying of sudden infant death syndrome. Note the bronchiole secretions and the marked interstitial inflammation and thickening that accompany this picture. The histologic picture certainly explains the observed bronchiolitis that is seen clinically. With the air trapping produced by the inflammation of the bronchiole, carbon dioxide is retained, which may, in part, lead to the process resulting in sudden death.

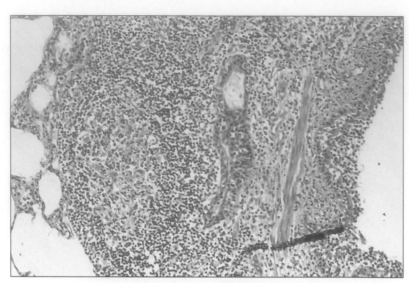

FIGURE 7-16 Histopathologic specimen from the lung of a baby dying of respiratory syncytial virus (RSV) pneumonia. Note the intense lymphocytic infiltration surrounding a disrupted bronchiole. This slide vividly demonstrates why the clinical presentation includes the wheezing and air trapping characteristic of this disease. Similar wheezing occurs in the elderly, and one of the most important causes of wintertime exacerbation of asthma is infection with RSV.

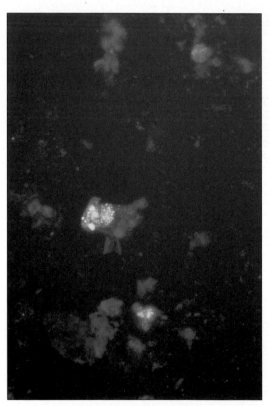

FIGURE 7-17 Rapid viral detection by respiratory syncytial virus (RSV) immunofluorescent assay (IFA). One important factor in RSV infection is that in babies, it is rarely accompanied by bacterial superinfection. Hence, rapid diagnosis is an important management aid. This slide shows immunofluorescing cells from a nasal specimen stained by anti-RSV antibody and then with anti-IgG tagged with an immunofluorescent label. In babies, a positive result in this test is as sensitive for infection as is culture. In adults, the IFA test is not nearly as sensitive as it is in infants, probably because of the differences in quantity of virus shed in the nasal secretions. In babies, the amount of virus per milliliter approaches 5 logs, but it is probably no more than 3 logs in adults. However, a positive result in both infants and adults is quite specific. If the clinician wishes to consider antiviral treatment with ribavirin, a positive result, which is available the same day, helps guide therapy, and it also allows the discontinuation of antibiotics that may have been initiated empirically. Most diagnostic laboratories have substituted the enzyme-linked immunosorbent assay test for IFA, but the sensitivity and specificity are similar to those of IFA.

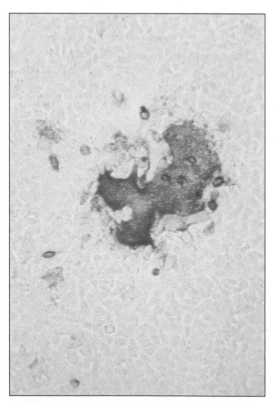

FIGURE 7-18 Cytopathic effect of respiratory syncytial virus (RSV) in HEp-2 tissue culture. Syncytium formation is clearly demonstrated. This finding leads to the unequivocal diagnosis of RSV infection. Staining is by immunoperoxidase method.

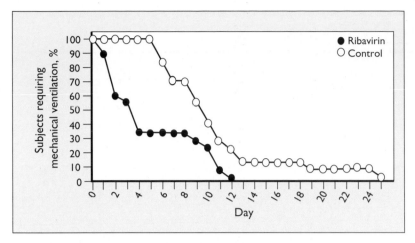

FIGURE 7-19 Rate of improvement in infants with proven respiratory syncytial virus infection given ribavirin treatment who required mechanical ventilation. Patients randomly received either inhaled ribavirin or a similar-appearing inactive substance. As indicated, 50% of ribavirin recipients no longer required mechanical ventilation after day 4, whereas placebo recipients did not obtain reduced level of ventilator use until day 8. Furthermore, 20% of placebo recipients still required ventilation on day 11, by which time all ribavirin recipients were breathing on their own.

Frequency of clinical findings in influenza vs RSV

	Influenza	RSV
Fever > 39.4° C	+++[†]	+
Myalgia	++++	++
Rhinorrhea	+	++++
Sore throat	+++	+
Asthma*	+++	++++
New wheezing	+	++++
COPD*	++++	++++
Diarrhea	–	–

*Exacerbation of these conditions.

[†]The frequency of occurrence and/or degree of severity is indicated, ranging from none (-) to uncommon/mild (+) to very frequent/severe (++++).

COPD—chronic obstructive pulmonary disease; RSV—respiratory syncytial virus.

FIGURE 7-20 Comparative frequencies of symptoms in elderly patients with proven influenza or respiratory syncytial virus (RSV) infection. Although both influenza and RSV infection can exacerbate asthma or chronic obstructive pulmonary disease, noticeable differences are apparent in the degree of fever (> 103° F), severity of nasal discharge, complaint of sore throat and precipitation of wheezing in an individual who had not previously wheezed. This clinical differentiation between influenza and RSV infection is important in at least two ways. First, in a long-term health care facility, where nearly 100% of the residents have been vaccinated against influenza, it tells physicians that RSV may be causing the outbreak and not be discouraged about their vaccine program. Second, it may forestall the use of an antiviral directed against influenza if the clinical presentation is more characteristic of RSV.

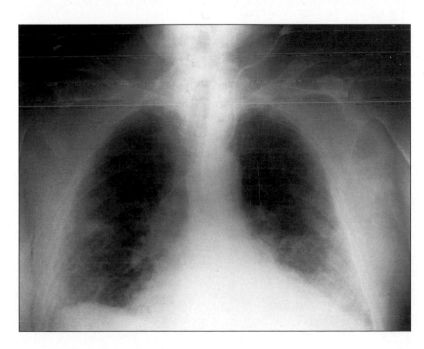

FIGURE 7-21 Chest radiograph showing respiratory syncytial virus (RSV) pneumonia in an elderly man. This elderly man presented with symptoms and chest findings consistent with congestive heart failure (CHF), but he was febrile. He was given standard therapy for CHF, but he failed to clear his lung fields and remained febrile. When RSV was isolated from a tracheal suction specimen, he was placed on inhaled ribavirin and improved promptly. Conclusions about the role of antiviral therapy in this setting are uncertain; however, in infants with congenital heart disease and unrelenting RSV infection, ribavirin appears to lead to improvement.

PARAINFLUENZA PNEUMONIA

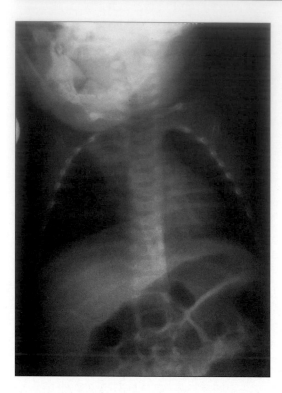

FIGURE 7-22 Chest radiograph showing upper lobe infiltrate in parainfluenza pneumonia. Parainfluenza virus infection of infants can mimic influenza or respiratory syncytial virus (RSV) infection. Most infants with parainfluenza infection present with upper respiratory disease, especially croup, but a small proportion have lower respiratory manifestations. In this infant, the right upper lobe infiltrate is partially obscured by the involuting thymus. The infant was hypoxic and febrile with a clinical picture of pneumonia. The patient presented outside the influenza/RSV season and thus was suspected of having infection with a virus other than influenza or RSV, which proved to be the case.

HANTAVIRUS PULMONARY SYNDROME

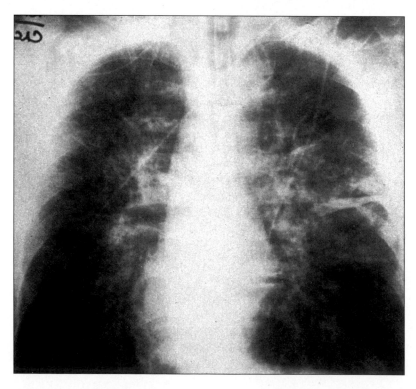

FIGURE 7-23 Chest radiograph of severe hantavirus pulmonary syndrome. Patients presenting with acute hantavirus pulmonary syndrome often are short of breath yet have a clear chest. Over the next several hours, they evolve rapidly, becoming hypoxic secondary to findings shown in this chest film. (*Courtesy of* G.J. Mertz, MD.)

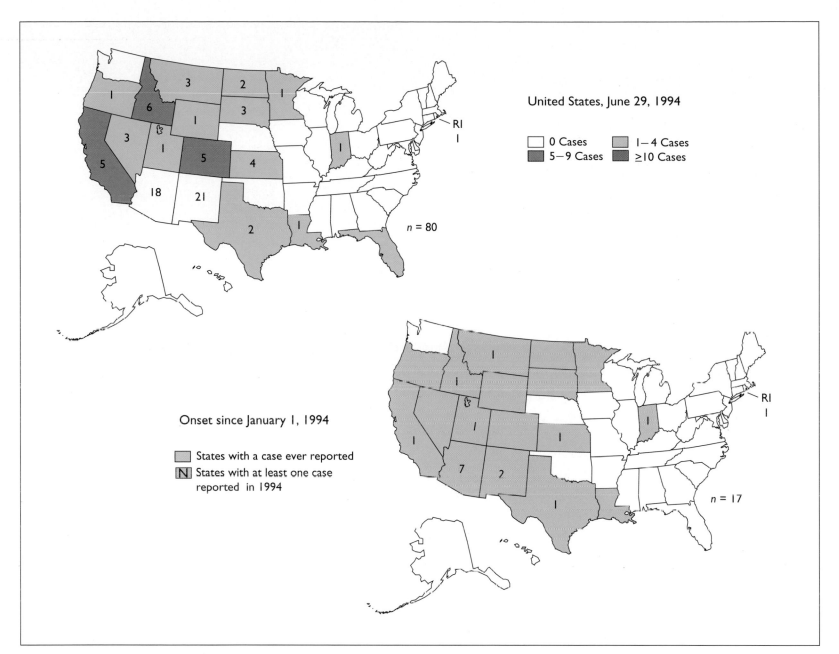

FIGURE 7-24 Reported cases of hantavirus pulmonary syndrome in the United States in 1994. The number of reported cases of hantavirus pulmonary syndrome has increased since the availability of serologic testing. Although the cases were originally assumed to be localized to the Four Corners area of the southwestern United States, further investigation has shown that cases have been documented in every region of the country. Because the disease is so rapidly fatal, the documented cases may represent the tip of the iceberg. If techniques directed at identifying the agent in secretions become widely available, a truer picture of the frequency of this infection will emerge. (*Courtesy of* the Centers for Disease Control and Prevention.)

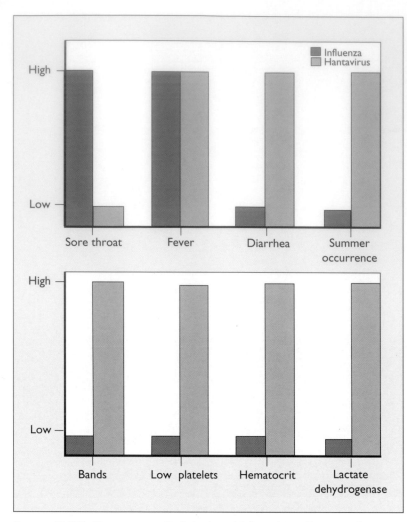

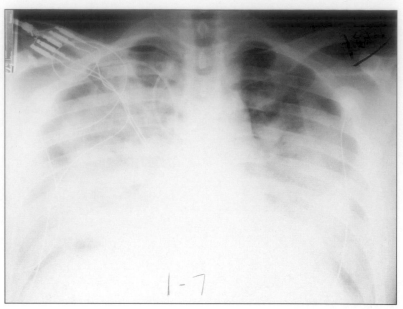

FIGURE 7-26 Chest radiograph showing pulmonary hemorrhage and edema in Korean hemorrhagic fever. Among the hantaviruses, there are different frequencies and different mechanisms of pulmonary abnormalities. Hantaan virus (which causes Korean hemorrhagic fever) produces a hemorrhagic syndrome with renal failure. As shown in this chest film, pulmonary manifestations, which are quite uncommon in Korean disease, are caused by fluid overload due to renal failure or to pulmonary hemorrhage. Pulmonary findings are even less common in the other Hantaan virus illnesses such as Puumala (occurs in Scandinavia and Europe), Seoul (worldwide), and other recognized milder forms of hantavirus-induced hemorrhagic fever/renal syndrome. By contrast, Sin Nombre virus, the cause of hantavirus pulmonary syndrome in the United States, virtually always causes a pulmonary syndrome that is inflammatory in type. Sin Nombre does not directly produce renal failure, and in it, renal dysfunction is a consequence of the severity of the systemic illness. However, the mode of spread of hantaviruses is similar for all, regardless of the syndrome that ensues, and is through rodents, but different rodents are responsible for spread of the respective viruses. For all, diagnosis is confirmed through serologic analysis. (*Courtesy of* E.D. Everett, MD.)

FIGURE 7-25 Frequency of clinical and laboratory features in influenza versus hantavirus pulmonary syndrome. Two viral infections, by hantavirus and influenza A virus, can cause very aggressive pulmonary disease. Aside from cough, fever, and dyspnea, which are features of both, there are distinct epidemiologic, clinical, and laboratory features that differentiate the two. The seasonal difference is the most striking feature. However, although influenza is rarely seen in the summer months, if and when another pandemic were to evolve, summer outbreaks of influenza might occur. Other findings are distinct as well. Diarrhea is very uncommon in influenza, and sore throat is not seen in hantavirus infection. To date, most documented cases of hantavirus infection have occurred in the Four Corners region of the US Southwest. With the availability of serologic testing, cases outside that area are being recognized.

VARICELLA PNEUMONIA

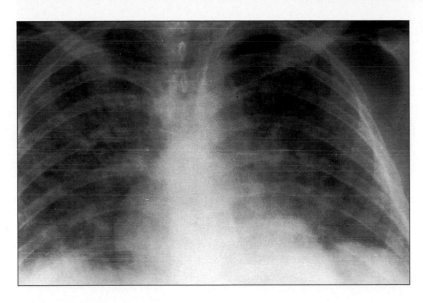

FIGURE 7-27 Typical diffuse reticulonodular infiltrates of varicella pneumonia in a pregnant woman. Varicella may be more severe in pregnancy. Early treatment with acyclovir has been shown to reduce fever and tachypnea in otherwise healthy adults with varicella pneumonia. (*From* Haake *et al.* [7]; with permission.)

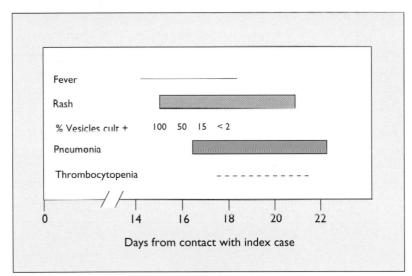

FIGURE 7-28 Clinical course of varicella pneumonia. Varicella pneumonia is a complication of primary varicella infection occurring in adults. Pregnancy or smoking seems to predispose. Dyspnea develops 48 hours after the onset of the rash, and radiographic changes are recognizable a day later. Self-limited thrombocytopenia usually accompanies the pneumonia. Although vesicles properly cultured at the onset of the rash almost invariably yield virus, vesicles cultured at the time pneumonitis is recognized will yield virus less frequently. Antiviral treatment in varicella pneumonia is of unproven value but is usually administered. The death rate in varicella pneumonia requiring hospitalization approximates 10%. Intravenous acyclovir is relatively safe, especially if the recipient is kept well hydrated. The significant death rate and safety of the drug are what dictate antiviral use. Hopefully, the recent availability of varicella vaccine will reduce the number of adults who remain susceptible to primary infection and thus reduce the incidence of varicella pneumonia. Women contemplating pregnancy who are susceptible are ideal candidates for the vaccine.

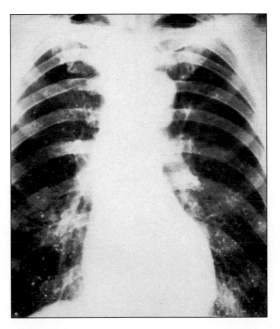

FIGURE 7-29 Chest radiograph showing diffuse pulmonary calcifications attributed to varicella. This chest film was taken 10 years after documented varicella pneumonia in a patient who was followed with serial radiographs after recovery. The calcified lesions are not associated with diminished pulmonary function. (*From* Knyvett [8]; with permission.)

VIRAL PNEUMONIA AND BONE MARROW TRANSPLANTATION

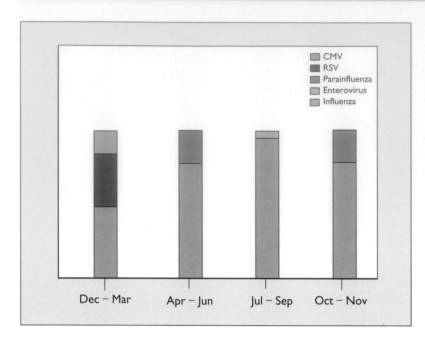

FIGURE 7-30 Etiology and seasonal occurrence of viral pneumonia in bone marrow transplant recipients. Patients undergoing chemotherapy are at great risk for viral pneumonia, but nowhere is the risk greater than in allogenic bone marrow transplant recipients. Because of complex pathophysiologic reasons, cytomegalovirus (CMV) is common in bone marrow recipients. However, respiratory syncytial virus (RSV), influenza, and parainfluenza also cause significant problems in these patients. Like viral pneumonia in normal children, these infections are very seasonal in their occurrence. Thus, CMV is virtually the only cause of viral pneumonia in the bone marrow unit in the summer, but it shares this role with the respiratory viruses in late fall to early spring. The transplant physician should consider a respiratory virus as a cause of pneumonia occurring in the appropriate season for two reasons. First, if the culture or rapid diagnostic test is positive, it explains the chest film findings and hypoxia, thus allowing the clinician to forgo further diagnostic intervention and/or antibacterial or antifungal therapy. Second, it is also reasonable to consider antiviral therapy directed at respiratory viruses.

REFERENCES

1. Betts RF: Influenza virus. *In* Mandell GL, Bennett EJ, Dolin R (eds.): *Principles and Practice of Infectious Diseases*, 4th ed. New York: Churchill Livingstone; 1995:1546–1567.

2. Glezen WP: *Options for Control of Influenza II*. Amsterdam: Elsevier-Exerpta Medica; 1993:11–13.

3. Louria DB, Blumenfeld HL, Ellis JT, *et al.*: Studies on influenza in the pandemic of 1957–1958: II. Pulmonary complications of influenza. *J Clin Invest* 1959, 38:213–265.

4. Kilbourne ED: *Influenza*. New York: Plenum Publishing; 1987.

5. Van Voris LP, Betts RF, Hayden FG, *et al.*: Successful treatment of naturally occurring influenza A/USSR/77 H1N1. *JAMA* 1981, 245:1128.

6. Little JW, Hall WJ, Douglas RG, *et al.*: Amantadine effect on peripheral airways abnormalities in influenza. *Ann Intern Med* 1976, 85:177.

7. Haake DA, Zakowski PC, Haake DL, Bryson YJ: Early treatment with acyclovir for varicella pneumonia in otherwise healthy adults: Retrospective controlled study and review. *Rev Infect Dis* 1990, 12:788–798.

8. Knyvett AF: The pulmonary lesions of chickenpox. *Q J Med* 1966, 35:313–323.

SELECTED BIBLIOGRAPHY

Englund JA, Sullivan CJ, Jordan C, *et al.*: Respiratory syncytial virus infection in immunocompromised adults. *Ann Intern Med* 1988, 109:203–208.

Falsey AR, Betts RF: Viral pneumonia, still a force to be reckoned with. *J Respir Dis* 1993, 14:31–54.

Falsey AR, Cunningham CK, Barker WH, *et al.*: Respiratory syncytial virus and influenza A infections in hospitalized elderly. *J Infect Dis* 1995, 172:389–394.

Greenberg SB: Viral pneumonia. *Infect Dis Clin North Am* 1991, 5(3):603–622.

CHAPTER 8

Protozoan and Helminthic Infections of the Lungs

John Froude

PROTOZOAN INFECTIONS

Protozoa causing lung disease in humans		
	Immunocompetent hosts	Immunocompromised hosts
Amebae		
Entamoeba histolytica	+	+
Flagellates		
Leishmania braziliensis	+	+
Trichomonas	—	AIDS
Coccidia		
Toxoplasma gondii	Rare	+
Cryptosporidium	—	AIDS
Sporozoa		
Plasmodium falciparum	+	Splenectomized patients
Babesia	+	at particular risk
*Pneumocystis carinii**	—	Especially AIDS

*May be reclassified as a fungus.

FIGURE 8-1 Protozoa causing lung disease in humans.

Amebiasis

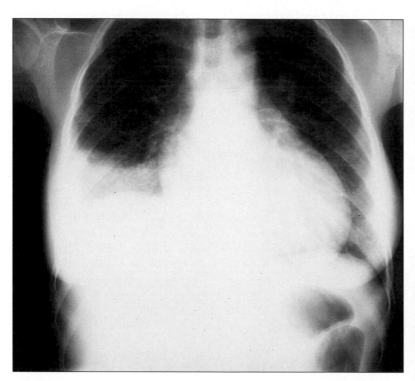

FIGURE 8-2 Chest radiograph of a patient with amebic liver abscess showing elevation of the right hemidiaphragm with pleural effusion. The incidence of pulmonary involvement in *Entamoeba histolytica* liver abscess ranges from 3% to 30%. When the abscess is adjacent to the diaphragm, it leads to its elevation, secondary atelectasis, and reactive pleural transudate. Pleuritic pain referred to the shoulder is typical, and pulmonary symptoms may dominate the clinical presentation. Effective treatment of the liver abscess leads to prompt resolution of the lung disease [1].

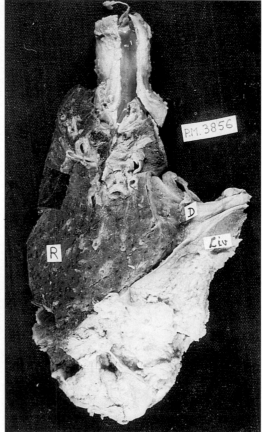

FIGURE 8-3
Pathologic specimen showing rupture of an amebic liver abscess through the diaphragm. This acute, life-threatening complication presents with shock, severe breathlessness, and chest pain with massive empyema and high mortality. Empyema occasionally develops more insidiously. It responds rapidly to intercostal intubation, as constricting visceral pleura does not develop without secondary bacterial infection [2]. (*Courtesy of* S.R. Bhusnurmath, MD.)

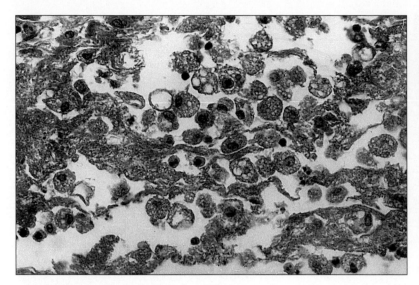

FIGURE 8-4 Photomicrograph of expectorated amebic pus from ruptured liver abscess. If an hepatobronchial fistula develops, the patient coughs out creamy white or, less commonly, chocolate-colored "anchovy paste" sputum. Left liver lobe abscesses may rupture into the left lung or pericardial sac. (*Courtesy of* S.R. Bhusnurmath, MD.)

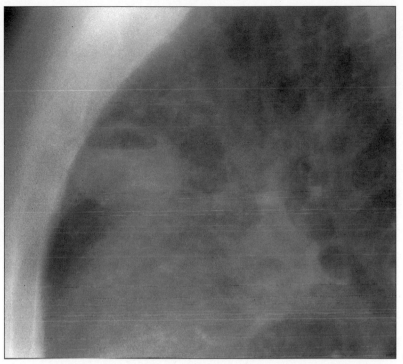

FIGURE 8-5 Chest radiograph showing an amebic lung abscess. Amebic lung abscesses may occur without liver disease. They are rare and usually seen in children. They are indistinguishable from pyogenic lung abscesses and have similar complications. Although amebae may be identified in the sputum, diagnosis is usually made by finding a high titer of amebic antibodies. It is assumed that trophozoites make their way from the colon to the lung via the inferior hemorrhoidal vein or through local lymphatic vessels to the inferior vena cava or thoracic duct.

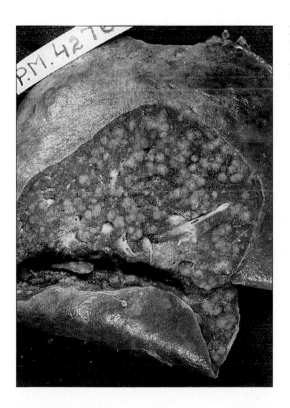

FIGURE 8-6 Pathologic specimen of lung showing amebic pneumonia. A 20-year-old Indian man presented with rapidly progressive fatal pneumonia due to *Entamoeba histolytica*. He had neither a recent history of dysentery nor evidence of liver disease. (*Courtesy of* S.R. Bhusnurmath, MD.)

Malaria and Babesiosis

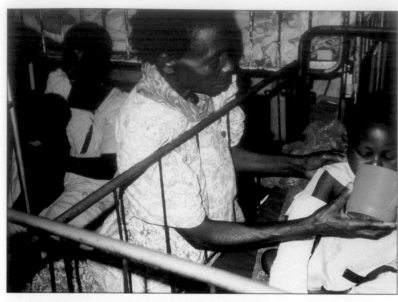

FIGURE 8-7 African child with malaria. Dry cough, moist crackles on auscultation, and small infiltrates on chest radiographs are nonspecific complications of malaria, particularly *Plasmodium falciparum* infection. Abnormalities of peak flow occur in most patients, and these alterations are more severe and take longer to recover in those with pulmonary symptoms. Coexistent bacterial or aspiration pneumonia may develop [3].

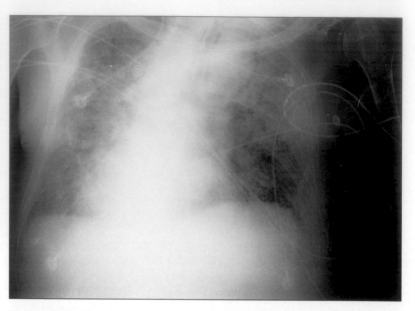

FIGURE 8-8 Chest radiograph showing acute respiratory distress syndrome (ARDS) in falciparum malaria. Unexplained ARDS should suggest the diagnosis of *Plasmodium falciparum* malaria in anyone who lives in or has traveled to an endemic area, regardless of whether they have taken antimalarial prophylaxis. It is characterized by abrupt onset and poor response to treatment and is present in nearly all fatal cases. It may occur at any point in the infection but tends to occur late, even after appropriate antimalarial chemotherapy has been started. It is particularly likely in patients with high parasitemia (> 10%) and pregnant women. Delay in diagnosis of imported cases in nonendemic zones has been catastrophic [4].

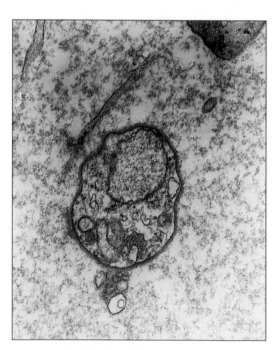

FIGURE 8-9 Electron micrograph of *Babesia microti*. The fuzzy border of the outer cell membrane is characteristic. Like falciparum malaria, babesiosis may present as adult respiratory distress syndrome. In both infections, pulmonary capillary wedge pressures are normal unless there is complicating fluid overload. Pathophysiologic mechanisms include marked increase in capillary membrane permeability with cytoadherence of endothelial cells and release of self-damaging inflammatory peptides, such as tumor necrosis factor and interleukin-1 [5]. (Original magnification, × 57,200.) (*Courtesy of* G. Siddhu, MD.)

Toxoplasmosis

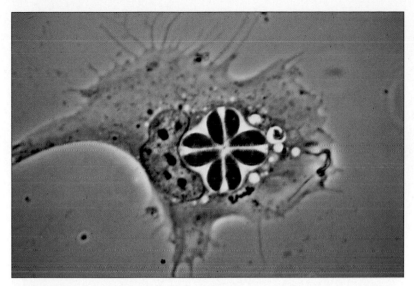

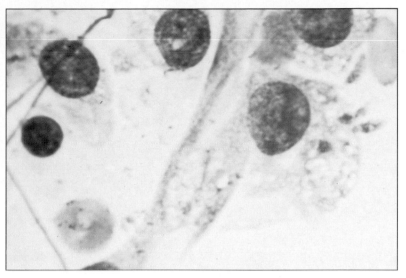

FIGURE 8-10 Trophozoite (tachyzoite) of *Toxoplasma gondii*. *T. gondii* is a sporozoa of the order Coccidia that infects almost all mammals and many birds. Fifty percent of adults living in the United States are seropositive by adulthood, but most acquired infections are asymptomatic. Localized lymphadenopathy can occur, sometimes accompanied by a mononucleosis syndrome. One percent of these patients will develop pneumonia, which is usually interstitial. Pneumonitis is also seen in congenital toxoplasmosis [6]. (*Courtesy of* H. Murray, MD.)

FIGURE 8-11 Tachyzoite of *Toxoplasma gondii* seen in bronchoalveolar lavage fluid. Toxoplasma pneumonia in AIDS and other immunocompromised patients is increasingly reported and remains underdiagnosed, as clinical features are nonspecific and histopathologic diagnosis is difficult. Interstitial pneumonia, indistinguishable radiologically from that caused by *Pneumocystis carinii*, progresses to parenchymal necrosis with respiratory failure. The sensitivity of histologic diagnosis is increased with the use of immunohistochemical stains [7]. (*Courtesy of* E.J. Bottone, PhD.)

Pneumocystosis

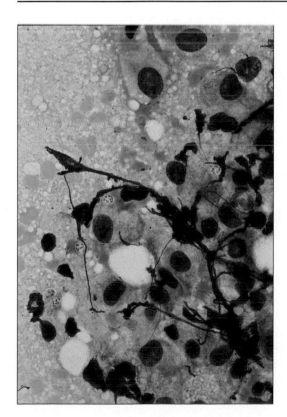

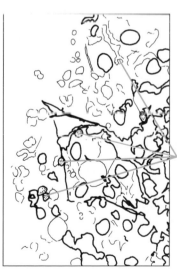

Cyst with intracystic bodies

FIGURE 8-12 Typical cysts and intracystic bodies (daughter trophozoites) of *Pneumocystis carinii* seen on a touch preparation of infected rat lung. *Pneumocystis* has been classified as a protozoan, but its ribosomal RNA sequence, the presence and composition of the cell wall, and other evidence strongly suggest that it is a fungus closely related to the Ascomycetes or yeasts such as *Candida*. The lack of a continuous *in vivo* culture system hinders research into some details of its life history, biochemistry, and ultrastructure [8]. (Giemsa stain.) (*Courtesy of* A. Clarkson, PhD.)

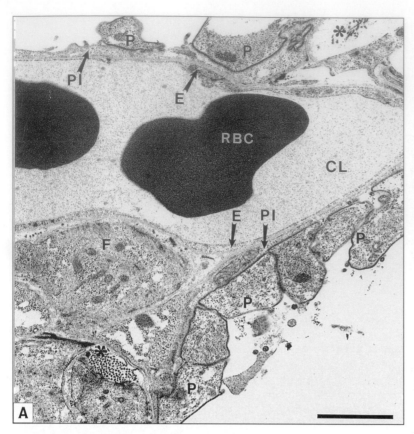

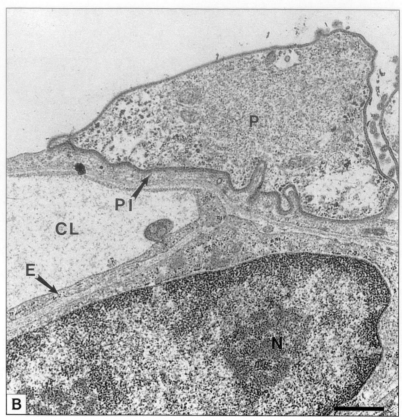

FIGURE 8-13 Electron micrograph showing *Pneumocystis carinii* trophozoites in rat lung specimens. **A,** *Pneumocystis* trophozoites (*P*) can be seen covering the alveolar surface of type 1 pneumocytes (*PI*). Two red blood cells (*RBC*) can be seen in the lumen of a lung capillary (*CL*). (Bar = 5 μm.) **B,** A higher-power view shows that trophozoites are closely apposed to and interdigitate with type 1 pneumocytes (*PI*). This leads to cell loss, increased permeability and leakage at the alveolar capillary barrier, reduced surfactant, intrapulmonary shunting, and decreased compliance with respiratory failure. Initiation of therapy may accelerate lung injury [9]. (Bar = 1 μm.) (E—endothelium; F—fibroblasts; N—nucleus of fibroblast.) (*Courtesy of* U. Frevert, PhD.)

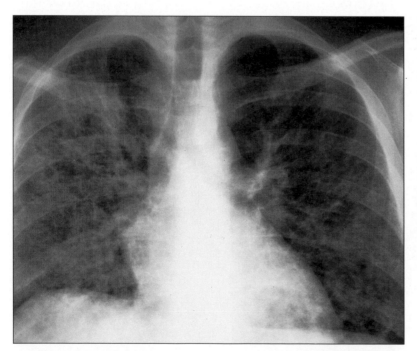

FIGURE 8-14 Chest radiograph showing bilateral interstitial infiltrates typical of acute *Pneumocystis carinii* pneumonia (PCP). Infection with pneumocystis is almost universal in the United States and occurs early in life. It causes acute disease in immunocompromised patients and is the most frequent AIDS-defining diagnosis, except in Africa where it is rare. Patients present with fever, dyspnea, and nonproductive cough, usually of insidious onset. The spectrum of disease is wide, however, and PCP should be considered in all patients with parenchymal lung disease and a CD4+ T-lymphocyte count < 300/mm³.

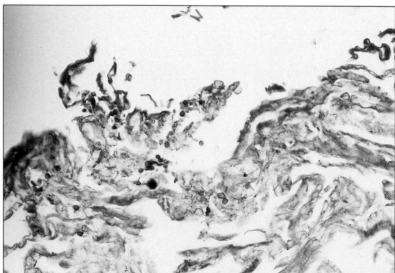

FIGURE 8-15 Transbronchial biopsy in *Pneumocystis carinii* pneumonia stained with methenamine silver. Three forms of *P. carinii* are recognized: cysts, cysts with intracystic bodies (*see* Fig. 8-12), and trophozoites. Methenamine silver is taken up only by the cyst wall. (*Courtesy of* J. Jagardir, MD.)

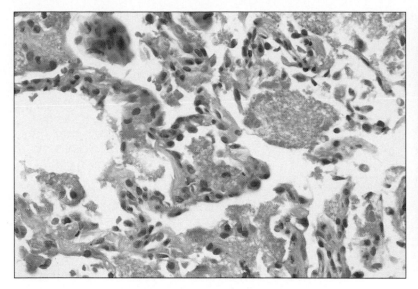

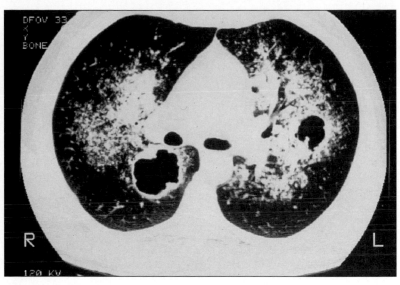

FIGURE 8-16 Transbronchial biopsy in *Pneumocystis carinii* pneumonia (PCP) stained with hematoxylin-eosin. The foamy alveolar cell exudate suggests PCP. The exudate consists of organisms, surfactant, and mucus. Dots in the exudate are trophozoites. (*Courtesy of* J. Jagardir, MD.)

FIGURE 8-17 Computed tomography scan showing cystic *Pneumocystis carinii* pneumonia (PCP). Cysts and pneumatoceles may complicate PCP. Rupture leads to pneumothorax and sometimes bronchopleural fistula. Pleural effusion and mediastinal adenopathy are rare in PCP and suggest other pathology.

Therapy for acute *Pneumocystis carinii* pneumonia

Drug	Mild disease	Moderate to severe disease
First choice		
Trimethoprim-sulfamethoxazole	5 mg/kg trimethoprim + 25 mg/kg sulfamethoxazole every 6–8 hrs orally or intravenously	5 mg/kg trimethoprim + 25 mg/kg sulfamethoxazole every 6–8 hrs intravenously
Trimethoprim-dapsone	300 mg trimethoprim every 8 hrs orally + 100 mg dapsone every 24 hrs orally	—
Alternatives		
Pentamidine	4 mg/kg every 24 hrs intravenously	4 mg/kg every 24 hrs intravenously
Clindamycin-primaquine	450 mg clindamycin every 6 hrs orally + 15 mg primaquine every 24 hrs orally	600 mg clindamycin every 6 hrs intravenously + 15–30 mg primaquine every 24 hrs orally
Atovaquone	750 mg every 8 hrs orally	—
Trimethoprim-leucovorin	—	45 mg/m² trimethoprim every 24 hrs intravenously + 20 mg/m² leucovorin every 6 hrs intravenously
Adjunctive therapy		
Prednisone or prednisolone	—	40 mg every 12 hrs orally or intravenously × 5 days, then 40 mg every 24 hrs orally or intravenously × 5 days, then 20 mg every 24 hrs × 11 days

FIGURE 8-18 Therapy for acute *Pneumocystis carinii* pneumonia (PCP). Trimethoprim-sulfamethoxazole (TMP-SMX) is the drug of choice for patients with PCP, but up to 30% of patients experience treatment-limiting toxicity. Pentamidine is the alternative for treatment failure but is also toxic. Trimethoprim-dapsone may be as effective as TMP-SMX and is less toxic. Limited data are available for newer agents and combinations. Adjunctive corticosteroids should be used if the patient's oxygen partial pressure on room air is < 70 mm Hg. (*Adapted from* Hopewell and Masur [9]; with permission.)

Primary and secondary prophylaxis for *Pneumocystis carinii* pneumonia	
Drug	**Dosage**
First choice	
Trimethoprim-sulfamethoxazole	160 mg trimethoprim + 800 mg sulfamethoxazole every day orally
Alternatives	
Aerosolized pentamidine	300 mg monthly by jet nebulizer
Dapsone	50 mg twice a day orally
Dapsone-pyrimethamine	200 mg dapsone + 75 mg pyrimethamine weekly orally
Atovaquone	(Unknown)

FIGURE 8-19 Primary and secondary prophylaxis for *Pneumocystis carinii* pneumonia (PCP). One double-strength tablet of trimethoprim-sulfamethoxazole daily is effective primary and secondary prophylaxis. It is superior to aerosolized pentamidine and dapsone in clinical trials. Primary prophylaxis should be given to patients with a CD4 count of < 200 cells/mm^3 or oropharyngeal candidiasis. Secondary prophylaxis is essential for all patients with a previous episode of PCP. Alternative agents are considered to be less effective. Prophylaxis should be maintained for life. (*Adapted from* Hopewell and Masur [9]; with permission.)

Leishmaniasis

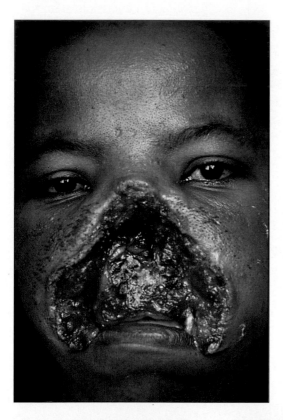

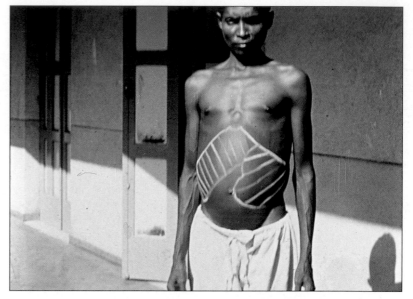

FIGURE 8-20 American mucocutaneous leishmaniasis. A small percentage of people infected with *Leishmania braziliensis* complex develop lesions of the oropharynx and larynx years after the characteristic skin lesions resolve. These mutilating lesions progress remorselessly to involve the larynx and trachea, and aspiration is a common terminal complication [10]. (*Courtesy of* F. Etges, PhD.)

FIGURE 8-21 Visceral leishmaniasis causing massive hepatosplenomegaly. Despite high levels of antibodies to leishmania antigens, patients with visceral leishmaniasis are severely immunocompromised with absent Th1-cell–mediated immunity. They become cachectic, and half of them develop severe bacterial infections [11].

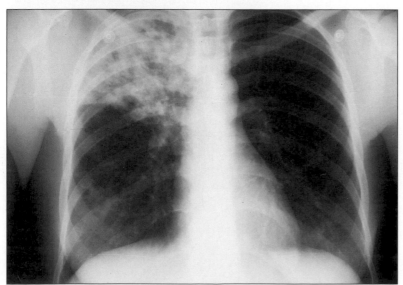

FIGURE 8-22 Chest radiograph showing tuberculosis complicating visceral leishmaniasis. Chest infections occur in about a quarter of patients with visceral leishmaniasis. This patient, shown in Figure 8-21, developed tuberculosis. Much of the morbidity and mortality of protozoan and helminthic disease is due to coinfections, malnutrition, anemia, and immunodeficiency.

HELMINTHIC INFECTIONS

A. Helminths causing lung disease in humans: Nematodes (roundworms)	
Clinical syndrome or finding	**Organism**
Löffler's syndrome/"asthma"	*Ascaris lumbricoides*
	Ancylostoma braziliensis (cutaneous larva migrans)
	Ancylostoma duodenale (hookworm)
	Necator americanus (hookworm)
	Strongyloides stercoralis
	Trichinella spiralis
	Toxocara canis, T. cati (visceral larva migrans)
Chronic cough	*Mammomonogamus* spp
Tropical eosinophilia	*Wuchereria bancrofti* (lymphatic filariasis)
	Brugia malayi
Coin lesion on chest radiograph	*Dirofilaria immitis* (dog heartworm)

B. Helminths causing lung disease in humans: Cestodes and trematodes	
Cestodes (tapeworms)	*Echinococcus granulosus* (hydatid disease)
Trematodes (flukes)	*Paragonimus westermani*
	Paragonimus spp
	Schistosoma mansoni
	Schistosoma haematobium
	Anisakis simplex (rare)

FIGURE 8-23 Helminths causing lung disease in humans. **A**, Nematodes (roundworms). **B**, Cestodes (tapeworms) and trematodes (flukes).

Immune Response to Helminthic Infection

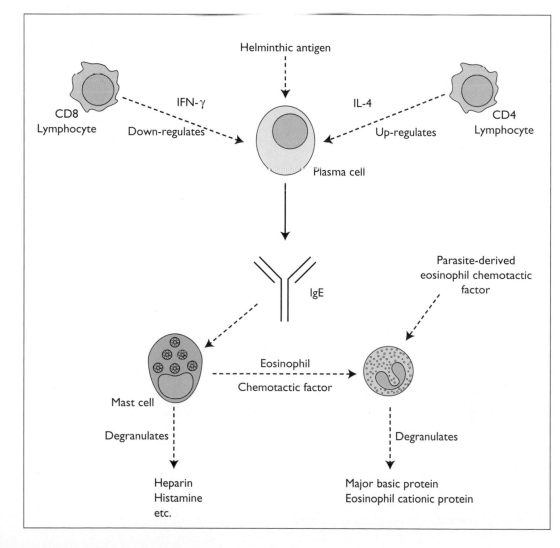

FIGURE 8-24 Simplified diagram of the cellular response to helminthic infection. Helminthic infection is associated with high levels of serum IgE, eosinophilia, and the recruitment of mast cells to the site of infection. This response is under T-cell control and is generated mostly by the larval or tissue invasive forms of the parasite [12]. (IFN-γ—interferon-γ; IL-4—interleukin-4.)

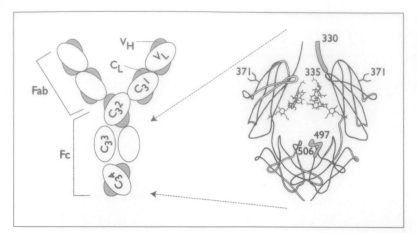

Figure 8-25 Diagram of an IgE molecule. IgE-secreting B cells are abundant in the gut, skin, and respiratory tract. This immunoglobulin, found only in mammals, elicits a range of cellular responses that lead to inflammation, itching, coughing, sneezing, lacrimation, bronchoconstriction, mucous secretion, vomiting, and diarrhea. (*From* Sutton and Gould [13]; with permission.)

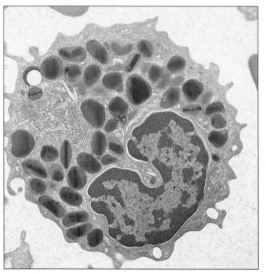

Figure 8-26 Electron micrograph of an eosinophil. Eosinophils defend against large nonphagocytable organisms. They bind by specific receptors to antihelminthic IgG, IgE, or C3B deposited on the worm's surface. Major basic protein and eosinophilic cationic protein are toxic to many helminths, especially in the larval stage. Toxicity is mediated to a lesser extent by oxidative products and acids generated by eosinophil peroxidase. Eosinophils are found in epithelial tissue in contact with the environment, such as the respiratory, gastrointestinal, and urinary tracts, where they are 1000-fold more plentiful than in peripheral blood [14]. (*Courtesy of* D. Muirhead.)

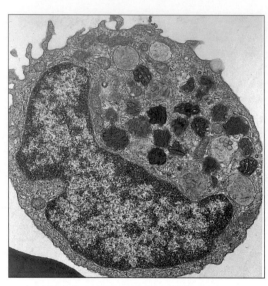

Figure 8-27 Electron micrograph of a mast cell. Mast cells and basophils have high-affinity receptors (FcεR1) for IgE. Their abundant cytoplasmic granules store many vasoactive compounds that produce the features of immediate hypersensitivity. They also secrete cytokines that orchestrate the infiltration of neutrophils [15]. (Original magnification, × 23,000.) (*Courtesy of* D. Zucker-Franklin, MD.)

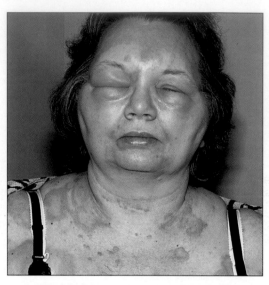

Figure 8-28 Severe urticaria. The immune response to helminthic infection does not always benefit the host. A similar response occurs in reaction to other environmental antigens in genetically susceptible individuals. In developed countries, physicians may overlook the fact that allergic disease, especially asthma and urticaria, can be caused by nematodes and other helminths. (*Courtesy of* H. Goodheart, MD.)

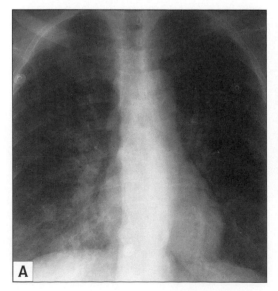

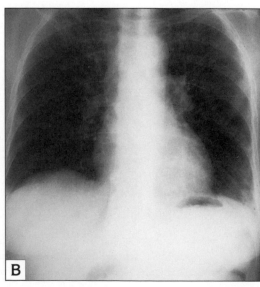

Figure 8-29 Chest radiographs showing Löffler's syndrome. Löffler's syndrome consists of intermittent, mild, nonproductive cough and wheeze that is often worse at night. It is associated with peripheral blood eosinophilia and fleeting migratory infiltrates on chest radiograph. **A** and **B**, Chest radiographs taken 2 months apart in a patient with *Ascaris lumbricoides* infestation [16].

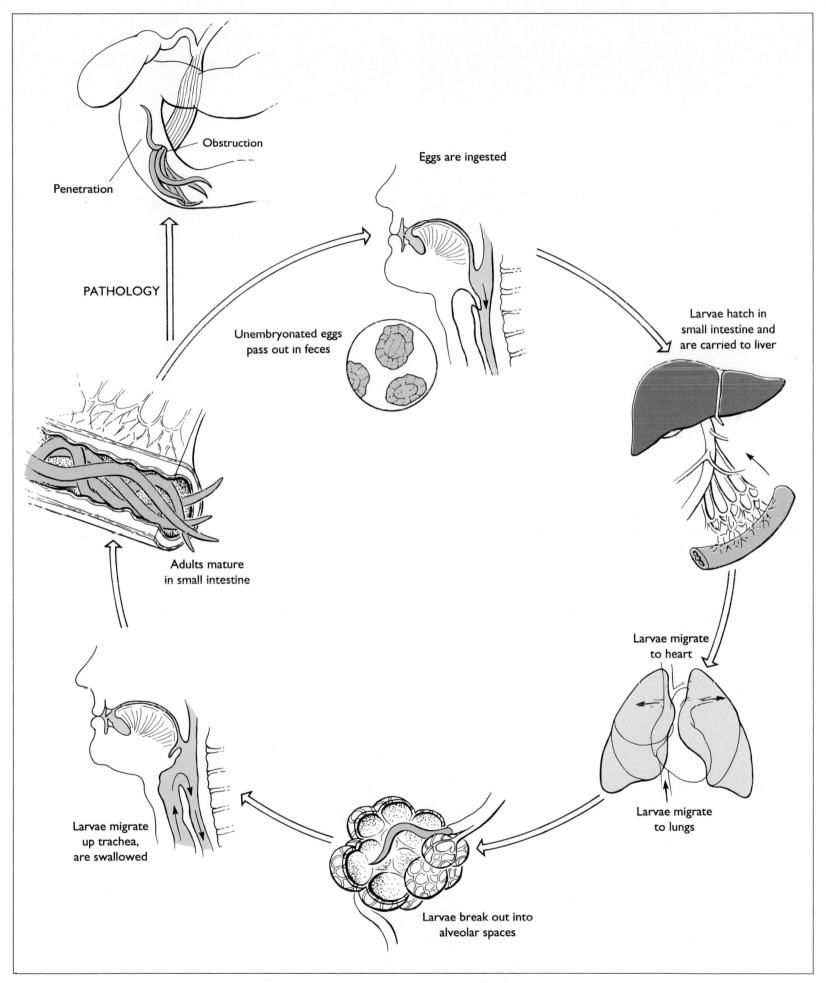

Obstruction

Penetration

PATHOLOGY

Eggs are ingested

Unembryonated eggs pass out in feces

Larvae hatch in small intestine and are carried to liver

Adults mature in small intestine

Larvae migrate to heart

Larvae migrate up trachea, are swallowed

Larvae migrate to lungs

Larvae break out into alveolar spaces

FIGURE 8-30 Diagram of nematode larval passage through the lung. Ascariasis, strongyloidiasis, hookworm, trichinosis, cutaneous larva migrans (particularly that due to *Ancylostoma braziliensis*), and visceral larva migrans (due to *Toxocara canis* and *T. catis*) are the commonest nematode infections with a larval stage that passes through the lung causing Löffler's syndrome. It is not known how or why these extraordinary journeys evolved. A similar syndrome may also be seen in schistosomiasis and paragonimiasis.

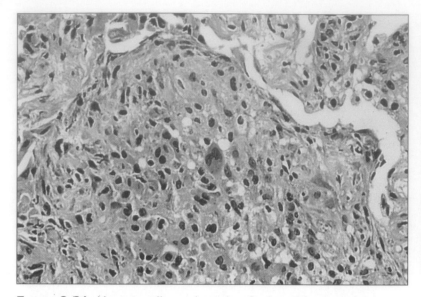

FIGURE 8-31 Hematoxylin-eosin stain of a lung biopsy specimen showing eosinophilic pneumonia in a patient with Löffler's syndrome. Many eosinophils are shown infiltrating airspaces and interstitial tissue. Eosinophils are also abundant in sputum and bronchoalveolar lavage samples. Nonhelminthic causes of Löffler's syndrome include bronchopulmonary aspergillosis, hypersensitivity pneumonitis, malignancy, and reaction to drugs including nonsteroidal anti-inflammatory drugs and minocycline. It has also been described in coccidioidomycosis, tuberculosis, and sarcoidosis.

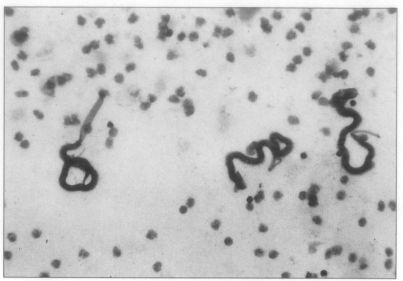

FIGURE 8-32 *Wuchereria bancrofti*, an arthropod-transmitted microfilaria, on blood smear. Tropical pulmonary eosinophilia is a term used to describe the syndrome of pulmonary infiltrates with eosinophilia caused by an anamnestic immunologic hyperresponsiveness to the filarial worms *Wuchereria bancrofti* and *Brugia malayi*. Patients are more symptomatic than those with Löffler's syndrome, reside in endemic areas, have very high levels of IgE and antifilarial antibodies, and respond to treatment with diethylcarbamazine or ivermectin. Worms are frequently absent from the blood. Repeated infection with inadequate therapy leads to progressive interstitial fibrosis [17]. (*Courtesy of* G.B. Craig, Jr, MD.)

NEMATODE INFECTIONS

Ascariasis

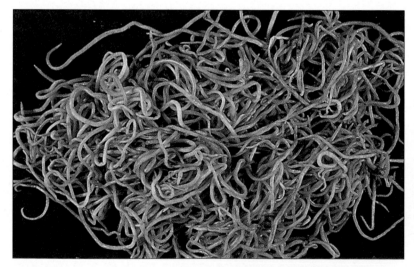

FIGURE 8-33 Tangle of adult *Ascaris lumbricoides*. It is estimated that 20% of the world's population is infected with this worm. In children of rural tropics, this figure may approach 100%. Globally, 10^{18} *Ascaris* eggs are extruded daily. Löffler's syndrome, which may occur within 2 weeks of initial infection, is seen in less than 1% of those infected. Because human infection depends on the ingestion of food or objects contaminated with feces, groups at risk include children, those living in overcrowded, unsanitary conditions, inmates of institutions, and people with pica. (*From* Daar and Mabogunje [18]; with permission.)

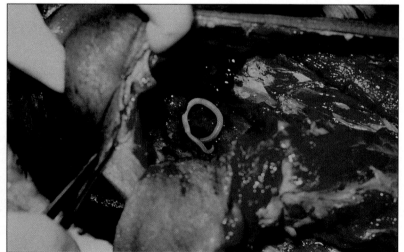

FIGURE 8-34 Respiratory obstruction by *Ascaris* causing death. Because adult helminths do not multiply in the human host, they cause disease only when the worm burden is high. (*From* Daar and Mabogunje [18]; with permission.)

Strongyloidiasis

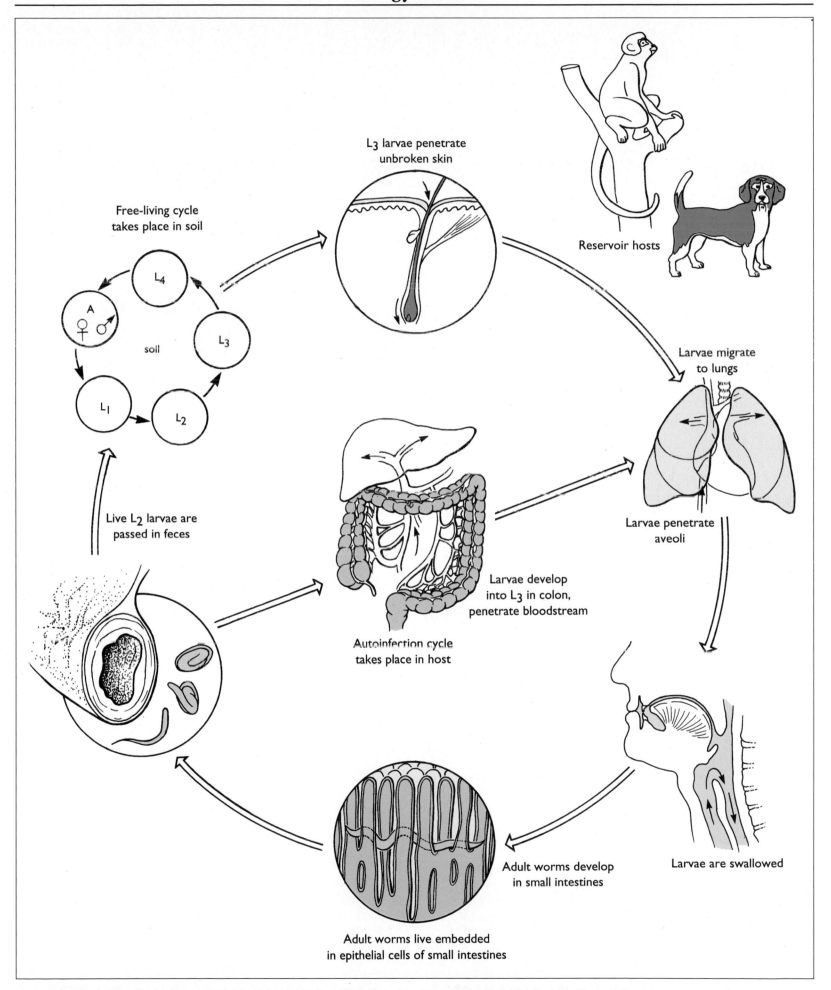

FIGURE 8-35 Life cycle of *Strongyloides*. Rhabditiform larvae mature directly to invasive filariform larvae, allowing autoinfec- tion through intestinal mucosa and perineal skin. Infection may therefore persist for decades [19].

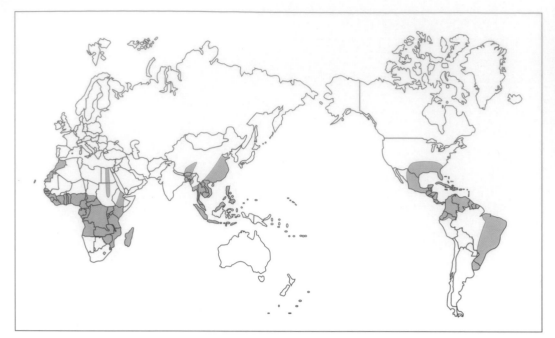

FIGURE 8-36 World distribution of strongyloidiasis. Strongyloides infection is seen in the United States in the following approximate order of frequency: imported cases from Southeast Asia, Latin America, and the Caribbean; people from rural southeastern United States, where the incidence may reach 3%; epidemics in mental institutions; World War II veterans from the Pacific theater, particularly prisoners of war; Vietnam veterans [20].

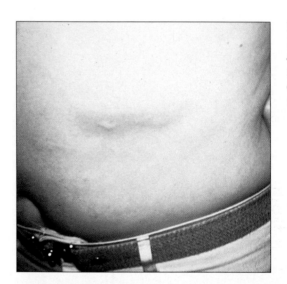

FIGURE 8-37 Urticarial lesions caused by filariform larvae of *Strongyloides stercoralis* (larva currens). Larvae travel 5 to 10 cm per hour under the skin to the lower abdomen and further sites. The lesions, persisting from hours to days, are recurrent over weeks or months and may be diagnosed as hives. The patients may also complain of nocturnal cough and wheeze and be considered asthmatic. If steroids are given for these misdiagnoses, the risk of disseminated strongyloidiasis is increased [21].

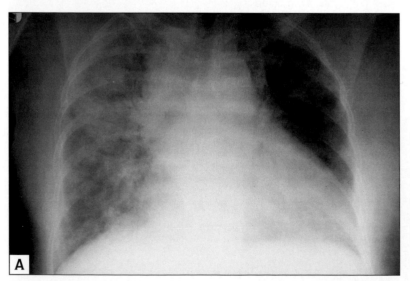

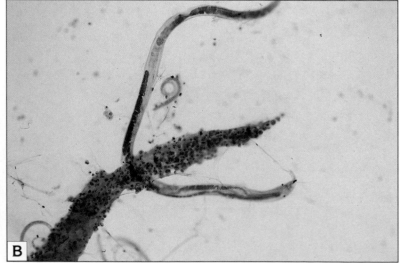

FIGURE 8-38 Disseminated strongyloides related to corticosteroid immunosuppression. **A**, Chest radiograph showing acute respiratory distress syndrome (ARDS). A 35-year-old Puerto Rican woman living in New York City who had not been home for 10 years had stage IV lymphoma treated with steroids and chemotherapy. She developed *Escherichia coli* septicemia, ARDS, and worsening diarrhea. *Strongyloides stercoralis* worms of every stage were found in her stool. **B**, Bronchoalveolar lavage (BAL) fluid showing an adult female worm and rhabditiform and filariform (invasive) larvae. Disseminated strongyloidiasis may occur in patients immunocompromised from any cause, particularly steroids or immunosuppressive drugs, and has an 85% mortality. It is characterized by ARDS, gram-negative septicemia with meningitis, and diarrhea. Larva currens or purpuric skin lesions in the flanks may be seen. Eosinophilia is absent. In disseminated disease, worms can be seen in BAL fluid and are easily detectable in stool samples [22].

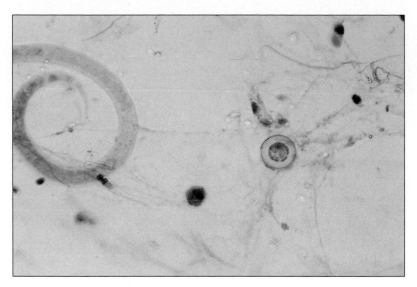

FIGURE 8-39 Bronchoalveolar lavage fluid in disseminated strongyloidiasis showing adult worms rhabditiform larvae, and ovum. Thiabendzole is the only effective treatment for strongyloidiasis, but disseminated disease requires the prolonged use of high doses with unsatisfactory levels of toxicity. Ivermectin is a promising therapy currently under evaluation. Disseminated disease has not been reported in renal transplant patients on cyclosporine, which has been shown to be antihelminthic *in vitro.* (*Courtesy of* J. Jagardir, MD.)

Dirofilariasis

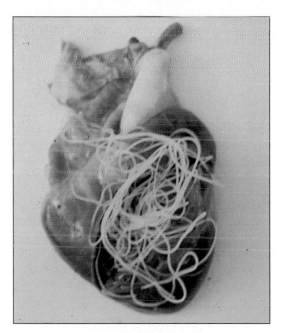

FIGURE 8-40 Dog heartworm, *Dirofilaria immitis*, in a dog heart. This filarial nematode is transmitted to humans from domesticated dogs by mosquitoes. Increasing numbers of cases are being reported in the United States, mostly from the southeastern states [23]. (*Courtesy of* H. Zaiman, MD.)

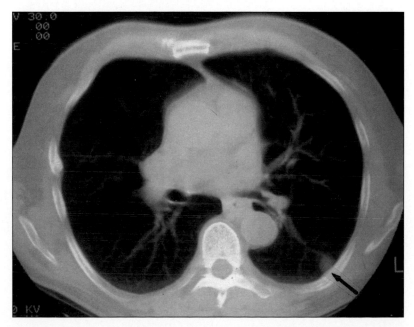

FIGURE 8-41 Computed tomography scan showing pleuropulmonary nodule of dirofilariasis (*arrow*). Immature filariae of *Dirofilaria immitis* migrate from the skin to the pulmonary circulation. Because they cannot mature (accidental infection) in humans, they die causing local vasculitis with pulmonary infarction; a granulomatous reaction may follow. Patients are usually asymptomatic. The coin lesions discovered on routine chest radiographs are frequently mistaken for malignancy. (*Courtesy of* K.L. Green, MD.)

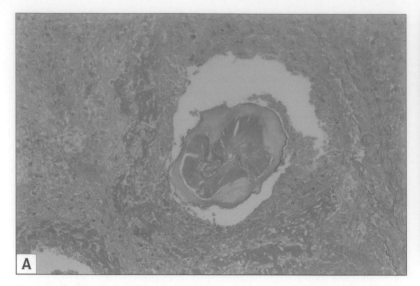

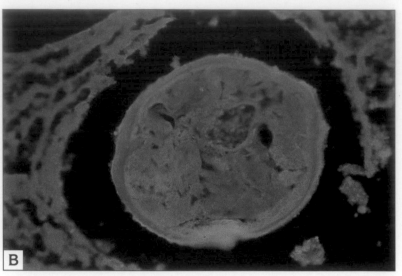

FIGURE 8-42 Lung biopsy showing cross-section of *Dirofilaria immitis*. **A**, Hematoxylin-eosin stain. Diagnosis of dirofilariasis is made by histologic examination of tissue obtained from thoracotomy or fine-needle aspiration. Parasites stain pale pink with hematoxylin-eosin and may be difficult to see against the background. (Original magnification, × 1000.) **B**, Fluorescent staining technique. Fluorescent whitener stains bind to the external chitin wall of the parasite, allowing rapid identification of even degenerated or fragmented organisms. The thick cuticle of the worm is evident, with lateral cords compressed between heavy muscle bands. (Tinobal CBS-X stain; original magnification, × 1000.) (Panel 42A *courtesy of* K.L. Green, MD; panel 42B *from* Green *et al.* [24]; with permission.)

Syngamosis

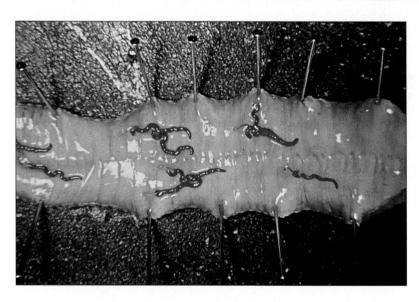

FIGURE 8-43 *Mammomonogamus laryngeus* in the trachea of a turkey. Gapeworms (genus *Syngamus*) infect birds and mammals. There have been about 80 infections in humans reported to date from Puerto Rico, other Caribbean islands, and Brazil. Patients have persistent dry cough and occasionally hemoptysis. Disease is usually confined to the larynx. The worms are seen in conjugal Y-shaped pairs at bronchoscopy, and removal leads to cure. Eggs are found in sputum or in feces if swallowed [25]. (*Courtesy of* H. Zaiman, MD.)

Therapy for Nematode Infections

Drug therapy for nematode-related lung disease in humans

Organism	First line	Alternatives
Ascaris lumbricoides *Necator americanus* *Ancylostoma duodenale*	Mebendazole, 100 mg orally twice a day × 3 days	Albendazole, 400 mg orally × single dose Pyrantel pamoate, 11 mg/kg daily × 3 days
Strongyloides stercoralis	Thiabendazole, 22 mg/kg orally twice a day × 2 days Hyperinfection: continue treatment for at least 2 wks	No proven alternative; consider ivermectin, 200 µg/kg × single dose Hyperinfection: consider ivermectin, 200 µg/kg on days 1, 2, 15, 16
Ancylostoma braziliensis	Thiabendazole, 22 mg/kg orally twice a day × 2 days	Albendazole, 400 mg orally twice a day × 3 days
Toxocara canis *T. cati*	Diethylcarbamazine, 2 mg/kg orally three times a day × 10 days	Albendazole, 400 mg twice a day orally × 5 days
Wuchereria bancrofti *Brugia malayi*	Diethylcarbamazine, 2 mg/kg orally three times a day × 21 days	Diethylcarbamazine, 6 mg/kg orally × single dose Ivermectin, 200 µg/kg × single dose
Dirofilaria immitis	No drug therapy indicated Surgical removal of worms where necessary	—

FIGURE 8-44 Drug therapy for nematode-related lung disease in humans. Ivermectin is useful therapy for several nematode infections, although it is not yet licensed in the United States. One report suggests it is therapeutically effective in the syndrome of disseminated strongyloidiasis [26].

CESTODES INFECTION

Echinococcosis

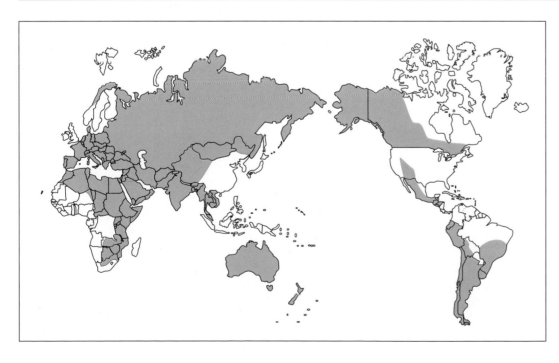

FIGURE 8-45 World distribution of echinococcosis. Echinococcosis, or hydatid disease, is usually found in temperate and subtropical zones where sheep are raised. Most cases seen in the United States are imported, but parts of Alaska and Canada are endemic for the disease [27].

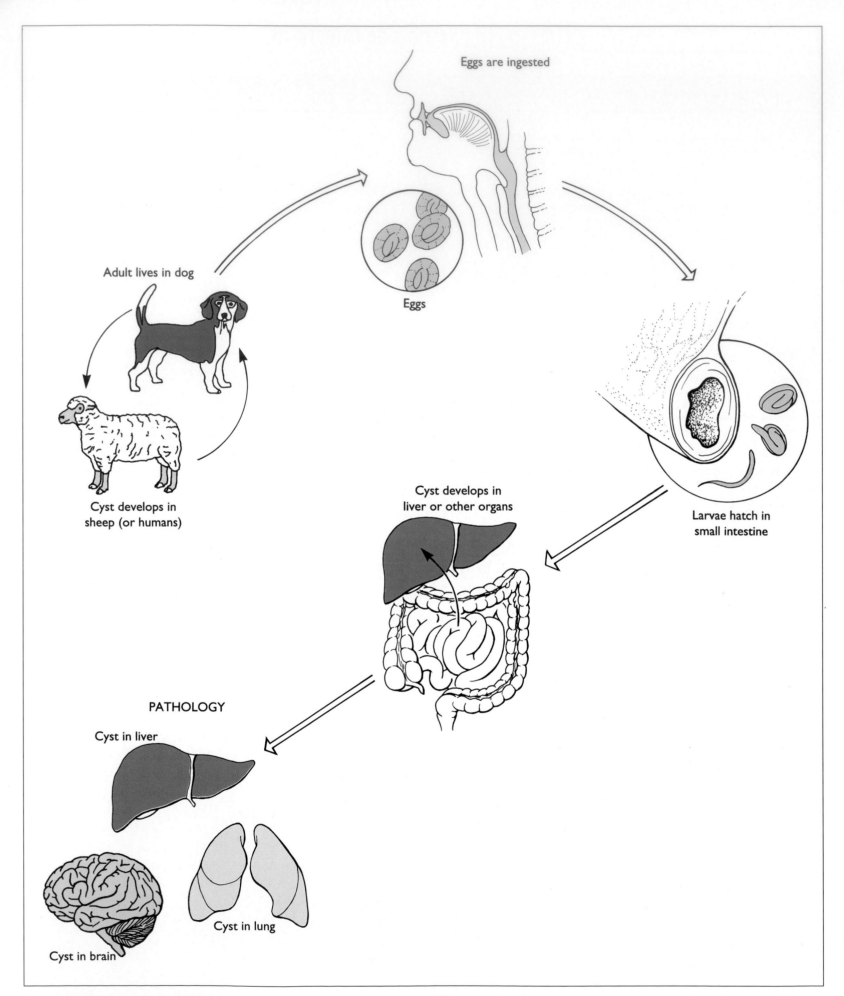

FIGURE 8-46 Life cycle of *Echinococcus granulosus*. In the pastoral form of echinococcosis, the dog is the definitive host, and sheep, cattle, swine, and humans are the intermediate hosts. In the sylvan form, the wolf is the definitive host, with caribou, moose, reindeer, the domestic dog, and humans as potential intermediate hosts. These differences in host/parasite adaptation are reflected in local differences in the disease characteristics; for example, lung cysts seen in Alaska follow a more benign course and are much more likely to be asymptomatic than those seen in the Middle East [28].

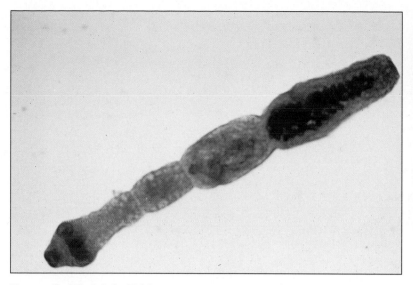

FIGURE 8-47 Adult *Echinococcus granulosus*. Children, shepherds, and farmers in close contact with dogs are particularly likely to become infected. The digestive juices of the intermediate host dissolve the coat of the egg, releasing larvae that burrow through intestinal mucosa into mesenteric venules and lymphatics. Most larvae lodge in the liver (65%–75%) or lung (25%–30%), but a few continue through the circulation to other organs.

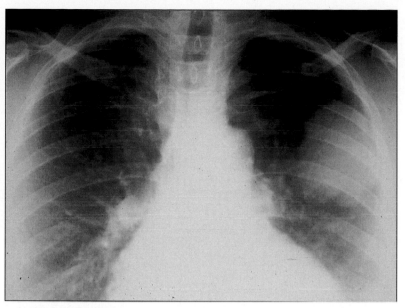

FIGURE 8-48 Chest radiograph showing hydatid cyst. If the larva is not destroyed, it develops into a tiny cyst, which grows from 1 to 3 cm per year depending on its location. It can remain indolent for decades. Most lung cysts (70%) are solitary, and the characteristic radiologic finding is of a well-circumscribed homogeneous opacity seen anywhere in the lung fields. Calcification in lung cysts is very uncommon, in contrast to liver cysts [29].

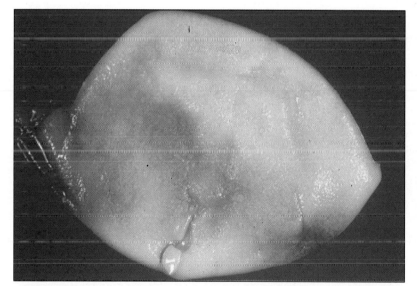

FIGURE 8-49 Intact unilocular hydatid cyst. Note the solid laminated ectocyst through which nourishment diffuses from the host to the inner germinal layer. Osmotic pressure within the cysts may reach 300 mm H_2O.

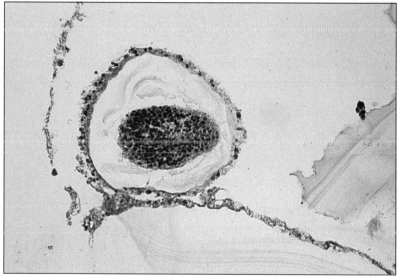

FIGURE 8-50 Tissue cross-section showing endocyst or germinal layer with brood capsule attached. In contrast to the ectocyst, which may reach 2 cm in width, the endocyst or germinal layer is one-cell-layer thick. When the brood capsule detaches from the germinal layer, it becomes a daughter cyst within the original. (*Courtesy of* W.N. von Sinner, MD.)

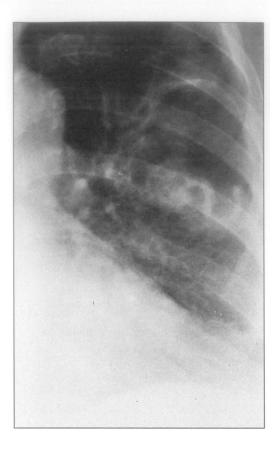

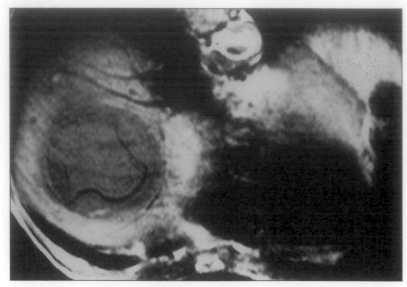

FIGURE 8-51 Chest radiograph showing ruptured hydatid cyst with water-lily or snake sign. This pathognomonic radiologic finding is seen when the cyst ruptures. A double line appears between the ectocyst and pericyst, and the collapsed hydatid membranes float on the surface of residual hydatid fluid and "sand." The patient complains of cough productive of watery sputum streaked with blood. Most tolerate this event, but 5% to 20% suffer anaphylactic shock or severe asthma and urticaria. (*From* von Sinner [30]; with permission.)

FIGURE 8-52 Magnetic resonance image (T2 weighted) of a ruptured hydatid cyst showing the pathognomonic "snake" sign. (*From* von Sinner *et al.* [31]; with permission.)

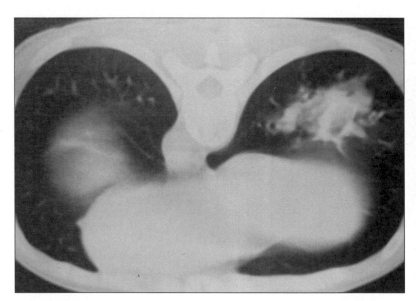

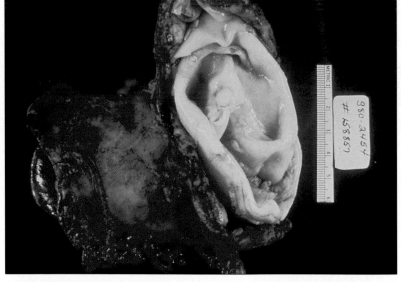

FIGURE 8-53 Computed tomography (CT) scan of a ruptured hydatid cyst showing "starburst" sign. (*From* von Sinner [32]; with permission.)

FIGURE 8-54 Ruptured hydatid cyst with contiguous tuberculous lymphadenopathy. The thickness of the ectocyst may partly explain the poor response to pharmacologic treatment of echinococcal cysts. Coincidentally, this patient had pulmonary tuberculosis. (*Courtesy of* W.N. von Sinner, MD.)

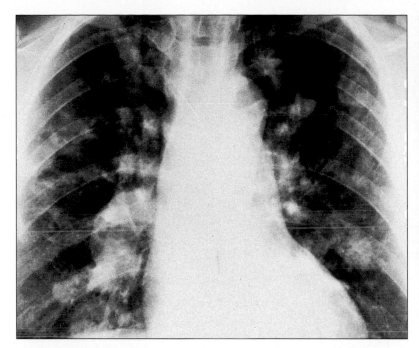

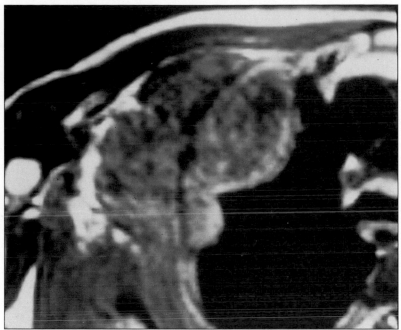

FIGURE 8-55 Chest radiograph showing multiple hydatid cysts mimicking metastatic lung disease. Another consequence of cyst rupture is the spillage of daughter cysts into the bronchial tree or pulmonary artery, leading to multiple metastatic cysts. The ectocyst induces a local fibrous capsule in the host called the *pericyst*. This may be compounded by leakage of hydatid fluid into the lung causing inflammation, further fibrosis, and pulmonary hypertension. (*Courtesy of* W.N. von Sinner, MD.)

FIGURE 8-56 Magnetic resonance imaging (MRI) scan showing hybrid mass involving the chest wall. The advent of ultrasonography, computed tomography, and MRI scanning has revolutionized the diagnosis, assessment, and posttreatment follow-up of hydatid cyst disease. This MRI shows multiple hydatid cysts involving the chest wall, which were found to contain 1.5 L of mucous material at surgery. (*From* von Sinner *et al.* [32]; with permission.)

FIGURE 8-57 Therapy for echinococcosis affecting the lung.

Therapy for echinococcosis causing lung disease	
Surgical excision of the cyst or tissue containing the cyst is the treatment of choice when feasible	
Albendazole	10 mg/kg orally in divided doses daily with meals for at least 3 months
	May be an alternative to surgery in uncomplicated lung cysts
	May be used adjunctively with surgery or palliatively in inoperable cases

TREMATODE INFECTIONS

Paragonimiasis

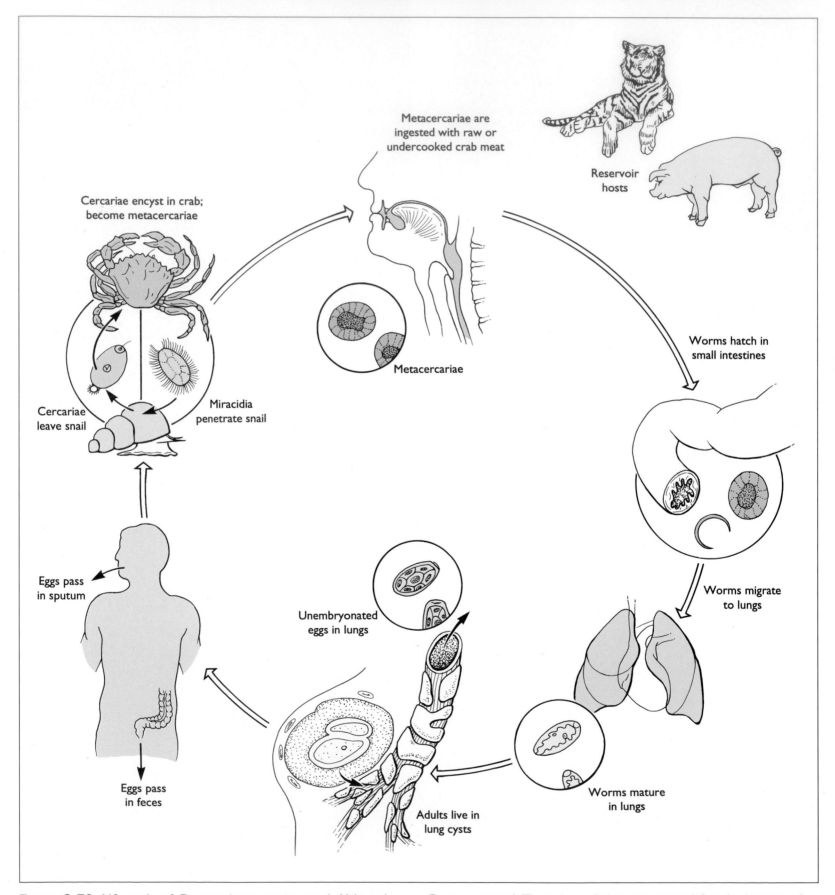

Metacercariae are
ingested with raw or
undercooked crab meat

Reservoir
hosts

Cercariae encyst in crab;
become metacercariae

Metacercariae

Worms hatch in
small intestines

Cercariae
leave snail

Miracidia
penetrate snail

Worms migrate
to lungs

Eggs pass
in sputum

Unembryonated
eggs in lungs

Worms mature
in lungs

Eggs pass
in feces

Adults live in
lung cysts

FIGURE 8-58 Life cycle of *Paragonimus westermani*. Although 10 of the 43 known trematode species of the genus *Paragonimus* infect humans, the great majority are caused by *P. westermani*. These lung flukes are named for the keeper of the Amsterdam Zoo, where they were first discovered in Bengal tigers in 1877 [33].

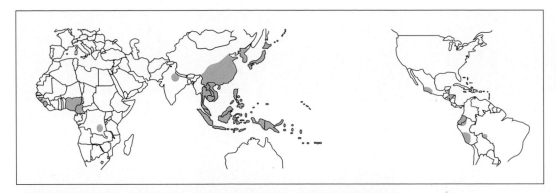

FIGURE 8-59 Geographic distribution of paragonimiasis. Carnivorous animals that eat crabs and crayfish may harbor the parasite. Cases are often imported into the United States. *Paragonimus kellacotti*, found only in North America, is reported to have caused four infections [34].

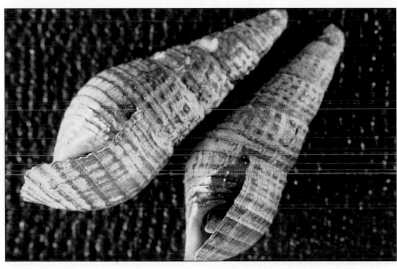

FIGURE 8-60 Shells of the *Semisulcospira bensoni* snail. *S. bensoni*, a freshwater snail, is one of several possible first intermediate hosts for *Paragonimus westermani*. Recent industrial pollution has reduced the number of these snails, with a corresponding decline in the incidence of paragonimiasis. Completion of the paragonimus life cycle is supported by the human host's appetite for raw or undercooked freshwater crustaceans. In Japan, infection is acquired mostly through the contamination of hands and utensils in the preparation of crab soup. (*Courtesy of* H. Zaiman, MD.)

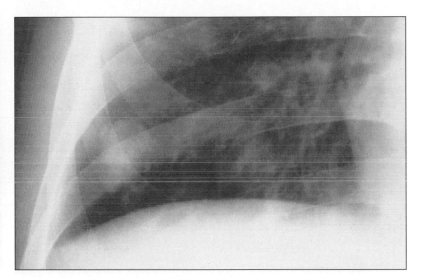

FIGURE 8-61 Chest radiographic features of paragonimiasis: Stage 1, migrating larvae. Patients with a large worm burden may complain of malaise, subcutaneous creeping tumors, chest or abdominal pain, and cough producing blood-streaked sputum 3 weeks after ingesting metacercaria in crustacea. Fluffy ill-defined infiltrates in the lower zones are typical, and, less frequently, pleural effusion and pneumothorax develop. Eosinophilia is seen in the peripheral blood. Most infected people, however, remain symptom-free or have vague symptoms and signs, complicating the diagnosis. In one series in an endemic zone, the correct initial diagnosis was made in only 25% of cases [34].

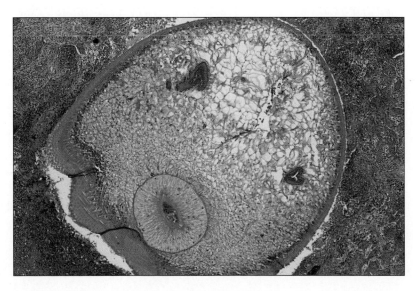

FIGURE 8-62 Cross-section of adult *Paragonimus* fluke in lung tissue. The adult fluke takes 1 to 27 months (average, 6) to become established in the lung. It is reddish brown, and preserved samples resemble coffee beans. The integument is covered with cuticular spines. The flukes lodge deep in the parenchyma near small bronchioles, where cystic cavities are formed in which they may live for 10 to 20 years. These cysts contain one to four worms and communicate with a bronchiole. (Hematoxylin-eosin stain.)

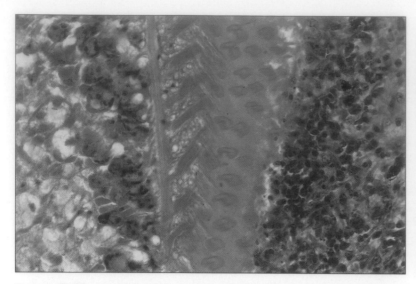

FIGURE 8-63 Longitudinal section of *Paragonimus westermani* in lung tissue, showing cuticular spines of the integument and surrounding inflammatory change. It is at this stage that patients most often present, complaining of persistent cough productive of gelatinous, tenacious, rusty-brown sputum. Fresh hemoptysis is common but irregular and rarely severe. Twenty percent of people complain of episodic pleuritic pain, and some may complain of wheezing. Most patients remain in good general health despite chronic infection. (Hematoxylin-eosin stain.) (*Courtesy of* Y. Yang, MD.)

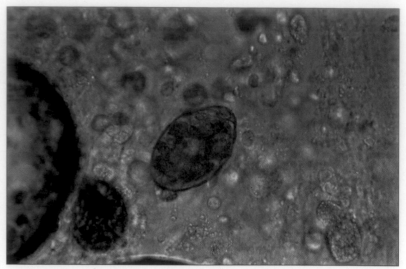

FIGURE 8-64 Ova of *Paragonimus westermani* in sputum. Up to 13,000 eggs a day are discharged into the sputum, from where they are coughed out or swallowed. The characteristic golden-brown, asymmetrical, operculate ova are unequivocal evidence of infection when found in sputum and should be looked for at the time of hemoptysis. An unstained smear should be examined, because the ova are destroyed by Ziehl-Neelsen stain. If worms are scanty, bronchioalveolar lavage or biopsy may be indicated. Stool examination is particularly helpful in diagnosing infected children. An enzyme-linked immunosorbent assay test for parago-nimus antibody is simple, quick, sensitive, and specific.

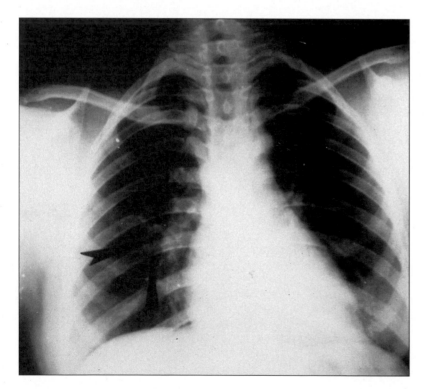

FIGURE 8-65 Chest radiographic features of paragonimiasis: Stage 2, adult worms. Radiographic features may not be conspicuous or extensive with adult flukes, but nodular, fibrotic, or bronchiectatic changes appear. Round or oval cysts varying in diameter from 0.5 to 4 cm are most often seen in the mid and lower zones bilaterally, close to the pleural surface. This is known as the "soap bubble" appearance. The cysts do not have fluid levels, and there is no mediastinal adenopathy. Pleural involvement with thickening or effusion is common, and bilateral hydropneumothorax suggests paragonimiasis in distinction to tuberculosis.

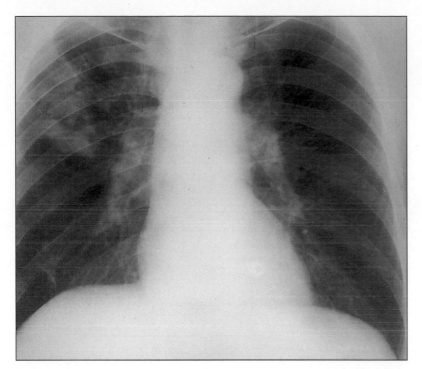

FIGURE 8-66 Chest radiographic features of paragonimiasis: Stage 3, recovery. After the death of the parasite, fibrosis follows, and the cysts disappear. Calcification may follow. The longer the duration of infection, the more extensive are the lesions. Reinfection leads to the superimposition of stages. Paragonimiasis is frequently mistaken for tuberculosis.

Schistosomiasis

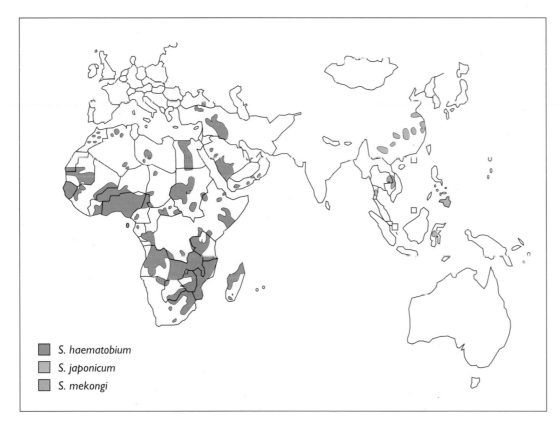

S. haematobium

S. japonicum

S. mekongi

FIGURE 8-67 Geographic distribution of schistosomiasis. Two hundred million people are currently infected with schistosomes, particularly in the agricultural communities of Africa, South America, and Asia, and the prevalence is increasing. In the United States, the absence of the intermediate snail host prevents transmission. Imported cases are not infrequent [35].

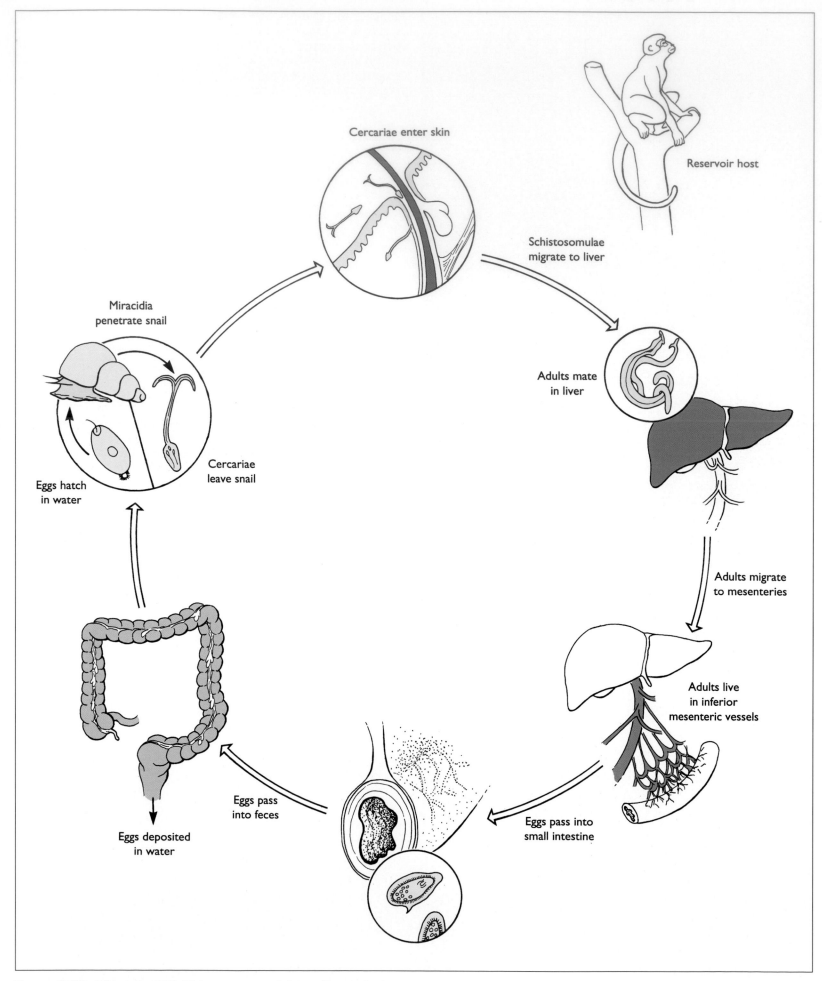

Figure 8-68 Life cycle of *Schistoma mansoni*. Lung disease is a complication of chronic infection with *S. mansoni*, and to a lesser extent *S. hematobium*.

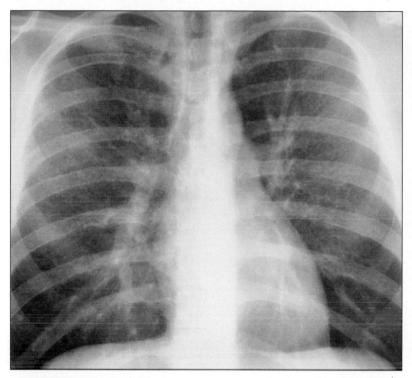

FIGURE 8-69 Chest radiograph in Katayama syndrome (acute schistosomiasis). By 4 to 8 weeks after schistosomal cercariae penetrate the skin, the worms have matured and oviposition begins. Katayama syndrome may then develop in travelers to endemic regions who are infected for the first time. It is characterized by acute onset of fever, headache, cough, abdominal pain, and diarrhea. Hepatosplenomegaly, lymphadenopathy, and marked eosinophilia are found. It is most severe after infection with *Schistosoma japonicum*, from which death has occurred. It has also been described following infection with *S. mansoni* but is rare with other species. Chest radiographs may show bilateral increase in interstitial markings and enlargement of hilar lymph nodes, which are abnormalities that may be exacerbated by treatment [36].

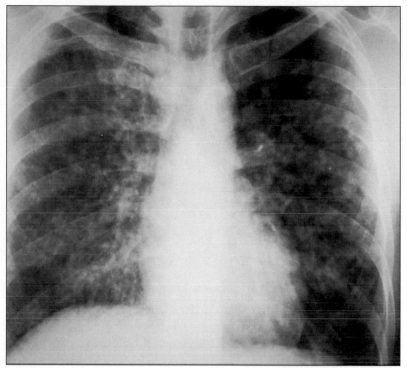

FIGURE 8-70 Chest radiograph showing miliary mottling in *Schistosoma mansoni* infection. Each pair of adult flukes in the mesenteric veins lives from 3 to 10 years and produces 200 to 3000 eggs daily. Most embolize to the liver, but some reach the pulmonary circulation, leading to obstruction to blood flow, arteritis, and granuloma formation followed by fibrous scarring. (*Courtesy of* G. McGuinness, MD.)

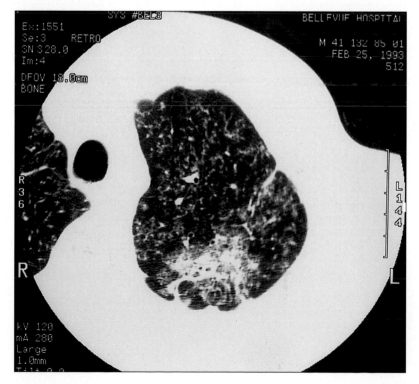

FIGURE 8-71 Computed tomography scan of the lung showing multiple *Schistosoma mansoni* granulomas. Tissue injury in chronic schistosomiasis is initiated by the egg-induced granulomas, which leads to collagen deposition and scarring, ultimately obstructing portal blood flow. (*Courtesy of* G. McGuinness, MD.)

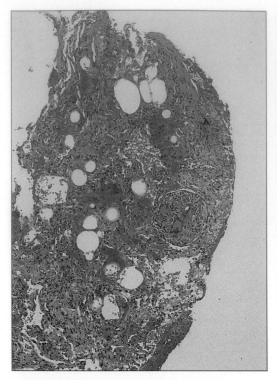

FIGURE 8-72 *Schistosoma mansoni* ova in lung tissue surrounded by granuloma. (Hematoxylin-eosin stain.) (*Courtesy of* J. Jagardir, MD.)

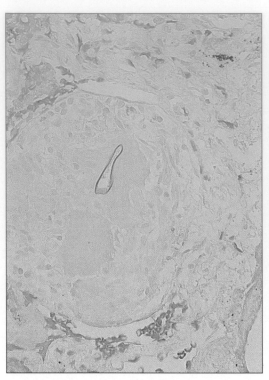

FIGURE 8-73 Acid-fast stain of *Schistosoma mansoni* granuloma. *Schistosoma hematobium* does not stain acid-fast. (*Courtesy of* J. Jagardir, MD.)

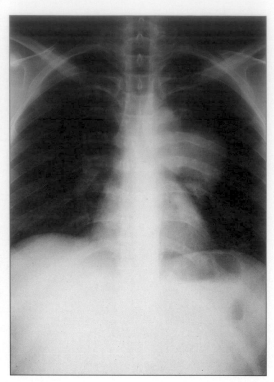

FIGURE 8-74 Chest radiograph showing a pulmonary artery aneurysm caused by *Schistosoma mansoni* infection.

Pentastomiasis (Porocephaliasis)

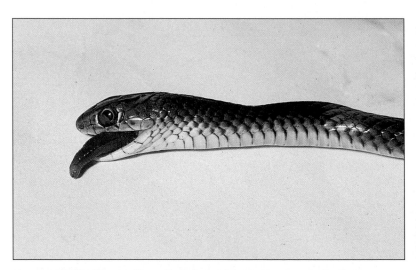

FIGURE 8-75 Papua New Guinean whip snake regurgitating a pentastomid. *Armillifer armillatus* is one of two genera of Pentasomida, or tongue worms, that cause human zoonotic disease. The adults, up to 20 cm long, live in the respiratory and digestive tracts of snakes. Ova are shed in nasal secretions and are picked up by herbivorous mammals. There, they may develop to the stage of nymphs but will only grow to adults in snakes [37]. (*Courtesy of* M. O'Shea, MD.)

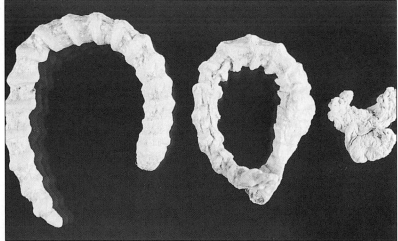

FIGURE 8-76 Adult *Armillifer armillatus* worms from the lungs of a gaboon viper. Humans ingest ova by drinking water contaminated by snakes or by eating living encysted larvae in raw or inadequately cooked snake meat. This infection has been reported in many tropical countries. (*Courtesy of* G.M. Ardran, MD.)

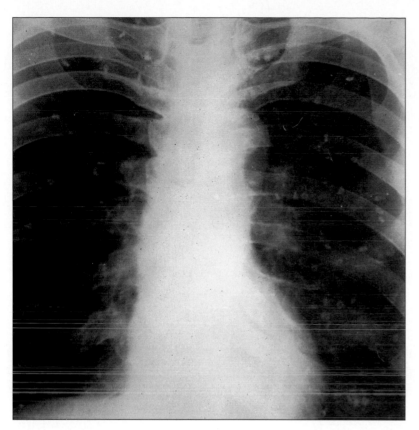

FIGURE 8-77 Chest radiograph showing calcified nymphs of *Armillifer armillatus* in the lung and soft tissue. Most infections are discovered by finding the characteristic discrete, crescent-shaped soft-tissue calcifications on radiographs of the chest and abdomen. In Ibadan, Nigeria, these shadows were seen in 2% of adult men and 4% of adult women. Inflammatory effects occasionally occur, and a number of fatal cases have been reported. (*Courtesy of* D.A. Warrell, MD.)

Therapy for Trematode Infections

Drug therapy for trematode-related lung disease in humans	
Paragonimus spp	Praziquantel, 25 mg/kg orally three times a day × 2 days
Schistosoma spp	
Katayama fever	Praziquantel, 25 mg/kg orally every 4 hrs with food × 3 doses
Established infection	Praziquantel, 20 mg/kg orally every 4 hrs with food × 2 doses

FIGURE 8-78 Drug therapy for trematode-related lung disease in humans.

REFERENCES

1. Lyche KD, Jensen WA, Kirsch CM, *et al.*: Pleuropulmonary manifestations of hepatic amebiasis. *West J Med* 1990, 153:275–278.

2. le Roux BT, Mohlala ML, Odell JA, Whitton ID: Suppurative diseases of the lung and pleural space: Part 1. Empyema thoracis and lung abscess. *Curr Probl Surg* 1986, 23:1–89.

3. Gozal D: The incidence of pulmonary manifestations during *Plasmodium falciparum* malaria in non-immune subjects. *Trop Med Parasitol* 1992, 43(1):6–8.

4. Warrell DA: Treatment of severe malaria. *J R Soc Med* 1989, 82(suppl 17):44–50.

5. Boustani MR, Lepore TJ, Gelfand JA, Lazarus DS: Acute respiratory failure in patients treated for babesiosis. *Am J Respir Crit Care Med* 1994, 149:1689–1691.

6. Pomeroy C, Filice GA: Pulmonary toxoplasmosis: A review. *Clin Infect Dis* 1992, 14:863–870.

7. Nash G, Kerschmann RL, Herndier B, Dubey JP: The pathological manifestations of pulmonary toxoplasmosis in the acquired immunodeficiency syndrome. *Hum Pathol* 1994, 25:652–658.

8. Kwon-Chung KJ: Phylogenetic spectrum of fungi that are pathogenic to humans. *Clin Infect Dis* 1994, 19(suppl I):S1–S7.

9. Hopewell PC, Masur H: *Pneumocystis carinii* pneumonia: Current concepts. *In* Sande MA, Volberding PA (eds.): *The Medical Management of AIDS*, 4th ed. Philadelphia: W.B. Saunders; 1995:367–401.

10. Pirmez C: Immunopathology of American cutaneous leishmaniasis. *Mem Inst Oswaldo Cruz* 1992, 87(suppl 5):105–109.

11. Andrade TM, Carvalho EM, Rocha H: Bacterial infections in patients with visceral leishmaniasis. *J Infect Dis* 1990, 162:1354–1359.

12. Wilson RA: Immunity and immunoregulation in helminth infections. *Curr Opin Immunol* 1993, 5:538–547.

13. Sutton BJ, Gould HJ: The human IgE network. *Nature* 1993, 366:421–428.

14. Weller PF: The immunobiology of eosinophils. *N Engl J Med* 1994, 324:1110–1116.

15. Galli SJ: New concepts about the mast cell. *N Engl J Med* 1993, 328:257–265.

16. Meeker DP: Pulmonary infiltrates and eosinophilia revisited. *Cleve Clin J Med* 1989, 56:199–211.

17. Otterson EA, Nutman TB: Tropical pulmonary eosinophilia. *Annu Rev Med* 1992, 43:417–424.

18. Daar AS, Mabogunje O: Ascariasis and other intestinal nematode infections. *In* Morris PJ, Malt RA (eds.): *Oxford Textbook of Surgery*. 1st ed. Oxford: Oxford University Press; 1995.

19. Liu LX, Weller PF: Strongyloidiasis and other intestinal nematode infections. *Infect Dis Clin North Am* 1993, 7(3):655–682.

20. Milder JE, Walzer PD, Kilgore G, *et al.*: Clinical features of *Strongyloides stercoralis* infection in an endemic area of the United States. *Gastroenterology* 1981, 80:1481–1488.

21. Davidson RA: Infection due to *Strongyloides stercoralis* in patients with pulmonary disease. *South Med J* 1992, 85:28–31.

22. Remington JS, Swartz MN (eds.).: *Current Clinical Topics in Infectious Disease*, vol 7. New York: McGraw-Hill, 1986:1.

23. Henry CJ, Dillon R: Heartworm disease in dogs. *J Am Vet Med Assoc* 1994, 204:1148–1151.

24. Green KL, Ansari MQ, Schwartz MR, *et al.*: Non-specific whiteners in the rapid recognition of pulmonary dirofilariasis: A report of 20 cases. *Thorax* 1994, 49:590–593.

25. de Lara T, de A Barbosa MA, de Oliviera MR, *et al.*: Human syngamosis: Two cases of chronic cough caused by *Mammomonogamus laryngeus*. *Chest* 1993, 103:264–265.

26. Torres JR, Isturiz R, Murillo J, *et al.* Efficacy of ivermectin in the treatment of strongyloidiasis complicating AIDS. *Clin Infect Dis* 1993, 17:900–902.

27. Kammerer WS, Schantz PM: Echinococcal disease. *Infect Dis Clin North Am* 1993, 7(3):605–618.

28. Pinch LW, Wilson JF: Nonsurgical management of cystic hydatid disease in Alaska: A review of 30 cases of *Echinococcus granulosus* infection treated without operation. *Ann Surg* 1972, 176:45–48.

29. Reeder MM, Palmer PS: Hydatid disease (echinococcosis). *In* Reeder MM, Palmer PS (eds.): *The Radiology of Tropical Disease*. Baltimore: Williams & Wilkins, 1981:157–223.

30. von Sinner WN: Ultrasound, CT and MRI of ruptured and disseminated hydatid cysts. *Eur J Radiol* 1990, 11:31–37.

31. von Sinner WN, Rifai A, teStrake L, Sieck J: Magnetic resonance imaging of thoracic hydatid disease: Correlation with clinical findings, radiology, ultrasonograpy, CT and pathology. *Acta Radiol* 1990, 31:59–62.

32. von Sinner WN: Radiographic CT and MRI spectrum of hydatid disease of the chest: A pictorial essay. *Eur Radiol* 1993, 3:62–70.

33. Nana A, Bovornkitti S: Pleuropulmonary paragonimiasis. *Semin Respir Med* 1991, 12:46–54.

34. Shim YS, Cho SY, Han YC: Pulmonary paragonimiasis: A Korean perspective. *Semin Respir Med* 1991, 12:35–45.

35. Mahmoud AAF, Abdel Wahab MF: Schistosomiasis. *In* Warren KS, Mahmoud AAF (eds.): *Tropical and Geographical Medicine*, 2nd ed. New York: McGraw-Hill, 1990:458–473.

36. Mahmoud AA: Schistosomiasis: An overview. *Immunol Invest* 1992, 21:383–390.

37. Warrell DA: Pentastomiasis (porocephalosis). *In* Morris PJ, Malt RA (eds.): *Oxford Textbook of Medicine*, 2nd ed. Oxford: Oxford University Press; 1987, vol 5, 603–605.

SELECTED BIBLIOGRAPHY

Maguire JH, Keystone J (eds.): Parasitic diseases. *Infect Dis Clin North Am* 1993, 7(3):467–738.

Mahmoud AAF (ed.): Section I: Diseases due to helminths. *In* Mandell GL, Bennett JE, Dolin R (eds.): *Principles and Practice of Infectious Diseases*, 4th ed. New York: Churchill-Livingstone; 1995:2525–2557.

Ravdin J (ed.): Section H: Protozoal diseases. *In* Mandell GL, Bennett JE, Dolin R (eds.): *Principles and Practice of Infectious Diseases*, 4th ed. New York: Churchill-Livingstone; 1995:2393–2524.

Reeder MM, Palmer PS (eds.): *The Radiology of Tropical Disease*. Baltimore: Williams & Wilkins; 1981.

Warren KS, Mahmoud AAF (eds.): *Tropical and Geographical Medicine*, 2nd ed. New York: McGraw-Hill; 1990.

CHAPTER 9

Pleural Effusion and Empyema

Christopher J. Salmon
Richard E. Bryant

ANATOMY

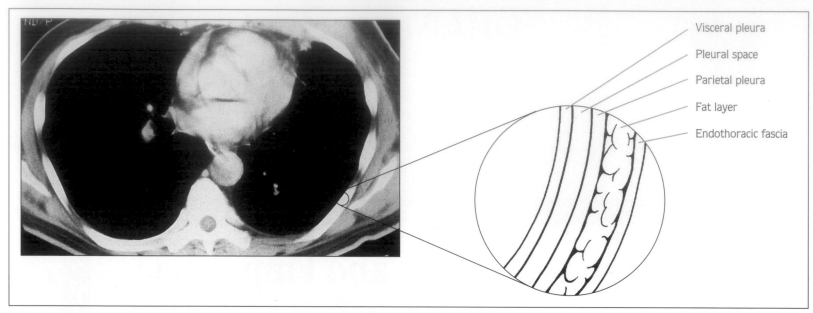

FIGURE 9-1 Anatomy of the normal pleura and surrounding tissues. The *visceral pleura* surrounds the individual pulmonary lobes and is contiguous with the subpleural pulmonary interstitium. It is approximately 200 µm thick and derives its blood supply from both pulmonary and systemic arteries, draining to the pulmonary veins. The *parietal pleura* consists of four layers, is slightly thinner than the visceral pleura and is supplied and drained by systemic vessels. It is surrounded by a layer of *fat* with a mean thickness of 250 µm. This extrapleural fatty layer may slightly thicken posterolaterally and laterally and can thus occasionally be visualized on computed tomography (CT) scans and chest radiographs of normal individuals. It commonly becomes diffusely thickened in the setting of pleural disease, especially empyema. It is not diffusely thickened in obese patients without pleural disease. The fatty layer is, in turn, surrounded by a layer of fibroelastic fascia, called the *endothoracic fascia*, that forms the boundary of the thoracic cavity. Anteriorly, this fascia is intimately related to the perichondrium of the costal cartilage. The endothoracic fascia lines the inner aspect of the ribs and intercostal muscles and forms a continuous sheath that posteriorly overlies the prevertebral fascia. The *pleural space* is interposed between the parietal and visceral pleura. It normally contains so little pleural fluid that it cannot be visualized by chest radiographs or CT scan. The thickness of the pleural space is normally about 20 µm. The pleural space and its contents effectively couple the lungs to the chest wall and diaphragm and lubricate the lungs to allow their movement relative to the chest wall and diaphragm.

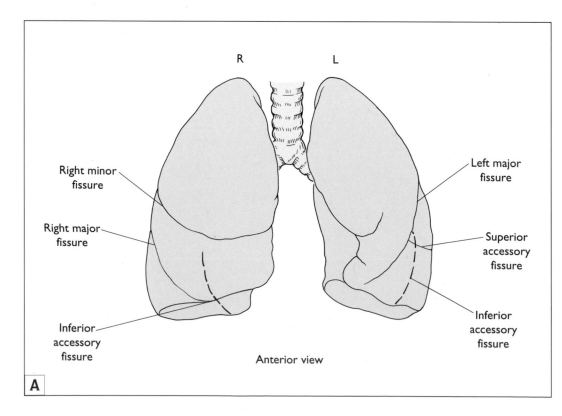

A

FIGURE 9-2 Accessory fissures. The pulmonary fissures are curved surfaces between two pulmonary lobes. They consist of the visceral pleura of the participating lobes, with a minute amount of interposed pleural fluid. **A,** Fissures commonly recognized on chest radiographs include the right major and minor fissures and the left major fissure. Anomalous pulmonary fissures are often noted at thoracotomy or postmortem examination but are less commonly appreciated on radiologic studies. Although fissures can occur between any adjacent bronchopulmonary segments, two particular variant patterns are commonly noted. The *inferior accessory fissure* separates the medial basal segment of the right lower lobe (or the medial subsegment of the anteromedial basal segment of the left lower lobe) from the rest of the lower lobe segments. The *superior accessory fissure* separates the superior segment of a right or left lower lobe from the basal segments of that lobe. Inferior and superior accessory fissures are present (at least incompletely) in about 40% to 50% and 30% of people, respectively. (*continued*)

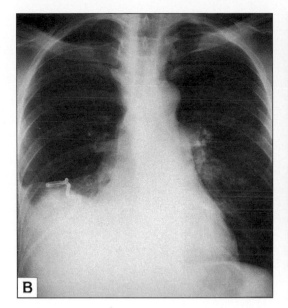

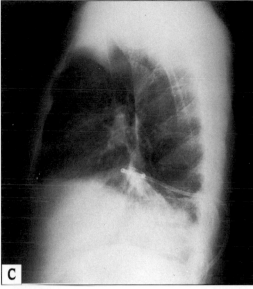

FIGURE 9-2 (*continued*) **B** and **C**, Posteroanterior and lateral chest radiographs show that a pleural drainage catheter, placed by a posterior approach for treatment of an empyema, has entered a right-sided superior accessory fissure, running in a horizontal plane.

DIAGNOSIS

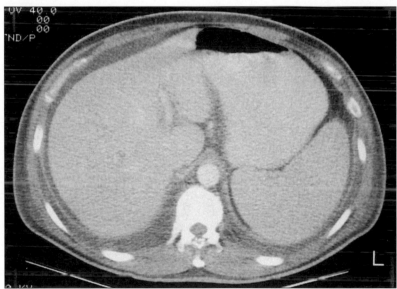

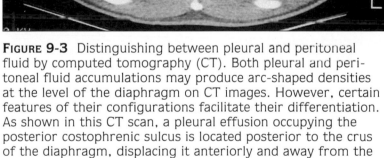

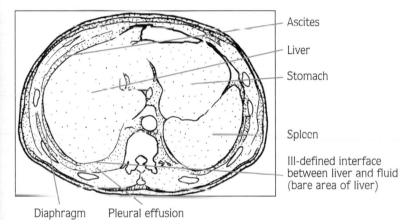

FIGURE 9-3 Distinguishing between pleural and peritoneal fluid by computed tomography (CT). Both pleural and peritoneal fluid accumulations may produce arc-shaped densities at the level of the diaphragm on CT images. However, certain features of their configurations facilitate their differentiation. As shown in this CT scan, a pleural effusion occupying the posterior costophrenic sulcus is located posterior to the crus of the diaphragm, displacing it anteriorly and away from the spine. Ascitic fluid is situated anterior to the diaphragmatic crus. The apparent interface between ascitic fluid and the dome of the liver is well-defined, whereas that between the hepatic dome and a pleural collection is ill-defined. Finally, because the posterior aspect of the liver attaches directly to the abdominal wall and diaphragm, this "bare area" (devoid of peritoneal covering) will not admit peritoneal fluid around it. Fluid presenting behind the liver is therefore pleural, located in the posterior costophrenic sulcus. In this patient, a 40-year-old man with AIDS, the pleural effusions are bilateral.

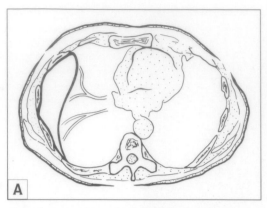 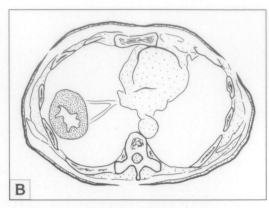

FIGURE 9-4 Distinguishing lung abscess from empyema by computed tomography (CT). Differentiating lung abscess from empyema is often impossible by chest radiography, but the CT findings are usually diagnostic. **A**, Empyemas usually are well defined, smooth, and round or elliptical in configuration. Their margins of inflamed visceral and parietal pleura enhance when radiographic contrast is given. These pleural leaves are separated by the interposed infected fluid collection, giving rise to the "split pleura sign." When air is introduced into them iatrogenically or spontaneously by a bronchopleural fistula, their inner margins are usually smooth. Empyema collections form acute or obtuse angles with the adjacent chest wall and displace subjacent lung. **B**, Lung abscesses are characteristically poorly defined and roughly spherical, surrounded by irregularly consolidated lung. They often contain multiple cavities with shaggy inner mural contours. When peripherally abutting the pleural surface, they form acute angles with the chest wall and rarely displace surrounding lung parenchyma and vessels.

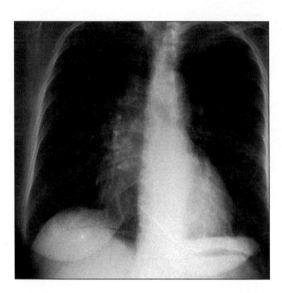 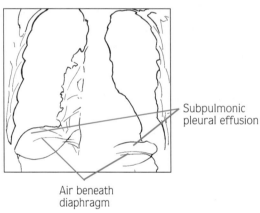

Subpulmonic
pleural effusion

Air beneath
diaphragm

FIGURE 9-5 Subpulmonic pleural effusions. Pleural effusions of significant size may collect principally in subpulmonic locations, without blunting of the costophrenic sulci on chest radiographs. In such cases, the configuration of the diaphragm provides a useful clue to the presence of the effusion: the apex of the affected hemidiaphragm appears to be displaced laterally. The moderate effusions in this patient illustrate this point. The subpulmonic pleural effusions are confirmed by the presence of free air under the diaphragm. The patient had recently undergone peritoneal dialysis.

FIGURE 9-6 Features differentiating exudative from transudative pleural effusion. Pleural effusion may be described as exudative or transudative according to Light's criteria, with an exudate satisfying one or both of the following criteria (and a transudate satisfying neither): 1) pleural fluid protein/serum protein ratio > 0.5, and 2) pleural fluid lactate dehydrogenase (LDH)/serum LDH ratio > 0.6.

Features differentiating exudative from transudative pleural effusion

	Transudate	Exudate
Appearance	Serous	Cloudy, bloody
Leukocyte count	< 10,000/mm³	Usually > 50,000/mm³
pH	> 7.2	< 7.2
Protein	< 3.0 g/dL	> 3.0 g/dL
LDH	< 200 IU/L	> 200 IU/L*
Fluid/serum LDH	< 0.6	> 0.6
Glucose	< 60 mg/dL	Usually < 60 mg/dL
Stained smears/cultures	No organisms	Pathogen

*May exceed 1000.
LDH—lactate dehydrogenase.

Differential diagnosis of exudative pleural disease effusion

Infection
Bacterial
Mycobacterial
Fungal
Parasitic
Mixed

Gastrointestinal disease
Esophageal perforation
Mediastinitis
Subdiaphragmatic infection

Other
Collagen-vascular disease
Malignancy
Uremia
Drug-induced disease
Pulmonary embolism
Abestosis
Sarcoidosis
Radiation injury
Trauma
Hemothorax
Chylothorax

FIGURE 9-7 Differential diagnosis of exudative pleural effusion. Once an effusion is classified as exudative, diagnostic considerations include many infectious and noninfectious diseases.

Disease associated with transudative pleural effusions

Heart, kidney, renal failure
Cirrhosis
Nephrotic syndrome
Pericardial disease
Myxedema
Sarcoidosis
Pulmonary emboli
Superior vena cava obstruction

FIGURE 9-8 Diseases associated with transudative pleural effusion. Differential diagnosis of transudative effusions subsumes a myriad of noninfectious causes.

A. Evaluation of empyema or complicated pleural effusion: Clinical risk assessment

Clinical presentation
Physical examination
Epidemiologic or host-specific disease susceptibility
Factors suggesting malignancy, rheumatologic disease, tissue injury from trauma or surgery, or contiguous infection
Severity of patient's infectious disease (the sickest and most susceptible need intervention most urgently)

B. Evaluation of empyema or complicated pleural effusion: Radiologic assessment

Routine posteroanterior and lateral views (< 1-cm meniscus usually treated with antibiotics)
Loculation assessed by:
Bilateral decubitus views
Ultrasound if volume is small
Computed tomography if site or volume is in question

FIGURE 9-9 Evaluation of empyema or complicated pleural effusion. **A** and **B**, Clinical assessment of infected pleural collections includes findings on history, physical examination, laboratory, and radiologic studies. **C**, Once a pleural collection is detected, fluid analysis is essential. Fluid may be obtained at the bedside with ultrasound guidance if needed, or under computed tomography guidance when the fluid is otherwise difficult to access or localize. The decision to place a chest tube is predicated on the character of the fluid obtained. (LDH—lactate dehydrogenase.)

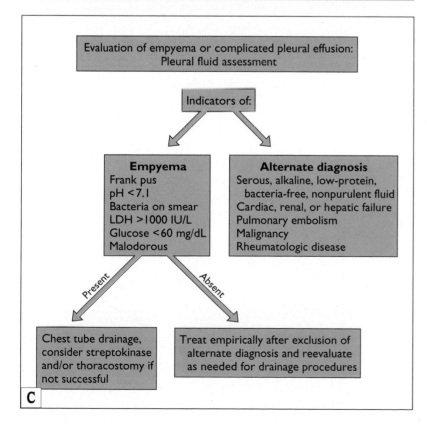

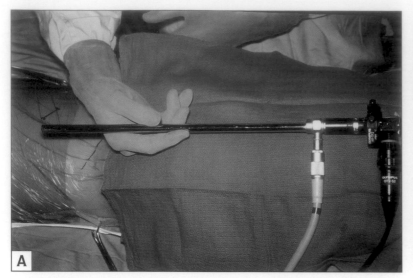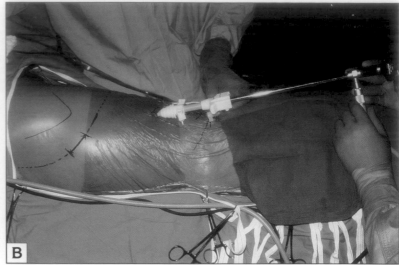

FIGURE 9-10 Video-assisted thoracoscopic surgery for pleural disease. The development of miniaturized video technology has allowed for less-invasive access to the pleural space for various surgical applications. **A,** The principal piece of equipment is the optical system, such as the rigid thoracoscope. The device uses a light-sensitive silicon chip to generate a real-time color image on a television screen. **B,** It is introduced into the pleural space through a cylindrical conduit. The ipsilateral lung is collapsed, while the other lung is selectively ventilated. Two additional 1.0- to 1.5-cm incisions are made to allow passage of surgical instruments to be used under thoracoscopic visualization. The morbidity of full thoracotomy is thus avoided. Besides its use for mediastinal and pulmonary disorders, thoracoscopy is often undertaken for diagnosis and therapy of pleural disease. Diagnostic procedures are generally done to exclude malignancy, with specific benign diagnoses not commonly made. Empyema and complicated (*ie*, loculated) parapneumonic effusions may be managed in part by thoracoscopy in selected patients. Lesions causing pneumothorax can be treated. Pleurodesis can also be performed under thoracoscopic guidance. (*Courtesy of* G. Ott, MD.)

EMPYEMA AND PARAPNEUMONIC EFFUSION

Bacteriologic findings in 217 cases of empyema				
Study	Aerobic or facultative only	Anaerobic only	Mixed aerobic/anaerobic	Sterile
Mandal *et al.*	44%	14%	20%	22%
Varkey *et al.**	40%	31%	8%	14%
Bartlett *et al.*	24%	35%	41%	NA[†]

*Includes 7% (mycobacteria or fungal infection).
[†]Excludes culture-negative cases.
NA—not applicable.

FIGURE 9-11 Bacteriology of empyema. Bacteriologic findings from three large published series of empyemas are summarized [1–3].

Incidence of pleural effusion and bacterial infection of the pleural space complicating pneumonia

	Incidence	
Infecting organism	Pleural effusion	Infected pleural space
Streptococcus pyogenes	75%	35%
Streptococcus pneumoniae	50%	3%
Staphylococcus aureus	40%	20%
Haemophilus influenzae	45%	20%
Escherichia coli	40%	80%
Klebsiella pneumoniae	10%	20%
Pseudomonas aeruginosa	50%	40%
Anaerobes	35%	90%
Legionella spp	40%	?
Mycoplasma pneumoniae	10%	NA
Viral, Q fever, psittacosis	Rare	NA

NA—not applicable.

FIGURE 9-12 Incidence of pleural effusion and bacterial infection of the pleural space complicating pneumonia. The frequencies of associated pleural effusion and infections are estimated in a variety of pneumonias. (*Adapted from* Light [4]; with permission.)

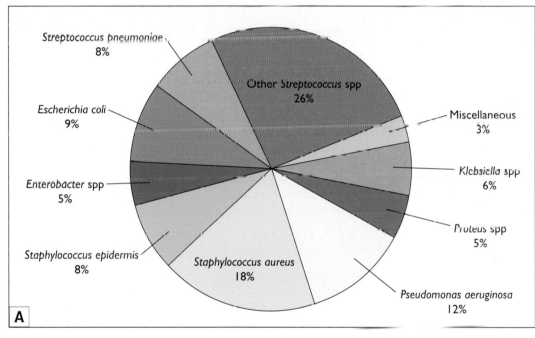

FIGURE 9-13 Pathogenic bacteria in empyema. **A**, Empyema caused by aerobic bacteria. **B**, Empyema caused by anaerobic bacteria. Cumulative data from three recent series are presented [1–3].

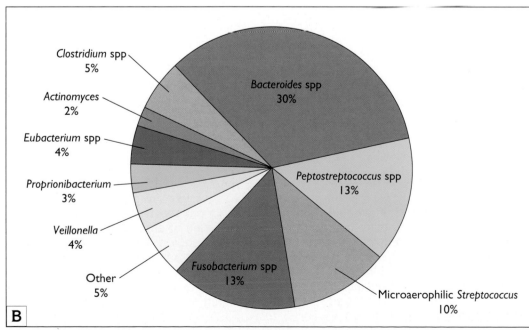

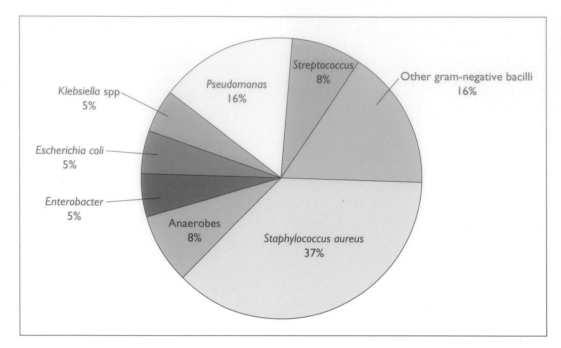

FIGURE 9-14 Causative bacteria in empyema following trauma. (*Adapted from* Caplan *et al.* [5]; with permission.)

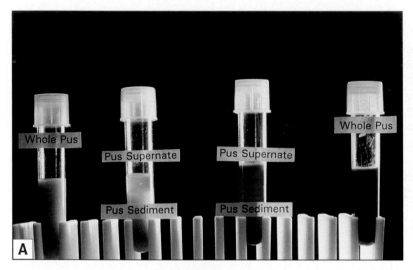

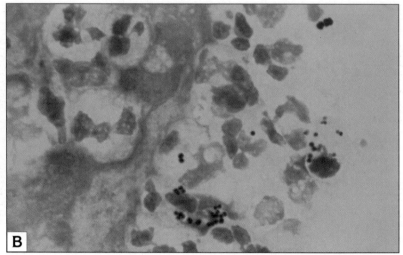

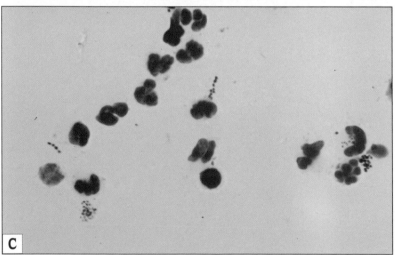

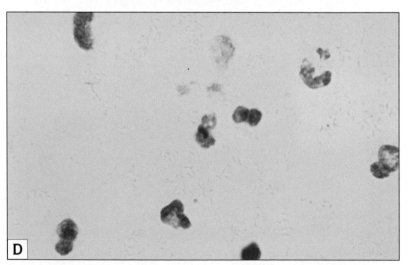

FIGURE 9-15 Microbiologic studies on pus samples obtained from empyemas. **A,** Nonhemorrhagic and darker hemorrhagic pus samples are shown in whole and centrifuged forms. The serous supernatant and the grumose, dependent debris from distinct phases in the centrifuged samples. Empyema fluid varies widely in appearance, chiefly due to its content of hemoglobin, cells, and debris. **B,** Gram stain demonstrates *Staphylococcus aureus* in empyema fluid at a concentration of approximately 10^8 bacteria/mL of pus, which greatly exceeds 100 microorganisms per high-powered microscopic field. Note the grouping of bacteria within phagocytic cells, indicating intracellular growth. **C,** Gram stain of empyema fluid reveals both *S. aureus* and streptococci, shown in clumps and chains, respectively. **D,** Empyema fluid shows high concentrations of pleomorphic gram-negative bacilli typical of *Haemophilus influenzae*. The extensive lysis of neutrophils may have contributed to the poor staining of the microorganisms. (Panels 15B–D *courtesy of* J.W. Rourke, Jr, MD.)

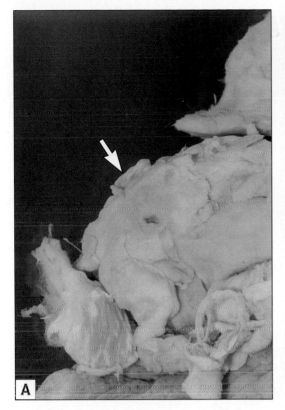

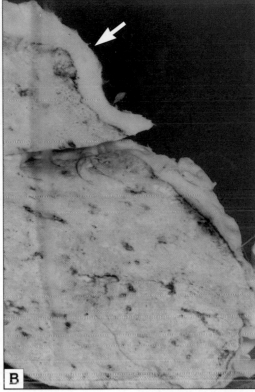

FIGURE 9-16 Pathologic specimen of organized empyema in a patient dying of cancer. **A**, An external view shows the lung covered by the organized empyema (*arrow*). **B**, Cross-sectional view of the lung and empyema reveals an 8-mm-thick fibrous peel (*arrow*). (*Courtesy of* N.R. Niles, MD.)

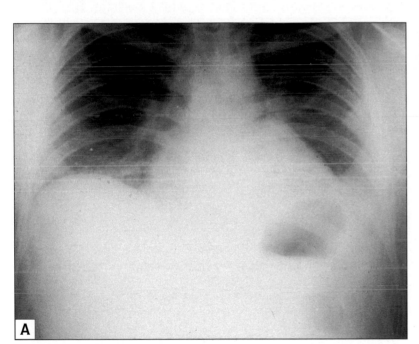

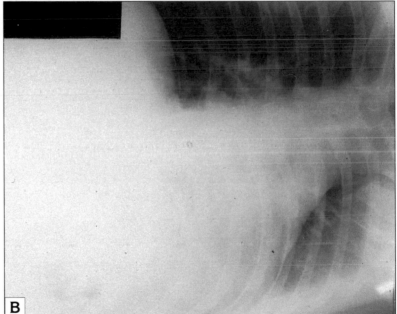

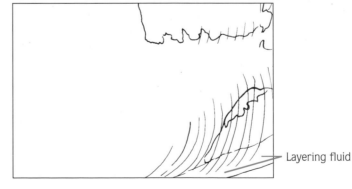

Layering fluid

FIGURE 9-17 Acute adenovirus pneumonia with associated parapneumonic effusion. **A** and **B**, Posteroanterior and left lateral decubitus radiographs demonstrate a mobile left pleural effusion. On the left lateral decubitus view, the fluid layer is interposed between aerated lung and the lateral ribs. A common pathogen in children, adenovirus occasionally causes atypical pneumonias in adults. Viral pneumonias may be associated with nonpurulent, exudative pleural effusions, and require no specific treatment.

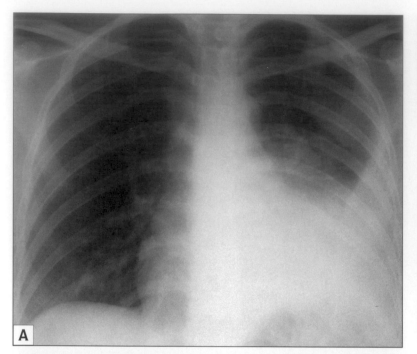

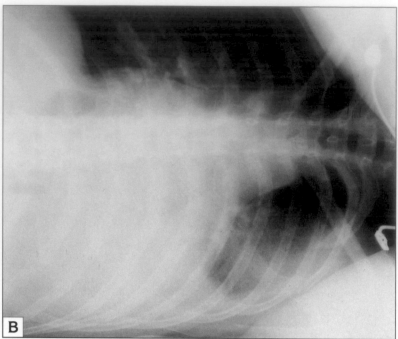

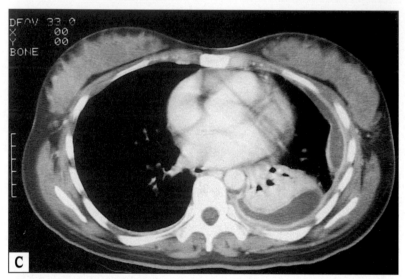

FIGURE 9-18 Acute community-acquired pneumonia with complicated parapneumonic effusion. **A,** Posteroanterior chest radiograph of a 30-year-old woman with fever and cough shows a left lower lobe consolidation. The lateral aspect of the density has the appearance of a pleural effusion, forming a meniscus. **B,** The left lateral decubitus view shows minimal alteration of the pleural shadow, indicating the presence of loculations. Ultrasound study (not shown) was not helpful in delineating the effusion. **C,** A computed tomography (CT) scan shows the loculated pleural effusion and subjacent pulmonary consolidation. The visceral and parietal pleural layers that envelop the pleural fluid collections are thickened and brightly enhance with intravenous contrast, indicating their inflamed, hyperemic character. Fat hyperplasia external to the parietal pleura is clearly visible in association with this effusion of < 1 week's duration. Pleural fluid was obtained by CT-guided diagnostic thoracentesis.

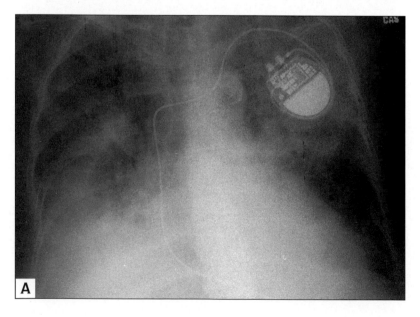

FIGURE 9-19 Bilateral parapneumonic pleural effusions. **A,** A radiograph taken with the patient supine shows extensive bilateral density. The element of diffuse "ground-glass" density over both lungs suggests that bilateral pleural effusions are present. The right costophrenic angle is also blunted, whereas the left angle was sharp in appearance. This finding implied a relatively larger effusion on the right side than on the left. (*continued*)

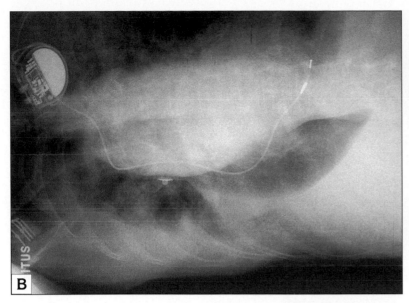

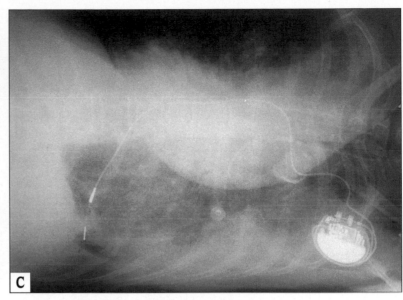

FIGURE 9-19 (*continued*) **B** and **C**, Right and left lateral decubitus views show freely flowing right and left pleural effusions. Bilateral upper lobe pneumonias are shown to much better advantage and are no longer obscured by the effusions. Approximate quantification of the pleural fluid is possible; a layer of fluid of 1 cm thickness is equal to about 400-mL volume in an adult patient.

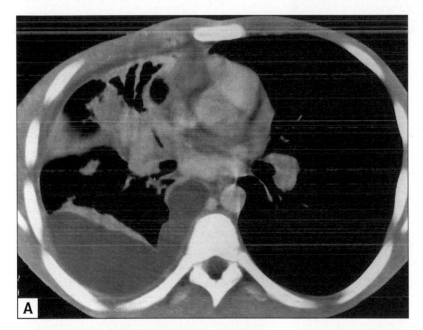

FIGURE 9-20 Pseudomonas empyema managed with intracavitary urokinase. An 18-year-old man with cystic fibrosis with Pseudomonas pneumonia of the right lung, complicated by effusion, had protracted fever despite appropriate antibiotic coverage. **A**, Contrast-enhanced computed tomography scan strongly suggests that the pleural collection, by its restricted configuration of fluid in nondependent locations, contains loculations. The individual septations are invisible because they have the same density as the pleural fluid. The pneumonia is visible anteriorly. **B**, Ultrasound of the pleural effusion reveals dependent, echogenic debris and a network of clearly defined limiting membranes, confirming the loculated nature of the collection. The brightly echogenic area in the lower portion of the image represents aerated lung. This image was used to select a percutaneous approach for catheter drainage, targeting the large loculation at the right. **C** and **D**, Posteroanterior and lateral chest radiographs were done following catheter placement and immediate removal of 150 mL of fluid. The catheter folds back upon itself within the pleural loculation, a configuration maintained for 24 hours with scant additional fluid output from the catheter. The patient remained febrile. Urokinase instillation through the catheter was then used to improve drainage. (*continued*)

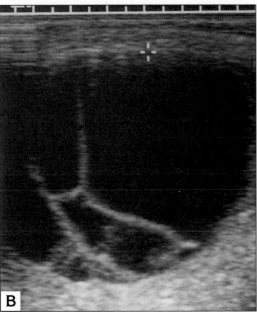

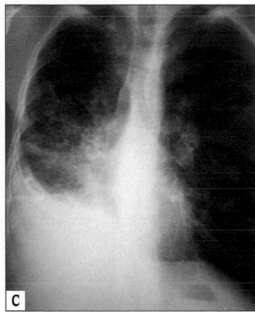

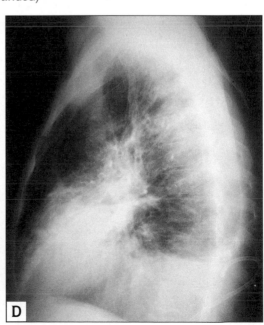

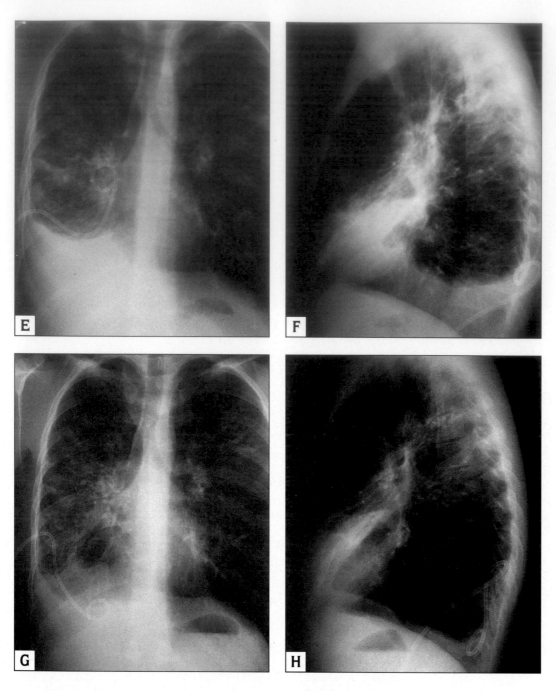

FIGURE 9-20 *(continued)* **E** and **F**, Chest radiographs obtained after the first urokinase instillation show that the walls of the loculation around the distal end of the catheter have been lysed, which permits the previously coiled catheter to uncoil. **G** and **H**, Serial urokinase installations and drainages were continued over a period of 48 hours, and the catheter was fluoroscopically repositioned. An additional 1200 mL of pleural fluid was removed with the aid of intracavitary urokinase. The patient defervesced within 24 hours of beginning urokinase use and subsequently responded fully to antibiotics.

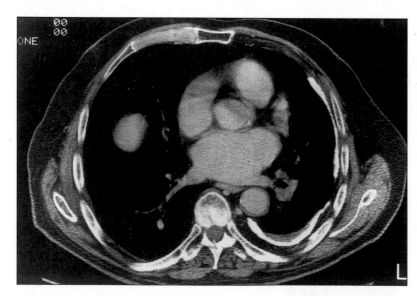

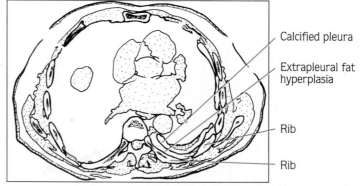

radiograph showed calcified "pleural thickening" typical of a healed tuberculous empyema. The computed tomography (CT) image reveals that pleural fibrosis and thickening actually constitute a relatively small proportion of the soft tissue external to the lungs and deep to the ribs. Most of the pleural thickening is due to extrapleural fat hyperplasia, seen as low-density tissue on CT. This condition was not generally appreciated before the advent of CT scanning. Note the similarity of its appearance to that of subcutaneous fat.

FIGURE 9-21 Chronic tuberculous empyema with extensive calcification. This patient had a remote history of tuberculosis, and his chest

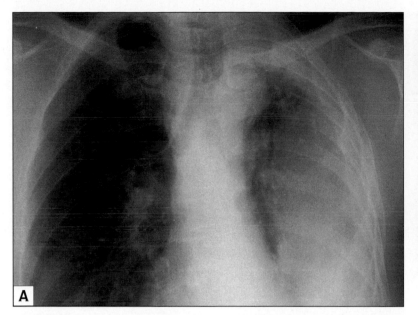

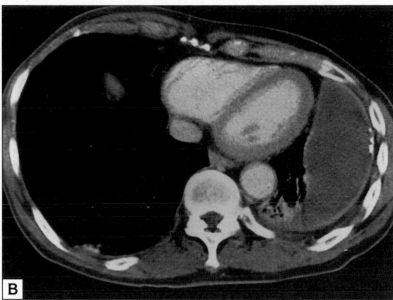

FIGURE 9-22 Large chronic tuberculous empyema. An asymptomatic 54-year-old man had a remote history of tuberculosis. **A,** The postcroanterior chest radiograph shows extensive thickening of the pleura laterally on the left side. Calcification is present. This radiographic appearance was unchanged during 10 years of observation. The differential diagnosis of unilateral thickened and calcified pleura includes a chronic empyema, most likely to be tuberculous, or a posttraumatic, organized hemothorax. The latter diagnosis is usually associated with healed ipsilateral rib fractures, not seen in the current case. **B,** Contrast-enhanced computed tomography image reveals a large chronic tuberculous empyema. The rib interspaces are narrowed, reflecting volume loss. Marked extrapleural fat hyperplasia is evident, deep to the ribs and superficial to the parietal pleura. Both parietal and visceral pleura are thickened and demonstrate contrast enhancement. Both layers also demonstrate focal calcification. Pleural collections due to tuberculosis can remain clinically quiescent and unchanged for many years. Drainage of such chronic collections is not indicated.

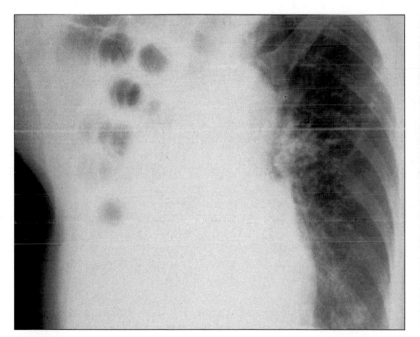

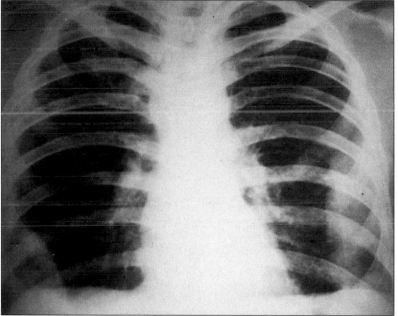

FIGURE 9-23 Lucite ball plombage for tuberculosis. Intrapleural placement of air-filled lucite balls was a commonly employed surgical therapy for pulmonary tuberculosis in the 1940s. Several complications were soon observed, and with the advent of effective chemotherapy, the technique was abandoned. Plombage was one of several mechanical approaches taken to collapse diseased lung and reduce oxygen availability to the aerobic mycobacteria. Other methods included pneumothorax, pneumoperitoneum, thoracoplasty, and phrenic nerve crushing. Chest radiographs showing the results of these procedures are rarely encountered in clinical practice. However, with the development of multidrug resistance and the increased incidence of tuberculosis in AIDS patients, surgical treatments will likely assume renewed importance.

FIGURE 9-24 Paragonimiasis. The chest film of a young man from Southeast Asia shows bilateral pleural effusions with an atypical configuration that suggests loculation. They did not layer freely on decubitus films. Analysis revealed an exudate with low glucose and low pH. There is a right upper lobe infiltrate with small areas of cystic lucency, often seen in paragonimiasis. Such cases may often be misdiagnosed initially as tuberculosis. Effusions are present in about half of paragonimiasis patients, sometimes as the only manifestation of disease.

DIFFERENTIAL DIAGNOSIS

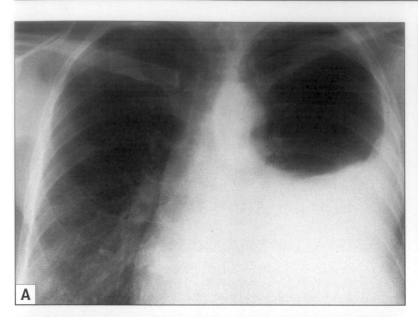

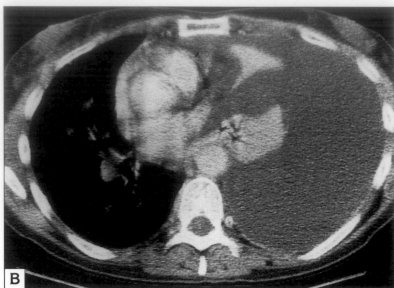

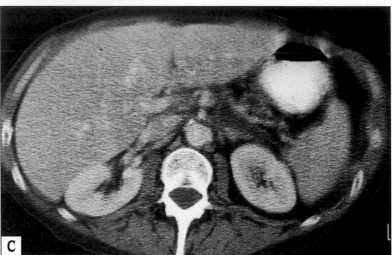

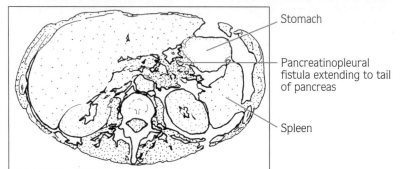

FIGURE 9-25 Large pleural effusion caused by a pancreaticopleural fistula. A 50-year-old woman with a history of alcohol use and bouts of pancreatitis presented with dyspnea, left-sided pleuritic pain, and nonproductive cough. **A,** The chest film showed a large left pleural effusion, with slight associated contralateral mediastinal shift, but was otherwise unremarkable. Thoracentesis yielded a bloody exudate. The amylase content of the fluid was > 5000 IU/L. The differential diagnosis of high-amylase pleural effusion includes esophageal rupture (amylase of salivary gland origin), neoplasm (< 10% of cases), and, rarely, pneumonia or ruptured ectopic pregnancy. **B** and **C,** Computed tomography images through the lower thorax and upper abdomen show the large left pleural effusion with compressive atelectasis of the underlying lung parenchyma. The abnormal fluid-density coursing contiguously from the pleural effusion to the tail of the pancreas corresponded to the pancreaticopleural fistula.

FIGURE 9-26 Sympathetic effusion secondary to subphrenic abscess. A 21-year-old woman developed intra-abdominal abscesses following rupture of an undiagnosed appendicitis. Her preceding clinical syndrome had been diagnosed as gastroenteritis while she traveled in Mexico. **A,** The chest radiograph shows the left pleural effusion. (*continued*)

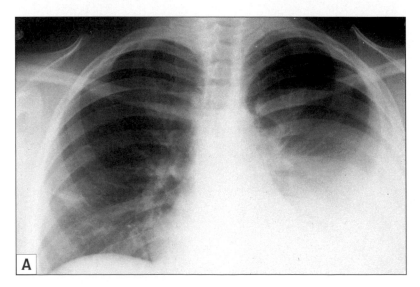

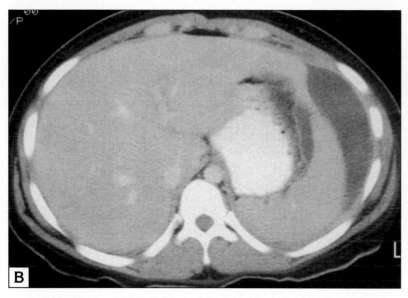

FIGURE 9-26 (*continued*) **B,** A computed tomography scan shows the pleural effusion extending inferolaterally in the costophrenic sulcus, displacing the spleen and a portion of the left hepatic lobe to the right. An abscess with an enhancing margin is present medial to the anterior portion of the spleen. Diagnostic thoracentesis revealed a sterile, serous exudate.

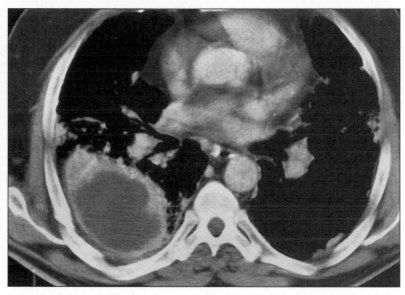

FIGURE 9-27 Lung abscess complicating pulmonary amyloidosis. The large infected fluid collection is intrapulmonary, as shown by the acute angles it forms with the adjacent chest wall and by the fact that it appears to occupy rather than displace lung tissue (*see* Fig. 9-4). The focal calcifications in the inner wall of the abscess represent areas of osseous metaplasia in lung tissue infiltrated by amyloid. Surgical and invasive interventional procedures carry increased risk in tissues involved by parenchymal amyloidosis, because the accompanying vasculopathy can frequently lead to excessive bleeding and air embolization. This abscess was successfully treated by percutaneous catheter drainage under computed tomography guidance. In general, a lung abscess may be drained percutaneously if it abuts a peripheral pleural surface and if normal lung does not occur along the course of the catheter.

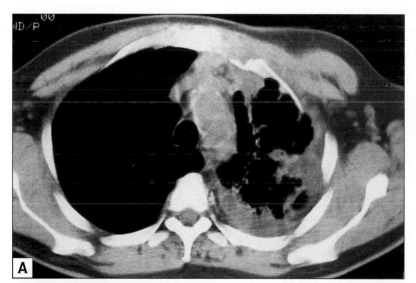

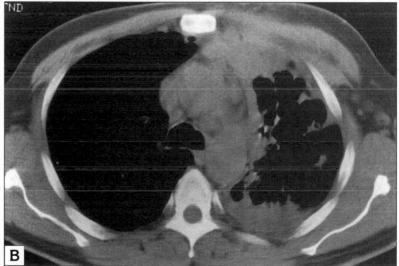

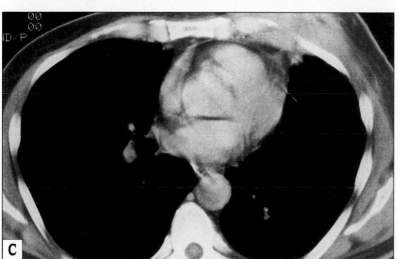

FIGURE 9-28 Thoracic actinomycosis with involvement of the pleural space, mediastinum, and chest wall. An alcoholic man presented with indolent weight loss, low-grade fever, and chest-wall tenderness and erythema. **A–C,** The computed tomography scan revealed a left upper lobe pneumonia spreading contiguously to involve the adjacent pleura, mediastinum, and chest wall. Edema and an inflammatory mass are evident in the subcutaneous tissues and musculature of the anterior chest wall. Involvement of an anterior rib is seen. Mediastinal lymphadenopathy and a small, dependently layering pleural effusion are also present. The diagnosis was established by fine-needle aspiration of the fluctuant subcutaneous abscess.

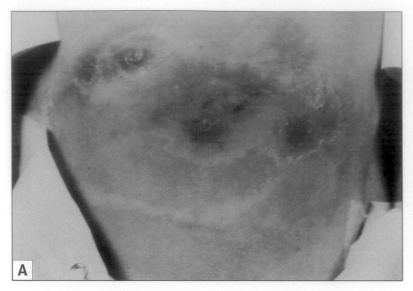

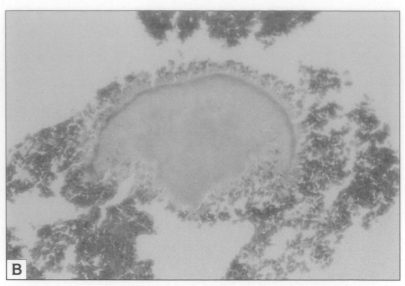

FIGURE 9-29 Thoracic actinomycosis. **A**, A different patient shows erythema on the lower flank and multiple draining sinuses of thoracic actinomycosis. **B**, Sulfur granules characteristic of *Actinomyces* were obtained from a draining sinus before antibiotic treatment was initiated. The grains have an eosinophilic coating derived from host protein and are surrounded by neutrophils. Intertwining filamentous bacteria are present in the periphery (Gram's stain; original magnification, × 100.)

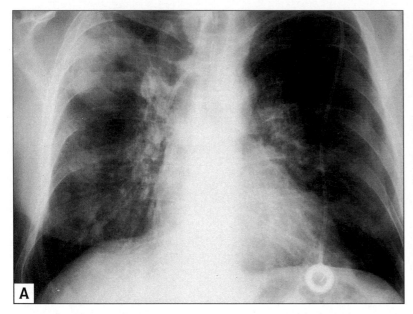

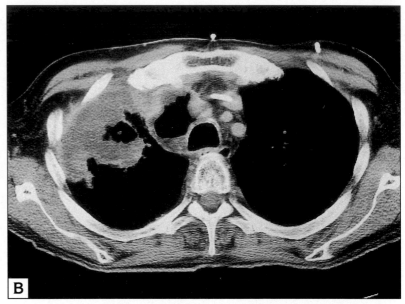

FIGURE 9-30 Nocardiosis. A 51-year-old man had recently received combination chemotherapy and prednisone for treatment of Hodgkin's disease. **A**, His chest radiograph demonstrates masslike consolidation in the right lung with cavity formation. There is an air-fluid level in the right paratracheal area. **B**, Computed tomography examination shows that the infection extends to the mediastinum, because the air-fluid level involves the innominate artery and superior vena cava. There is extensive liquefaction in both the pulmonary infiltrate and mediastinal disease.

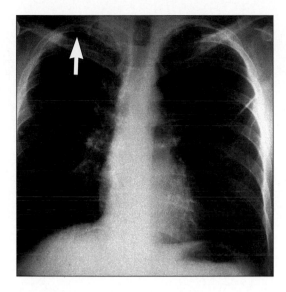

FIGURE 9-31 Invasive aspergillosis invading the chest wall, mimicking a superior sulcus carcinoma (Pancoast tumor). A 32-year-old man with AIDS presented with right shoulder pain and ipsilateral ulnar neuropathy. His chest radiograph revealed a right apical pulmonary density, a so-called apical cap (*arrow*). Invasion of the masslike lesion into the posterior limb of the brachial plexus was demonstrated by magnetic resonance imaging (not shown). Diagnosis was established by fine-needle biopsy.

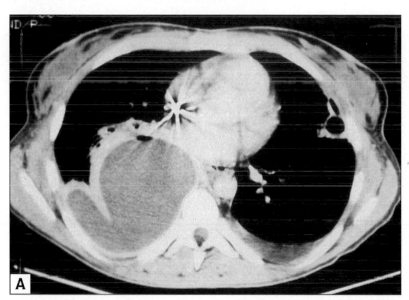

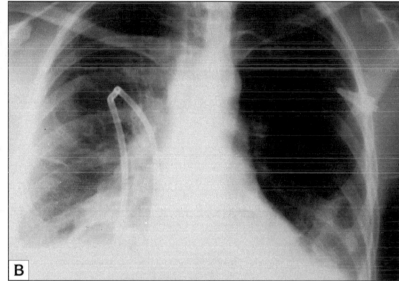

FIGURE 9-32 Bilateral lung abscesses and bronchopleural fistulas in an intravenous drug abuser with fever. **A**, Contrast-enhanced computed tomography image shows a loculated right-sided pleural collection that compresses and displaces lung parenchyma anteri-

orly. An air-fluid level is present within the empyema. Blood cultures were positive for *Staphylococcus aureus*. **B**, Chest radiograph after placement of drainage catheter into the right empyema. The bronchopleural fistula and air leak resolved over several days.

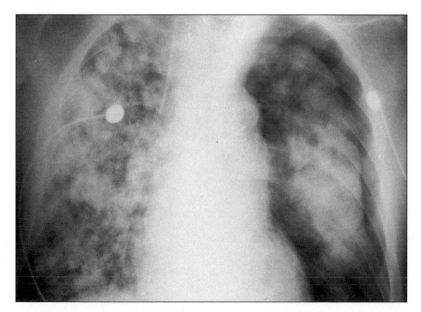

FIGURE 9-33 Acute cavitary coccidioidomycosis resulting in acute pneumothorax. A 53-year-old man had progressive multifocal coccidioidal pneumonia that led to cavitation and pneumothorax by the 6th day after presentation. The chest film reveals air-containing cavities that were not seen on previous films. (*Courtesy of* D. Lucas, MD.)

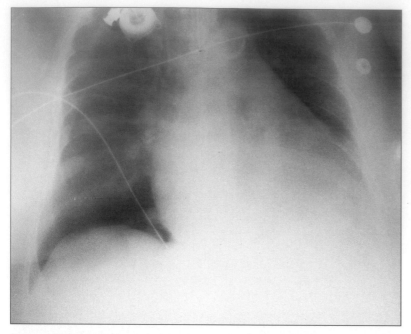

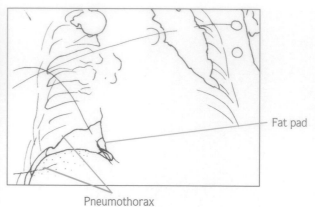

Fat pad

Pneumothorax

FIGURE 9-34 Subtle pneumothorax in a supine patient. Pleural air collections tend to occur in the least-dependent portion of the pleural space. When the patient is upright, pneumothorax can be identified at the apex of the affected hemithorax, and a pleural line of the retracted lung is easily visualized. However, when the patient is supine, the anteroinferior aspect of the pleural space is the least dependent, and when air collects here, a more subtle set of radiographic features results. The ipsilateral hemidiaphragm is often relatively "lucent," with the zone of increased transradiancy conforming to the anteroinferior costophrenic recess (obliquely oriented, with greater caudal extension in moving from medial to lateral). The lateral costophrenic sulcus is often abnormally distended (deep sulcus sign). Structures in the cardiophrenic angles, such as fat pads, are often discriminated with abnormal clarity. Ill-defined lucency may also be seen to parallel the hemidiaphragm or heart border. Unlike the situation when the patient is erect, a pleural line is only rarely detected. This patient had required intubation for severe asthma, initially responding well, then precipitously worsening with rapidly diminishing oxygen saturation. The portable, supine radiograph showed no pulmonary edema or new infiltrate but showed a halo of abnormally low radiodensity in the region of the right hemidiaphragm, the inferior limits of which corresponded to the inferior extent of the anterior costophrenic sulcus. The periepicardial fat pad at the right cardiophrenic angle had a nodular appearance. A left decubitus radiograph (not shown) confirmed the pneumothorax.

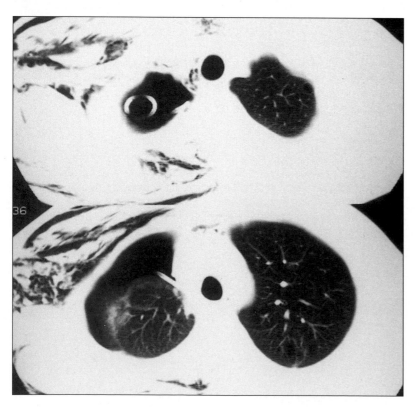

FIGURE 9-35 Pneumothorax and subcutaneous emphysema. During catheter placement for treatment of a persistent bronchopleural fistula, which followed a segmental pulmonary resection, two computed tomography images show the distal portion of a curved catheter placed in the pleural space. There is marked subcutaneous air from a prior chest tube placement. Air is noted to dissect between fascial planes, highlighting the pectoral muscles.

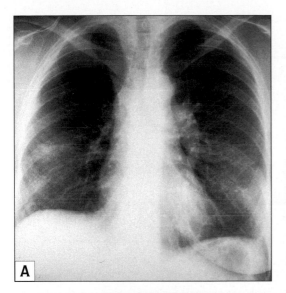

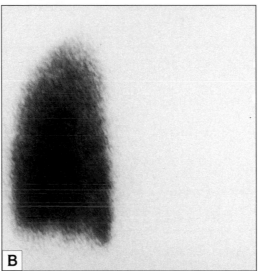

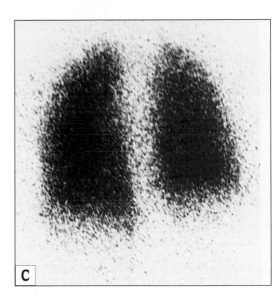

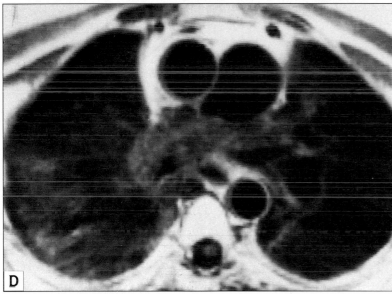

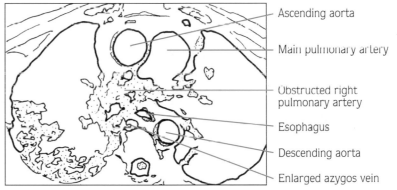

facial plethora consistent with superior vena cava syndrome, which was self-limited. The left pulmonary artery is greatly enlarged, and the right pulmonary artery diminutive. There is abnormal calcification in the region of the superior vena cava. **B**, Radionuclide perfusion scan (posterior view) demonstrates normal perfusion of the left lung and complete absence of right lung perfusion. **C**, The ventilation radionuclide scan was normal in both lungs. **D**, T1-weighted magnetic resonance image in the axial plane shows obliteration of the superior vena cava and the right pulmonary artery by an infiltrative process of intermediate signal intensity. The azygos vein is dilatated, transmitting collateral flow in the setting of caval obliteration.

FIGURE 9-36 Histoplasmosis with fibrosing mediastinitis. **A**, Postero-anterior chest radiograph was performed in a 50-year-old woman, former inhabitant of an area endemic for histoplasmosis, who complained of mild dyspnea on exertion. She had previously experienced

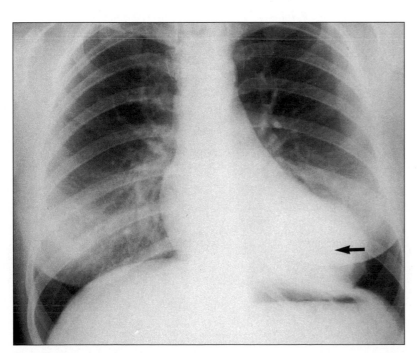

FIGURE 9-37 Cardiac echinococcosis. Intrathoracic echinococcosis is usually pulmonary in origin and is seen in approximately one fourth of cases. Much less frequent is pleural or cardiac involvement. This 24-year-old Greek woman, who emigrated to the United States 2 years previously, had symptoms of congestive heart failure and a pericardial friction rub. At thoracotomy, a 6.3-cm-diameter echinococcal cyst was found along the surface of the posterolateral left ventricular wall, adherent to the pericardium (*arrow*). (*Courtesy of* J. Rosch, MD.)

REFERENCES

1. Bartlett JG: Anaerobic bacterial pleuropulmonary infections. *Semin Respir Med* 1992, 13:158–166.

2. Mandal AK, Thadepalli H: Treatment of spontaneous bacterial empyema. *J Thorac Cardiovasc Surg* 1987, 94:414–418.

3. Varkey B, Rose HD, Kutty K, Politis J: Empyema thoracis during a 10 year period. *Arch Intern Med* 1982, 141:1771–1776.

4. Light RW: *Pleural Diseases*. Philadelphia: Lea & Febiger, 1983.

5. Caplan ES, Hoyt NJ, Rodriguez A, Cowley RA: Empyema occuring in the multiply-traumatized patient. *J Trauma* 1984, 24:785–788.

SELECTED BIBLIOGRAPHY

Bryant RE: Pleural effusion and empyema. *In* Mandell GL, Bennett JE, Dolin R (eds.): *Principles and Practice of Infectious Diseases*, 4th ed. New York: Churchill Livingstone; 1995:637–641.

Light RW: Management of empyema. *Semin Respir Med* 1992, 13:167–176.

Light RW: Pleural Diseases. Philadelphia: Lea & Febiger, 1983.

Light RW: Pleural effusion. *In* Murray JF, Nadel JA (eds.): *Textbook of Respiratory Medicine*, 2nd èd. Philadelphia: W.B. Saunders; 1994:2164–2192.

Sahn SA: Management of complicated parapneumonic effusions. *Am Rev Respir Dis* 1993, 148:813–817.

CHAPTER 10

Pneumonias in Cancer Patients

Donald Armstrong

Immune defects in patients with neoplastic disease

Defect	Type of patient
Integument	Indwelling intravenous catheters
	Cytotoxic chemotherapy (especially leukemia, lymphoma)
	Mycosis fungoides
Neutrophil	Cytotoxic chemotherapy (especially leukemia, lymphoma)
	High-dose corticosteroids
T-helper cell	High-dose corticosteroids
Mononuclear phagocyte	Acute lymphocytic leukemia
	Hodgkin's disease
	Hairy cell leukemia
Postsplenectomy	Hodgkin's disease (staging in past)
	Chronic myelogenous leukemia
	Hairy cell leukemia
B-cell defect	Chronic lymphocytic leukemia
	Multiple myeloma
	Some lymphomas
	Long-term cytotoxic chemotherapy
Local tissue damage	Radiation therapy
	Cytotoxic chemotherapy

FIGURE 10-1 Immune defects in patients with cancer.

A. Causes of pneumonias complicating a neutrophil defect

Bacteria	Fungi	Parasites	Viruses
Streptococcus spp	*Aspergillus* spp		
Staphylococcus spp	Mucoraceae		
Enterobacteriaceae	*Trichosporon* spp		
Pseudomonas aeruginosa	*Fusarium* spp		
Bacillus spp	*Candida* spp		
	Pseudallescheria boydii		

B. Causes of pneumonia complicating a T-lymphocyte/mononuclear phagocyte defect

Bacteria	Fungi	Parasites	Viruses
Mycobacterium spp	*Cryptococcus neoformans*	*Pneumocystis carinii*	Cytomegalovirus
Nocardia asteroides	*Histoplasma capsulatum*	*Toxoplasma gondii*	Varicella-zoster virus
Legionella spp	*Coccidioides immitis*	*Strongyloides stercoralis*	Measles virus
Rhodococcus equi	*Candida* spp		Adenovirus
Chlamydia pneumoniae	*Penicillium marneffii*		Respiratory syncytial virus

FIGURE 10-2 Causes of pneumonias complicating cancer. **A.** Neutrophil defect (*eg*, cytotoxic chemotherapy, acute leukemia, transplantation). **B.** T-lymphocyte/mononuclear phagocyte defect (*eg*, Hodgkin's disease, transplantation, HIV infection). (*continued*)

C. Causes of pneumonia complicating a globulin or splenic defect

Bacteria	Fungi	Parasites	Viruses
Streptococcus pneumoniae		*Pneumocystis carinii*	
Haemophilus influenzae			
Neisseria meningitidis			

FIGURE 10-2 (*continued*) **C**, Globulin or splenic defect (*eg*, multiple myeloma, chronic lymphocytic leukemia, transplantation, splenectomy).

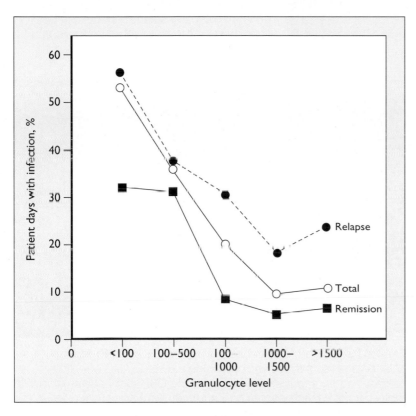

FIGURE 10-3 Incidence of infection as related to leukocyte count in acute leukemia. The incidence of infection rises as absolute granulocyte (neutrophil) count is reduced. (*From* Bodey *et al.* [1]; with permission.)

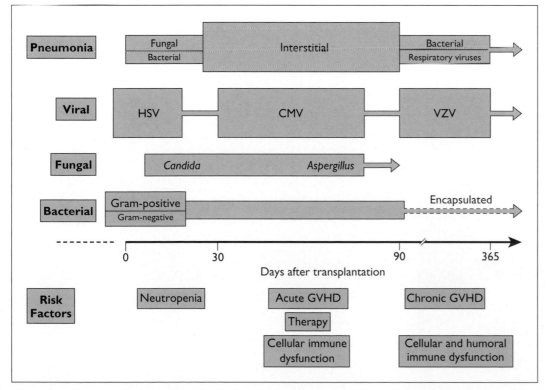

FIGURE 10-4 Common infections and risk factors after bone marrow transplantation. (CMV—cytomegalovirus; GVHD—graft-versus-host disease; HSV—herpes simplex virus; VZV—varicella-zoster virus.) (*Adapted from* Winston [2]; with permission.)

BACTERIAL PNEUMONIAS

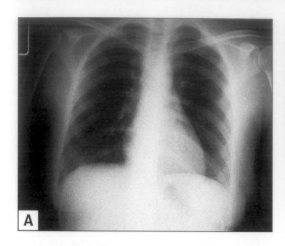

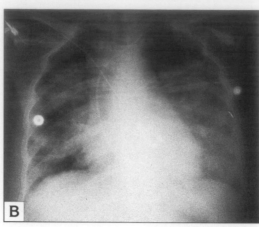

FIGURE 10-5 Chest radiographs of typical pneumococcal lobar pneumonia following bone marrow transplantation. The patient was postbone marrow transplant for > 1 year when she developed shaking chills, fever, and leukocytosis. **A** and **B**, The first chest radiograph (*panel 5A*) was negative, but within 24 hours, the second chest film (*panel 5B*) showed extensive bilateral infiltrates. The blood culture was positive for > 1000 colony-forming units of *Streptococcus pneumoniae* per mL. The B-cell defect in bone marrow transplant patients can last for years despite return of marrow function. The patient died of overwhelming sepsis.

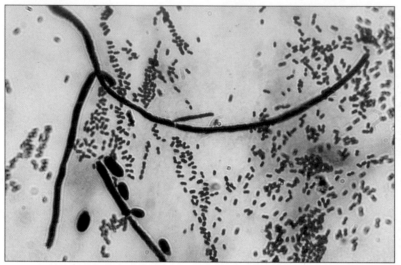

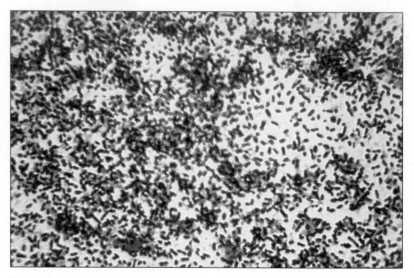

FIGURE 10-6 Sputum Gram stain from a patient with chronic lymphocytic leukemia (CLL) and a lobar pneumococcal pneumonia. Note the lack of polymorphonuclear cells (the patient was neutropenic due to chemotherapy), gram-positive diplococci, and yeast forms and pseudohyphae. The patient was on adrenocorticosteroids, and his mouth was colonized with *Candida*. Treatment with penicillin alone resulted in a response. Patients with hypogammaglobulinemia due to CLL or multiple myeloma develop less severe pneumococcal or haemophilus infections than those following bone marrow transplantations or splenectomies. In either case, treatment today would require vancomycin to cover penicillin-resistant pneumococci in addition to ceftriaxone.

FIGURE 10-7 Gram stain of cerebrospinal fluid (CSF) from a splenectomized patient with Hodgkin's disease. Although the patient had no apparent pneumonia, the CSF shows gram-positive diplococci of *Streptococcus pneumoniae*. Similar severe disease may be seen in bone marrow transplant patients.

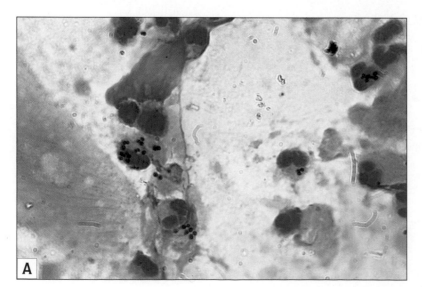

FIGURE 10-8 *Staphylococcus aureus* pneumonia in a neutropenic patient following cytotoxic chemotherapy. **A**, Sputum Gram stain showing large gram-positive cocci in clusters typical of *S. aureus*. *S. aureus* rarely causes pneumonia in normal hosts, except following influenza. In neutropenic patients, it may cause a primary pneumonia with cavitation or empyema. (*continued*)

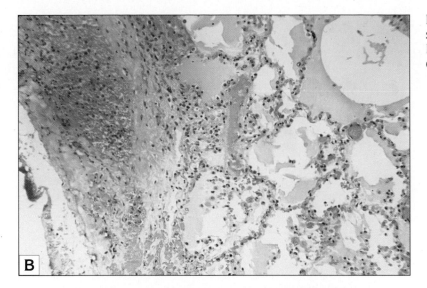

FIGURE 10-8 (*continued*) **B**, Biopsy specimen of lung and pleura showing acute inflammation and necrosis due to *S. aureus*. Hematogenous spread to the lungs causes bilateral thin-walled cavities. The source may be an intravenous catheter.

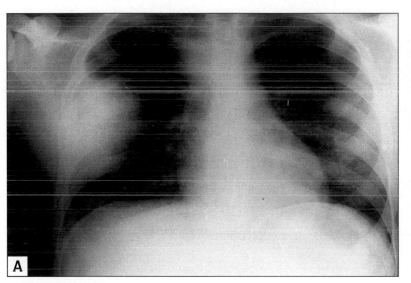

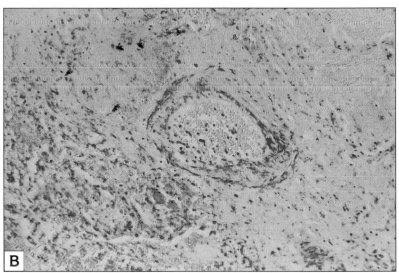

FIGURE 10-9 *Pseudomonas aeruginosa* pneumonia in a neutropenic patient. **A**, A chest radiograph shows a typical wedge-shaped infiltrate. Sputum samples in neutropenic patients do not show polymorphonuclear cells, and thus a representative sputum should show the absence of epithelial cells, normal oral flora, and the presence of multiple gram-negative rods. **B**, Histopathologic specimen of the lung shows clotting of vessels due to invasion by *P. aeruginosa*, which results in infarction and wedge-shaped infiltrates. The clotting of arteries and arterioles makes it difficult for antibiotics to reach the area of infection.

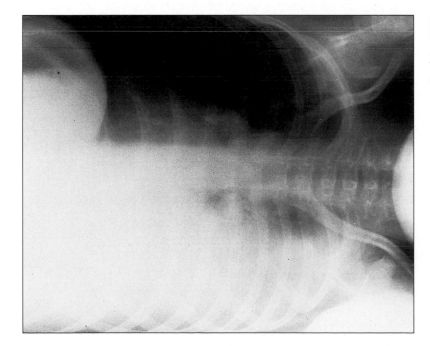

FIGURE 10-10 Decubitus chest radiograph of a child with acute leukemia, neutropenia, and *Bacillus cereus* pneumonia. Even *B. cereus* can cause invasive disease in neutropenic patients. In this child, a meningitis also developed due to this usually innocuous organism.

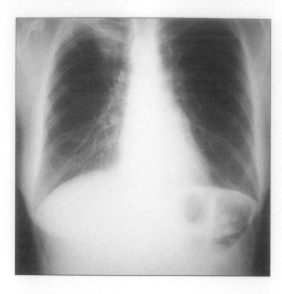

FIGURE 10-11
Chest radiograph of a patient with Hodgkin's disease and *Rhodococcus equi* pneumonia. *R. equi* pneumonia can mimic tuberculosis. This organism takes advantage of a CD4 or T-helper cell defect. It often causes skin ulcers as well as lung lesions. There may be a history of exposure to farm animals, such as horses.

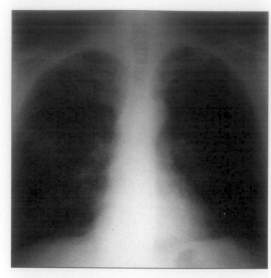

FIGURE 10-12
Chest radiograph of a patient with Hodgkin's disease and *Nocardia asteroides* pneumonia. This organism can also cause pulmonary disease mimicking tuberculosis. It complicates T-helper cell defects and may cause skin lesions varying from cold abscesses to ulcers to cellulitis.

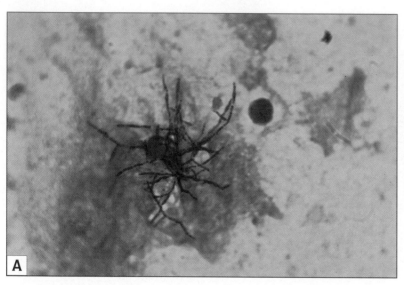

A

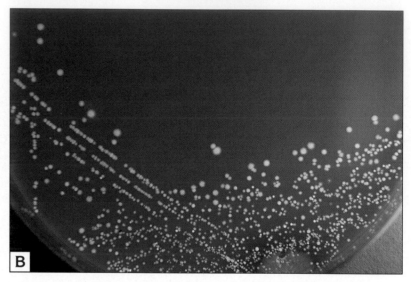

B

FIGURE 10-13 *Nocardia asteroides* pneumonia. **A**, Sputum Gram stain shows filamentous, beaded, branching, gram-positive rods. They usually take the acid-fast stain, which helps to rapidly differentiate them from *Actinomyces*. *Actinomyces* is an obligate anaerobe, so culture characteristics can result in early differentiation. **B**, Dry, white colonies of *N. asteroides* growing on chocolate agar.

Repeated specimens may be necessary to yield positive smears or cultures, and specimens may be positive for one but not the other. Cultures should be kept for at least 5 days to allow this slow-growing organism to appear. The microbiology laboratory should be notified when *Nocardia* infection is suspected.

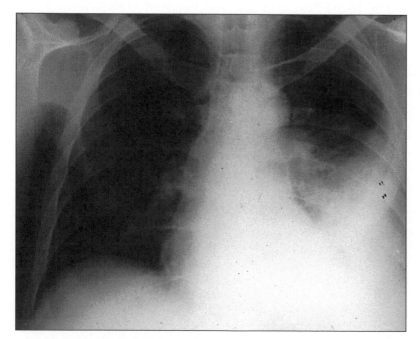

FIGURE 10-14 Chest radiograph of a patient with lymphoma, neutropenia, and a T-cell defect (*Mycobacterium tuberculosis* infection). Acute pneumonia considered to be gram-negative bacillary because of neutropenia turned out to be tuberculosis because of a T-cell defect. Multiple immune defects must be considered in some patients according to underlying disease and types of chemotherapy.

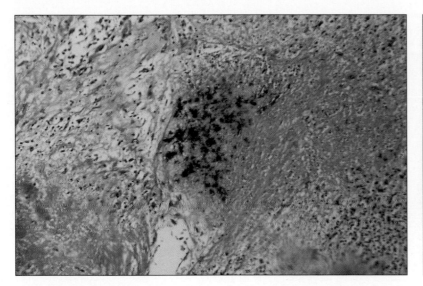

FIGURE 10-15 Acid-fast stain of a lymph node specimen from a patient with hairy cell leukemia, neutropenia, and a negative chest radiograph (extrapulmonary *Mycobacterium tuberculosis* infection). This type of leukemia is accompanied by a severe T-cell defect, and *M. tuberculosis* may disseminate from undetectable pulmonary lesions.

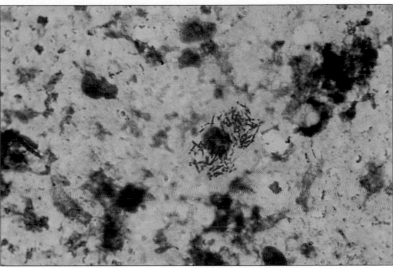

FIGURE 10-16 Acid-fast stain of a spleen specimen from a patient with severe combined immunodeficiency disease and bone marrow transplantation, showing *Mycobacterium avium* infection. In patients with severe T-cell defects, especially those with AIDS, *M. avium* appears to disseminate from the gastrointestinal tract and involves the lungs by hematogenous spread.

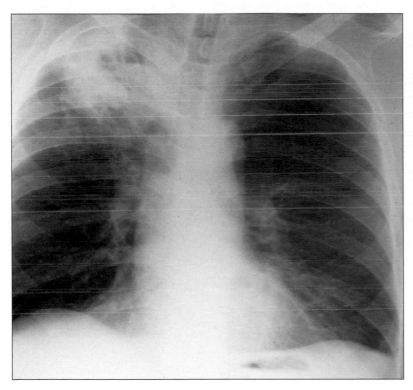

FIGURE 10-17 Chest radiograph of a patient with lymphoma, a T-cell defect, and *Mycobacterium kansasii* pneumonia. This organism may also mimic tuberculosis.

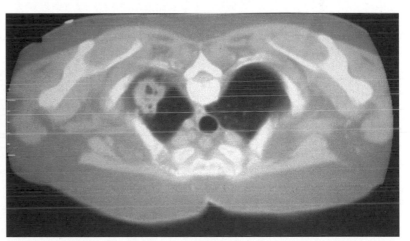

FIGURE 10-18 Computed tomography scan from a bone marrow transplant patient showing a cavitary lesion considered to be tuberculosis. Transthoracic needle aspiration yielded *Legionella pneumophila*.

FUNGAL PNEUMONIAS

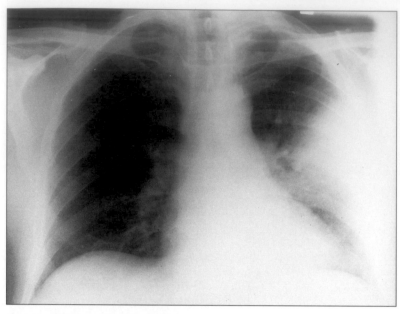

FIGURE 10-19 Chest radiograph of a patient with neutropenia following cytotoxic chemotherapy, complicated by invasive aspergillosis. The large wedge-shaped infiltrate looks similar to that produced by *Pseudomonas aeruginosa*, and the pathogenesis is similar. Invasion of vessels with clotting and infarction is common with *Aspergillus* species or Mucorales infections in neutropenic patients.

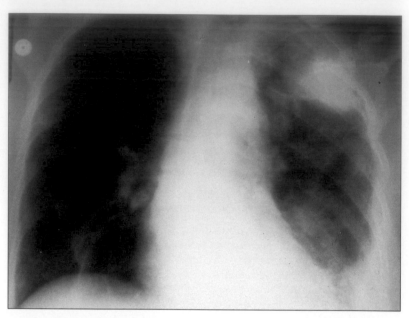

FIGURE 10-20 Chest radiograph of a neutropenic patient with invasive aspergillosis. Chest radiographs can vary considerably among patients, and some may even be negative despite acute, diffuse disease.

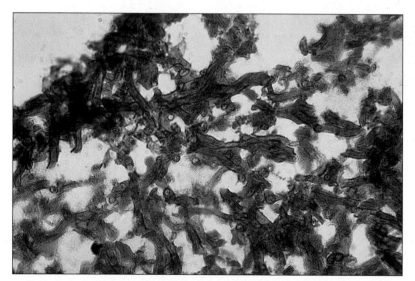

FIGURE 10-21 Tracheal biopsy specimen from a neutropenic patient with invasive aspergillosis due to *Aspergillus flavus*. Tracheal and/or bronchial invasion may occur in neutropenic patients, especially after bone marrow transplantation.

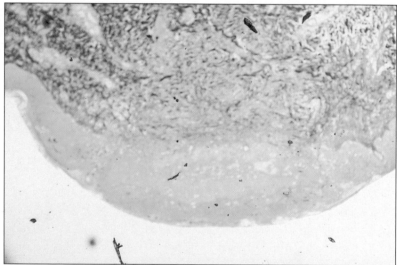

FIGURE 10-22 Biopsy specimen of a skin lesion yielding *Aspergillus flavus*. Biopsy of a skin lesion from the patient shown in Figure 10-21 yielded the same organism. Skin lesions offer easily accessible sites for biopsy, whereas sputum specimens are usually repeatedly negative.

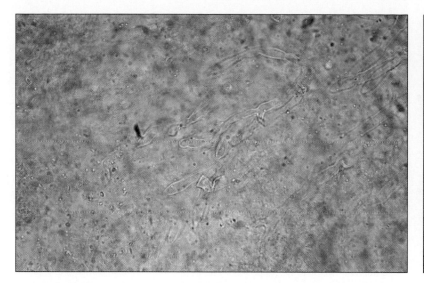

FIGURE 10-23 Potassium hydroxide wet mount of an open lung biopsy specimen from a neutropenic, leukemic patient with invasive aspergillosis. Acutely branching septate hyphae can be seen. Sputum specimens are usually negative on wet mounts. Positive cultures of sputum specimens may be due to colonization, but in neutropenic patients are considered an indication for therapy.

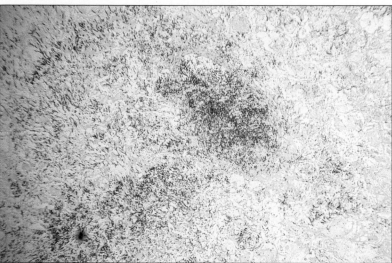

FIGURE 10-24 Methenamine silver stain of a lung biopsy specimen showing the hyphae of *Aspergillus* species. Even with the advent of bronchoalveolar lavage, the diagnosis of aspergillosis may require an open lung biopsy. Presently, amphotericin B is empirically added to treatment when a pulmonary infiltrate appears in a neutropenic patient already on broad-spectrum antibacterial therapy.

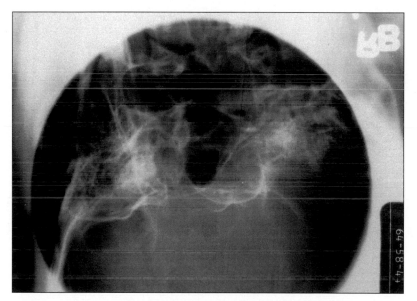

FIGURE 10-25 Computed tomography scan of the sinuses showing invasive mucormycosis. The Mucoraceae also invade local blood vessels, causing infarction that leads to black, necrotic lesions of the nasopharynx or sinuses. The broad, nonseptate, ribbonlike hyphae are often seen by merely swabbing such lesions. A deeper biopsy may be necessary in some cases. Rhinocerebral mucormycosis, first described in diabetics, is seen in a minority of neutropenic or transplant patients. More commonly, the Mucoraceae cause pulmonary lesions, less often brain lesions, and occasionally both. *Aspergillus* species can also cause rhinocerebral mucormycosis.

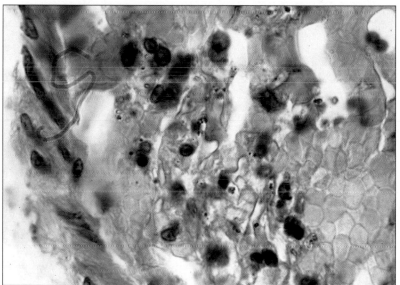

FIGURE 10-26 Hematoxylin-eosin stain of a skin biopsy in invasive mucormycosis. The Mucoraceae can cause skin lesions after hematogenous spread, just as other fungi may. Also, just as with aspergillosis, skin lesions show a dark necrotic center. This skin biopsy specimen was obtained from the patient with sinusitis and pneumonitis seen in Figure 10-25.

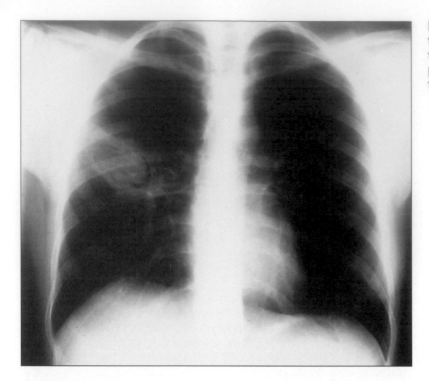

FIGURE 10-27 Chest radiograph of pulmonary mucormycosis. In this patient, pulmonary lesions suggestive of aspergillosis proved to be due to mucormycosis on open lung biopsy. Progressive pulmonary lesions due to either fungus result in fungus balls in the cavitary lesions.

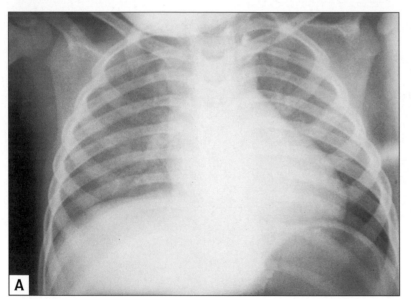

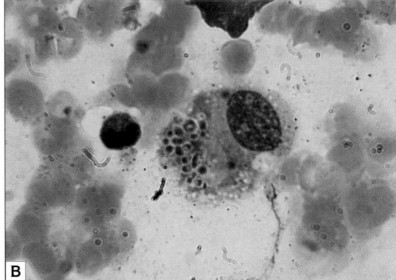

FIGURE 10-28 Histoplasmosis in a child with acute lymphatic leukemia (ALL) and a T-cell defect. **A**, A chest radiograph shows diffuse pulmonary lesions and a widened mediastinum due to histoplasmosis. The histoplasmosis had been asymptomatic and was reactivated when the patient received chemotherapy for ALL in a nonendemic area. **B**, Hematoxylin-eosin stain of a bone marrow aspirate from this patient shows the yeast forms of *Histoplasma capsulatum* within a macrophage. This remains the quickest, readily available method of diagnosis. Skin lesions from this patient also revealed the organism.

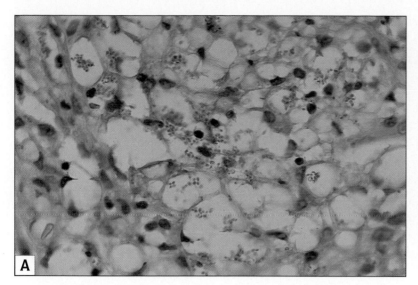

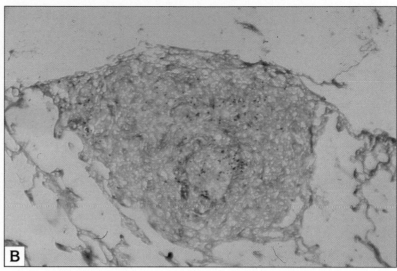

FIGURE 10-29 Lung biopsy of reactivated histoplasmosis. **A,** Hematoxylin-eosin stain showing small budding yeasts. **B,** Methenamine silver staining of the same slide readily shows the small yeast forms. An enzyme-linked immunosorbent assay test to detect antigen in urine and serum appears sensitive and specific but is not widely available.

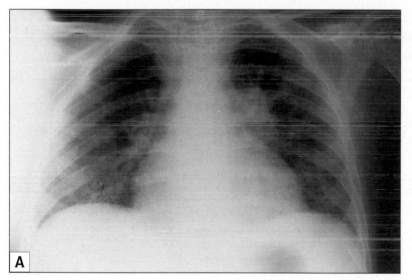

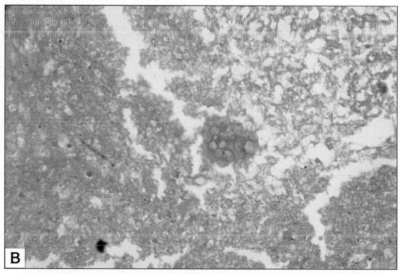

FIGURE 10-30 Reactivated coccidioidomycosis in a patient under treatment for acute myelogenous leukemia. **A,** A chest radiograph shows disseminated infiltrates due to coccidioidomycosis. Although the patient was neutropenic, it was a T-cell defect that permitted reactivation of this disease in a nonendemic area. **B,** Histopathologic examination of a lung biopsy specimen shows encysted spherules of *Coccidioides immitis*. Sputum specimens are only variably positive, and tissue from skin or lung biopsies may be necessary to yield a diagnosis.

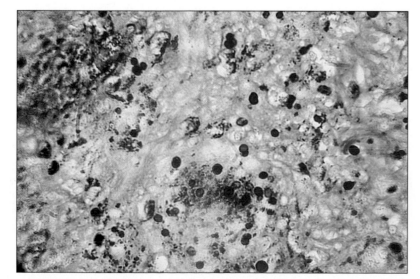

FIGURE 10-31 Methenamine silver stain of an open lung biopsy showing cryptococcal pneumonia in a patient with a T-cell defect. *Cryptococcus neoformans* may cause pneumonia in patients with T-cell defects due to neoplastic disease or following transplantation, but far less often than in HIV-infected patients. Originally, the diagnosis was made by open lung biopsy by microscopy with methenamine silver stain and culture. Now, extensive disease can be diagnosed by detecting cryptococcal antigen in serum. Bronchoalveolar lavages also can be tested for antigen.

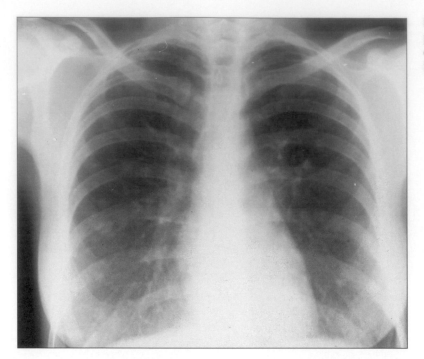

FIGURE 10-32 Chest radiograph from a leukemic, neutropenic patient with candidemia. The radiograph shows the typical pattern of hematogenous spread, which is the usual way *Candida* species invade the lungs. Primary pneumonia due to *Candida* is unusual.

PARASITIC PNEUMONIAS

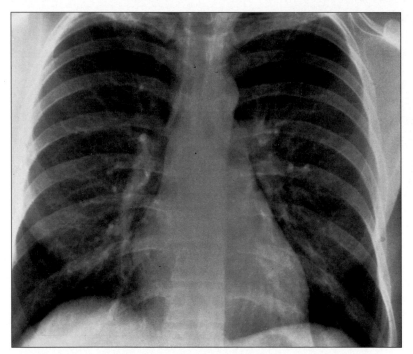

FIGURE 10-33 Chest radiograph of *Pneumocystis* pneumonia. Pneumocystosis usually presents as a pneumonia. It may also present in a disseminated form, including primarily gastrointestinal symptoms and signs. The pneumonias can be quite variable. The chest radiograph depicted represents recurrent *Pneumocystis* pneumonia with upper lobe disease and pneumothorax. The patient responded to therapy but died of multiple infections and had disseminated pneumocystosis at autopsy.

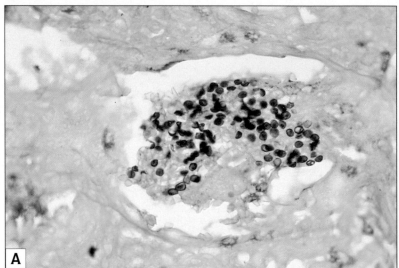

FIGURE 10-34 Stains for *Pneumocystis carinii*. **A**, Classic methenamine silver stain. (*continued*)

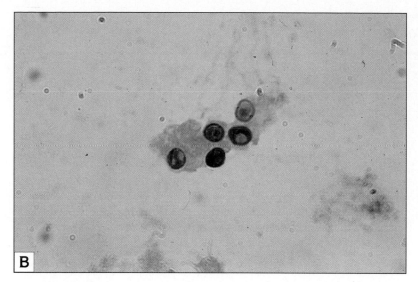

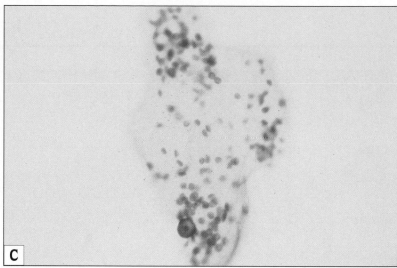

FIGURE 10-34 (*continued*) **B,** Gram-Weigart stain. **C,** Toluidine blue stain. Expectorated sputum should be examined first, and if negative, then bronchoalveolar lavage and, when possible, transbronchial biopsy should be done. All specimens should be examined for concomitant infections, ranging from *Streptococcus* *pneumoniae* or *Staphylococcus aureus* to cytomegalovirus. Direct fluorescent antibody studies have been found productive in some laboratories, as have Giemsa stains. Both are more likely to detect the smaller, but harder to recognize, trophozoites.

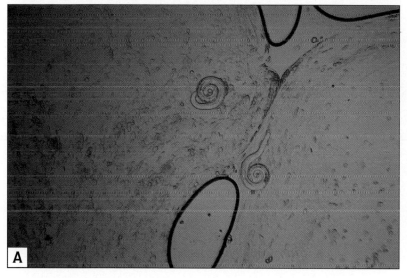

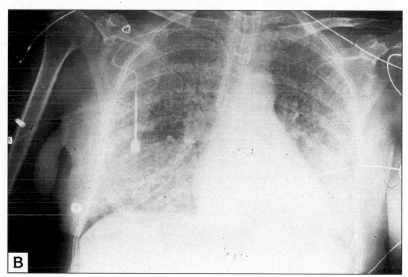

FIGURE 10-35 Disseminated strongyloidiasis. Disseminated strongyloidiasis or the hyperinfection syndrome with pneumonia is unusual in patients with T-cell defects but is eminently treatable, especially if diagnosed early. Polymicrobic sepsis should suggest the diagnosis, especially in a person with a T-cell defect who is not neutropenic or does not have an indwelling intravenous catheter. **A,** Sputum wet mount shows the organism and is the most direct, but late, method of diagnosis. **B,** Chest radiograph showing diffuse pulmonary infiltrates. Typically, diffuse alveolar and interstitial infiltrates appear on the radiograph. The patient responded to therapy.

VIRAL PNEUMONIAS

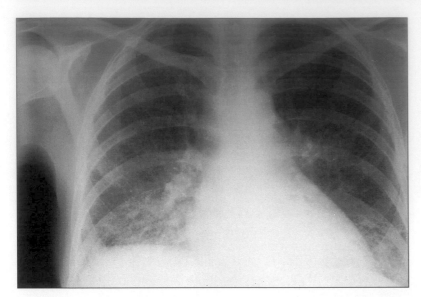

FIGURE 10-36 Chest radiograph showing a diffuse infiltrate due to cytomegalovirus (CMV) pneumonia in a bone marrow transplant patient. A lung biopsy specimen revealed "owl's eye" inclusions characteristic of CMV infection plus coinfection by *Toxoplasma*. Cancer patients are often susceptible to dual infections because of a specific immune defect, such as a T-cell defect in this patient, but also they often have multiple immune defects broadening their susceptibility. Clinicians must be alert to the possibility of dual infection, and if less invasive procedures do not answer the clinical question, more invasive procedures such as bronchoalveolar lavage or lung biopsy are warranted at the earliest opportunity.

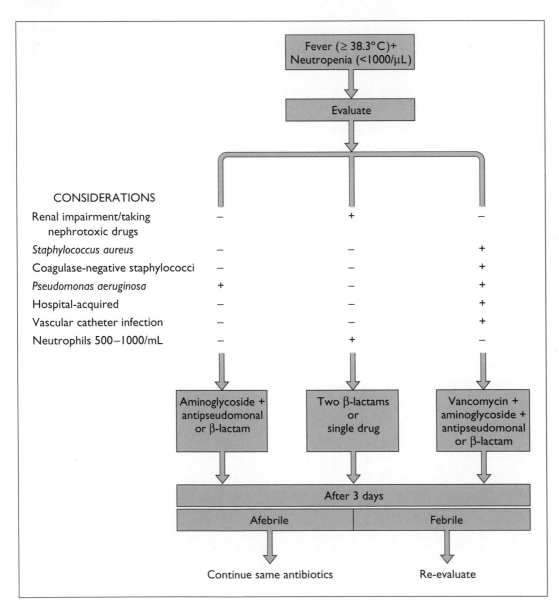

FIGURE 10-37 Initial management of the febrile neutropenic patient. According to guidelines issued by the Infectious Diseases Society of America in 1990 [3], high-dose, parenteral, broad-spectrum antibiotics should be begun empirically in any febrile patient with a neutrophil count < 1000/μL. Among the regimens that have been used, most support combination therapy with an aminoglycoside plus an antipseudomonal penicillin or β-lactam, with or without vancomycin, or two β-lactam drugs. In selecting among the four antibiotic regimens, consideration must be given to the local prevalence of bacterial virulence and antibiotic resistance, as well as specific patient factors such as allergy or coexisting renal or hepatic failure. If a causative agent is identified, therapy should be modified to provide optimal susceptibility, but broad-spectrum coverage should be maintained. (*Adapted from* Armstrong [4]; with permission.)

Fever (≥ 38.3°C)+
Neutropenia (<1000/μL)

Evaluate

CONSIDERATIONS			
Renal impairment/taking nephrotoxic drugs	–	+	–
Staphylococcus aureus	–	–	+
Coagulase-negative staphylococci	–	–	+
Pseudomonas aeruginosa	+	–	+
Hospital-acquired	–	–	+
Vascular catheter infection	–	–	+
Neutrophils 500–1000/mL	–	+	–

Aminoglycoside + antipseudomonal or β-lactam	Two β-lactams or single drug	Vancomycin + aminoglycoside + antipseudomonal or β-lactam

After 3 days

Afebrile	Febrile
Continue same antibiotics	Re-evaluate

REFERENCES

1. Bodey GP, Buckley M, Sathe YS, *et al.*: Quantitative relationships between circulating leukocytes and infection in patients with acute leukemia. *Ann Intern Med* 1966, 64:328–340.

2. Winston DJ: Infections in bone marrow transplant recipients. *In* Mandell GL, Bennett JE, Dolin R (eds.): *Principles and Practice of Infectious Diseases*, 4th ed. New York: Churchill Livingstone; 1995:2718.

3. Hughes WT, *et al.*: Guidelines for the use of antimicrobial agents in neutropenic patients with unexplained fever. *J Infect Dis* 1990, 161:381–396.

4. Armstrong D: Management of fever and sepsis in the immunocompromised host. *Hosp Formul* 1994, 29(suppl 3):8–22.

SELECTED BIBLIOGRAPHY

Armstrong D, Brown AE (eds.): Controversies in the management of infectious complications of neoplastic diseases. *Rev Inf Dis* 1989, 11(Suppl 7).

Brown AE, White MH (eds.): Controversies in the management of infections in immunocompromised patients. *Clin Inf Dis* 1993, 17(Suppl 2).

Wiernick PH, *et al.* (eds.): *Neoplastic Diseases of the Blood*, 3rd ed. New York: Churchill Livingstone; 1996.

CHAPTER 11

Respiratory Infections in Transplant Recipients

Jay A. Fishman
Robert H. Rubin

APPROACH TO THE PATIENT

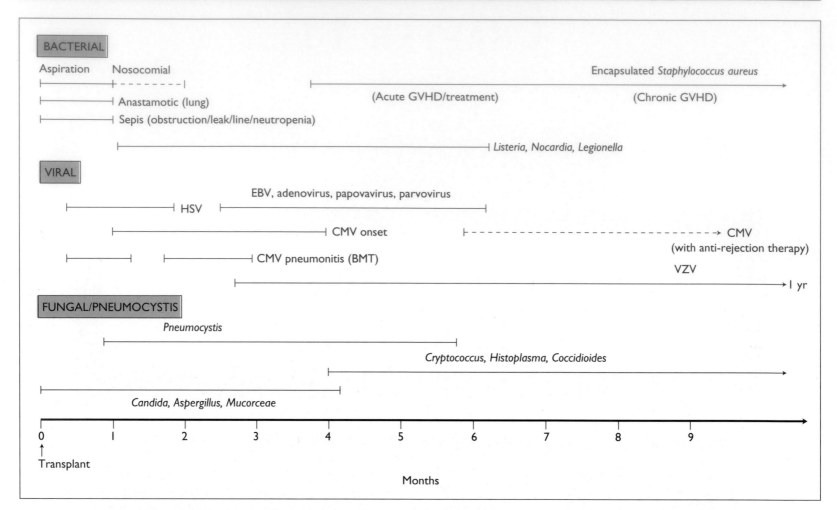

FIGURE 11-1 Timetable for pulmonary infections following transplantation. Patients' greatest risk for specific infections occurs in a specified sequence after transplantation. Patients who deviate significantly from this pattern may represent increased epidemiologic exposure to a given pathogen or a unique susceptibility (*eg*, increased immune suppression or tissue injury). Technical problems, such as anastomotic leaks or infections of hematomas, are associated with infection in the first month following transplantation but become a source of recurrent disease if uncorrected. (BMT—bone marrow transplant; CMV—cytomegalovirus; EBV—Epstein-Barr virus; GVHD—graft-vs-host disease; HSV—herpes simplex virus; VZV—varicella-zoster virus.) (*Modified from* Rubin *et al.* [1]; with permission.)

Potential infectious causes of pulmonary disease in transplant recipients

Community-acquired bacteria
  Streptococcus pneumoniae
  Haemophilus influenzae
  Staphylococcus aureus
  Escherichia coli
  Klebsiella pneumoniae
  Mycoplasma pneumoniae
  Legionella spp
  Mixed flora (aspiration)

Nosocomial bacteria
  Enteric gram-negative bacilli
  Pseudomonas aeruginosa
  Staphylococcus aureus (methicillin-resistant)

Other bacteria
  Nocardia spp
  Rhodococcus equi
  Mycobacterium tuberculosis
  Multidrug-resistant *Mycobacterium avium* complex

Viruses
  Cytomegalovirus
  Influenza virus
  Adenovirus
  Herpes simplex virus
  Respiratory syncytial virus

Fungi
  Aspergillus fumigatus
  Histoplasma capsulatum
  Cryptococcus neoformans
  Coccidioides immitis
  Candida spp
  Fusarium spp
  Mucoraceae
  Pneumocystis carinii

Parasites
  Strongyloides stercoralis
  Toxoplasma gondii

FIGURE 11-2 Potential infectious causes of pulmonary disease in organ transplant recipients. A broad range of pathogens has been described as affecting the organ transplant recipient. The incidence of specific pulmonary pathogens is related to the specific institution, geographic location, intensity of immune suppression, and presence or absence of rejection.

Testing of clinical specimens from the immunocompromised host

Organism	Fresh material tests	Histopathology	Culture technique	Time of growth
Aspergillus	KOH	H-E, PAS, silver	Blood agar, Sabourand, L-C	1–2 wks
Candida	Wet mount	H-E, PAS, silver	Blood agar, Sabouraud, L-C	1–14 days
Cryptococcus neoformans	India ink, serum crytococcal antigen	H-E, PAS, silver, mucicarmine	Sabouraud	4–7 days
Cytomegalovirus	Wright-Giemsa, Tzanck prep, antigenemia assay, PCR	H-E, antibody	Cell culture, shell vial, IF	2–14 days
Herpes simplex virus	Antibody/IF, Tzanck prep	H-E, Papanicolaou, antibody, DNA	Cell culture, IF	1–7 days
Legionella	IF, urinary antigen	Dieterle, acid-fast, antibody	BCYE	3–5 days, up to 10 days
Mucoraceae	KOH	H-E, silver	Blood agar, Sabouraud	1–2 wks
Mycobacterium tuberculosis	Acid-fast, IF	Acid-fast, DNA	Löwenstein-Jensen, Middlebrook, BACTEC*, L-C, DNA	2–6 wks
Nocardia	Modified acid-fast, Gram	Gram stain, modified acid-fast	Blood agar, BCYE, Sabouraud	5 days—4 wks
Pneumocystis	IF, silver, Giemsa, toluidine, PCR	Silver, H-E	Cell culture (fibroblasts)	Not useful
Respiratory syncytial virus	IF	H-E, antibody	HEp-2, HeLa cells, IF	Hours—5 days

*Becton-Dickinson, Sparks, MD.
BCYE–buffered charcoal yeast extract; DNA—nucleic acid hybridization; H-E—hematoxylin-eosin; IF—immunofluorescent stain; KOH—potassium hydroxide; L-C—lysis-centrifugation; PAS—periodic acid–Schiff; PCR—polymerase chain reaction.

FIGURE 11-3 Testing of clinical specimens from the immunocompromised host. The proper use of microbiologic specimens is important to the rapid diagnosis of opportunistic infections in the transplant recipient. The specific tests selected vary depending on the likelihood of specific infections (ie, epidemiologic risk), type of specimen, and diagnostic techniques available to the clinician.

Epidemiologic exposures of importance to transplant recipients

Exposure before transplantation	Community-acquired exposure after transplantation	Nosocomial epidemiologic exposure
Mycobacterium tuberculosis	Influenza	*Aspergillus* spp
Hepatitis B and C virus	Primary varicella-zoster infection	*Candida krusei*
HIV	Nontyphoidal salmonellosis	*Torulopsis glabrata*
Herpes simplex virus	*Mycobacterium tuberculosis*	*Legionella* spp
Varicella-zoster virus	Geographic mycoses	*Pseudomonas aeruginosa* and Enter-
Histoplasma capsulatum	*Legionella* spp	obacteriaceae
Coccidioides immitis	*Nocardia asteroides*	Methicillin-resistant *Staphylococcus*
Blastomyces dermatitidis	*Cryptococcus neoformans*	Vancomycin-resistant enterococci
Pneumocystis carinii	Respiratory syncytial virus	
Toxoplasma gondii	*Pneumocystis carinii*	
Strongyloides stercoralis	Cytomegalovirus (primary)	

FIGURE 11-4 Epidemiologic exposures of importance to transplant recipients. Identification of epidemiologic exposures of the immunocompromised host often allows the selection of appropriate diagnostic tests and effective empiric therapies in advance of the availability of microbiologic data. Data on the local infectious risks in the community and hospital environments are central to the management of the transplant recipient.

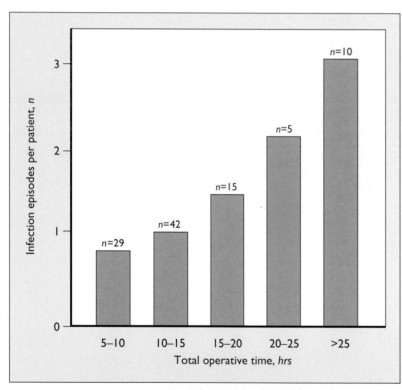

FIGURE 11-5 Frequency of severe infections in relation to time spent in liver transplantation surgery. In the first month following transplantation surgery, infections are most often due to anatomic defects related to patient management, including the incision, hematomas, urinary and vascular catheters, assisted ventilation, nosocomial pathogens, and adverse drug reactions. The duration of surgery and the absence of anastomotic or other anatomic sites for infection are factors in the development of early infection. (*From* Kusne *et al.* [2]; with permission.)

Potential noninfectious causes of pulmonary disease

Adult respiratory distress syndrome
Pulmonary edema
Pulmonary emboli
Leukoagglutinin reaction
Drug-induced pneumonitis
Pulmonary hemorrhage
Pulmonary fibrosis
Radiation pneumonitis
Tumor (especially lymphoma or hepatoma)

FIGURE 11-6 Common noninfectious causes of pulmonary disease. The transplant recipient is subject to many of the noninfectious causes of significant pulmonary disease. Dual processes, both infectious and noninfectious, are common.

Radiologic approach to opportunistic infections in transplant recipients

Abnormality	Rate of progression	
	Acute	**Chronic**
Consolidation	Bacteria	Fungi
	Pulmonary edema, edema	TB, *Nocardia*, PCP
	Hemorrhage	
Interstitial infiltrate	Pulmonary edema	Virus, PCP
	Leukoagglutinin	Radiation, drug
	Drug (bacteria)	(Tumor, TB, fungi)
Nodular infiltrate	Bacteria, edema (cytomegalovirus, VZV)	Tumor, fungi
	BOOP, Wegener's	*Nocardia*, TB, PCP
		Bacteria

BOOP—bronchiolitis obliterans with organizing pneumonia; PCP—*Pneumocystis carinii* pneumonia; TB—tuberculosis; VZV—varicella zoster virus.

FIGURE 11-7 Radiologic approach to opportunistic pulmonary infection in the immunocompromised host. The radiographic pattern and rate of progression of pulmonary abnormalities often provide clues to the etiologic agent. Pulmonary infiltrates appearing during the weaning of immunosuppressive drugs or following neutropenia may appear rapidly, regardless of etiology.

Antimicrobial prophylaxis in transplant recipients

Agent	Prevents/Reduces
TMP-SMX	PCP, *Listeria monocytogenes*, *Nocardia*, *Haemophilus*, many bacteria
Quinolines	Gram-negative bacillary infections
Fluconazole	Many *Candida* infections
G-CSF, GM-CSF	Granulocytopenia, leukopenia
IVIG	Graft-vs-host disease, interstitial pneumonia, septicemia
CMV-negative blood products	CMV infection in CMV-seronegative patient
Ganciclovir (intravenously, orally)	CMV disease
Acyclovir	Herpes simplex virus infection
Pentamidine (aerosol, intravenously)	PCP
Atovaquone suspension	PCP, *Toxoplasma gondii*
CMV-hyperimmune globulin	Intensity/incidence (?) of CMV infection

CMV—cytomegalovirus; G-CSF—granulocyte colony-stimulating factor; GM-CSF—granulocyte-macrophage colony-stimulating factor; IVIG—intravenous immune globulin; PCP—*Pneumocystis carinii* pneumonia; TMP-SMX—trimethoprim-sulfamethoxazole.

FIGURE 11-8 Antimicrobial prophylaxis in transplant recipients. Many antimicrobial agents are available for the prevention of infection in the transplant recipient. The selection of specific agents depends on the epidemiologic risks to the patient (*see* Fig. 11-4) and the identification of infection either in a latent state (*ie*, cytomegalovirus, *Toxoplasma gondii*) or prior to surgery (from the donor or recipient).

Drugs associated with pneumonitis

With eosinophilia	Without eosinophilia
Aminosalicylic acid	Azathioprine
Bleomycin sulfate	BCG
Carbamazepine	Busulfan
Chlorpropamide	Chlorambucil
Cromolyn	Colchicine
Furosemide	Cyclophosphamide
Gold compounds	Cytarabine
Hydralazine	Gold compounds
Imipramine	Hydroxyureas
Nitrofurantoin	Ibuprofen
Para-aminosalicyclic acid	Mechlorethamine
Penicillins	Melphalan
Phenytoin	Methotrexate
Procarbazine	Mitomycin
Sulfanilamide	Nitrosoureas
Sulfasalazine	Penicillamine
Sulfonamides	Procarbazine hydrochloride
Tetracycline	

BCG—bacille Calmette-Guérin.

FIGURE 11-9 Drugs associated with pneumonitis. Drug toxicities and interactions are common in the transplant recipient. The use of corticosteroids may mask eosinophilia (particularly to sulfonamides) in an otherwise allergic patient.

Pretransplantation laboratory testing of the organ recipient*

Bacteria
  Mycobacterium tuberculosis (skin test)
  Antibiotic-resistant bacteria (susceptibility data; *eg, Pseudomonas* or *Staphylococcus* spp in lung transplantation)
  Treponema pallidum
  Legionella spp
Parasites
  Toxoplasma gondii (also test heart donors)
  Strongyloides stercoralis[†]
  Stool (ova and parasites)[†]
Fungi
  Aspergillus spp (*eg*, in nares or sinuses in bone marrow or lung transplantation)
  Geographic mycoses (*Histoplasma capsulatum, Coccidioides immitis*)
Viruses
  HIV-1 and 2 (also test donors)
  Epstein-Barr virus
  Cytomegalovirus (also test donors)
  Human T-cell leukemia virus 1
  Measle, mumps, rubella
  Varicella-zoster virus
  Hepatitis viruses (A, B, C) (also test donors)
  Herpes simplex virus type 1 and 2

*Serologic tests (IgG) unless indicated. Not all tests are necessary in all patients. Serum samples should be stored against future clinical indication.
[†]From endemic region.

FIGURE 11-10 Pretransplantation laboratory testing of the organ recipient. Based on the specific epidemiologic exposures at each institution (*see* Fig. 11-4) and on evidence of latent infection in the transplant recipient, a prophylactic regimen can be individualized for the transplant recipient. Because of the risk of vaccination with live vaccines following transplantation, candidates should receive such agents before surgery. Empiric treatment for *Strongyloides stercoralis* may be useful in patients with epidemiologic exposure, even in the absence of evidence of active infection.

PNEUMOCYSTOSIS AND FUNGAL INFECTIONS OF THE LUNGS

Coccidioidomycosis

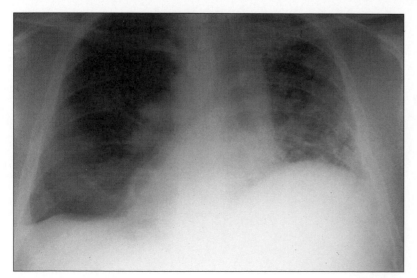

FIGURE 11-11 Chest radiograph of a lung transplant recipient with pulmonary coccidioidomycosis. *Coccidioides immitis* is found in the soil of the southwestern United States and Central and South America. Pulmonary infection is generally associated with asymmetric lymphadenopathy and with eosinophilic or granulomatous infiltration of the lymph nodes. Segmental or lobar infiltrates are most common, but diffuse disease may occur in the immunocompromised host (as seen here) or in the presence of prior pulmonary disease. (*Courtesy of* F. Patterson, MD.)

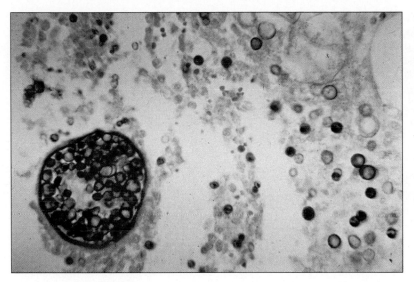

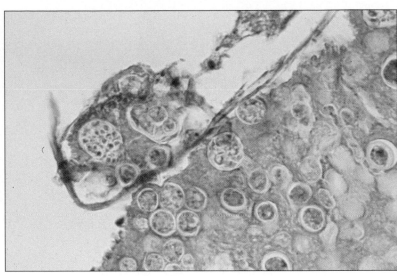

FIGURE 11-12 Periodic acid–Schiff stain of a diagnostic thick-walled spherule of *Coccidioides immitis* containing numerous endospores. Generally, growth of the organism in culture is rapid (3–4 days) from infected tissues. Hematoxylin-eosin (*see* Fig. 11-13) and methenamine silver (*see* Fig. 11-14) stains or fluorescent antibodies are also useful. Hyphae are often found in pulmonary cavities and in granulomatous lesions. (*Courtesy of* T.F. Patterson, MD.)

FIGURE 11-13 Hematoxylin-eosin stain of pulmonary coccidioidomycosis shows thick-walled spores and prominent endospores.

FIGURE 11-14 Methenamine silver stain of pulmonary coccidioidomycosis demonstrating mature spherule in pulmonary tissue.

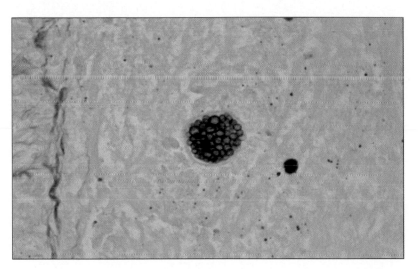

Aspergillosis

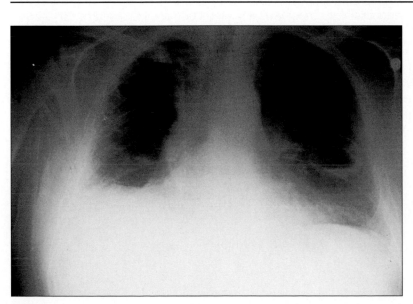

FIGURE 11-15 Left cavitary lung disease due to invasive pulmonary aspergillosis (*Aspergillus fumigatus*) in a lung transplant recipient. The *Aspergillus* species are ubiquitous environmental molds. In the transplant recipient, anastomotic sites (tracheal anastomosis) and the use of antilymphocyte antibodies are associated with infection. Tropism for vascular structures may result in pulmonary infarction and/or hemoptysis. (*Courtesy of* T.F. Patterson, MD.)

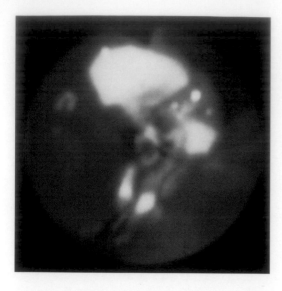

FIGURE 11-16 Bronchoscopic view of an obstructed mainstem bronchus in a lung transplant recipient with *Aspergillus* ulcerative tracheobronchitis. Mucosal ulceration, broad-spectrum antibiotics, and immunosuppression contribute to the development of invasive local disease in the trachea. Surgical excision and antifungal therapies are recommended for localized disease; the transplanted lung is often poorly responsive to antifungal therapy alone. (*Courtesy of* S.M. Levine, MD.)

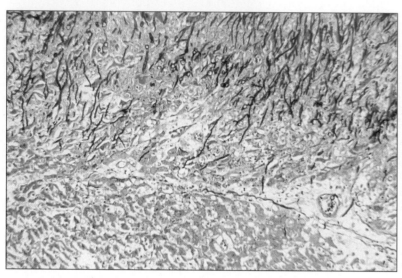

FIGURE 11-17 Extensive lung tissue invasion due to *Aspergillus fumigatus* in a lung transplant recipient. Invasion through the tracheal mucosa into parenchyma, blood vessels, or cartilage is less common than distal invasion with hemorrhagic infarction. Invasive disease due to *Aspergillus* species has been reported in 2% (renal) to 4% to 17% (liver) of organ recipients [3]. (Methenamine silver stain.) (*Courtesy of* T.F. Patterson, MD.)

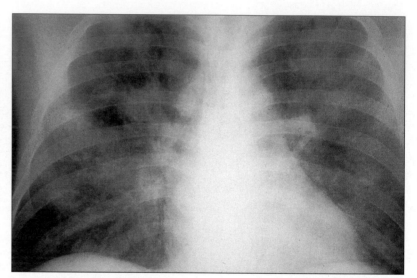

FIGURE 11-18 Diffuse pulmonary infiltrates in a bone marrow transplant recipient due to invasive pulmonary aspergillosis. The incidence of diffuse invasive *Aspergillus* infection is as high as 20% at some institutions following bone marrow transplantation or during prolonged neutropenia after chemotherapy. High-energy particulate air or laminar flow air filtration has significantly reduced the incidence of nosocomial aspergillosis. Disease may emerge during the acute treatment of organ rejection (pulse corticosteroids) or during the tapering of high-dose immunosuppressive therapy. Graft-vs-host disease, pulmonary hemorrhage, and viral (cytomegalovirus) coinfection are risk factors for the development of this disease. (*Courtesy of* T.F. Patterson, MD.)

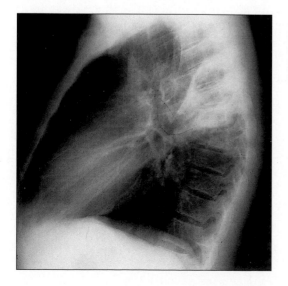

FIGURE 11-19 Lateral chest radiograph of a renal transplant recipient following pulmonary embolus with *Aspergillus* abscess in infarcted tissue. Sputum cultures are often negative in the setting of significant pulmonary infection with *Aspergillus*. Atypical presentations of noninfectious processes (emboli, drug toxicity, pulmonary edema) often necessitate invasive diagnostic procedures in the immunocompromised host.

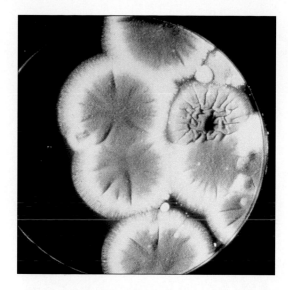

FIGURE 11-20 Culture of *Aspergillus fumigatus* showing typical blue-green colonies. Single colonies from surveillance cultures or respiratory secretions should not be considered contaminants in the immunocompromised host until the absence of parenchymal disease is demonstrated. Each clinical mycology laboratory should document the incidence of potential fungal contaminants and of clusters of infection in order to recognize increased nosocomial risks (*eg*, associated with construction).

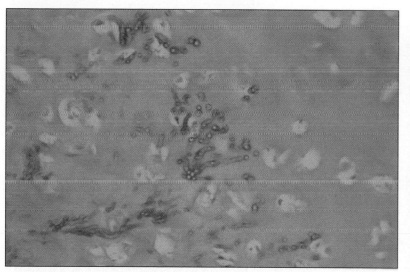

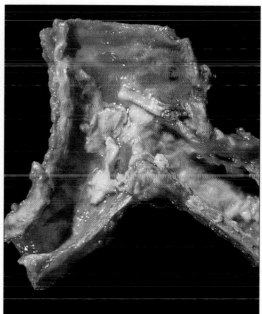

FIGURE 11-22 Necrotizing tracheobronchitis with pseudomembrane formation due to aspergillosis in a lung transplant recipient. Bacterial superinfection may mask the presentation of *Aspergillus* infection.

FIGURE 11-21 Biopsy of an area of inflammation surrounding the tracheal anastomosis of a lung transplant recipient with recurrent *Aspergillus* infections. *Aspergillus fumigatus* was detected in an area of scar tissue by periodic acid–Schiff stain. Gross examination of the specimen showed normal findings, and fungal cultures were negative. Infection may be detected during the evaluation of an unexplained air-leak or bleeding following lung transplantation. (*Courtesy of* R. Kradin, MD.)

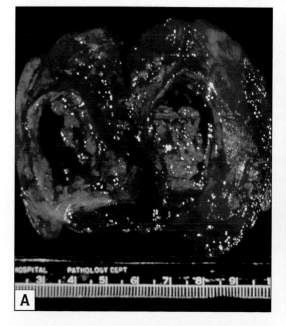

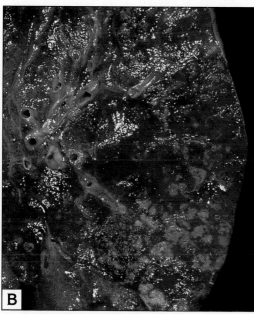

FIGURE 11-23 Colonization versus invasive *Aspergillus* infection. **A**, Gross examination of a lung cavity containing a fungus ball of *Aspergillus* (aspergilloma). Traditional distinctions between colonization and invasive *Aspergillus* infection break down in the immunocompromised host. Minimally invasive disease may produce fungemia and disseminated infection in the transplant recipient, as occurred in this liver transplant patient. **B**, Invasive pulmonary aspergillosis in a liver transplant recipient.

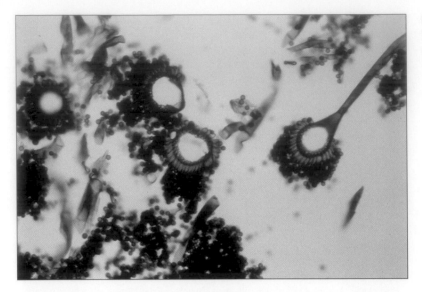

FIGURE 11-24 *Aspergillus fumigatus* from lung cavity of a renal transplant patient. (Methenamine silver satin.) (*Courtesy of* M. Joseph, MD, S. Salman, MD, and M. Goodman, MD.)

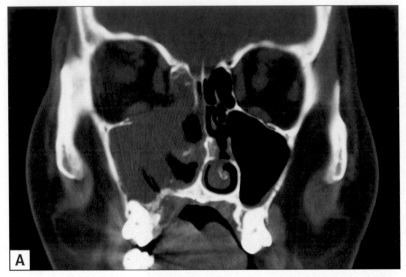

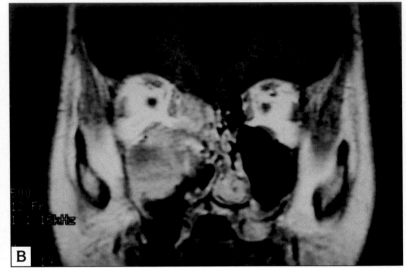

FIGURE 11-25 A and **B**, Coronal computed tomography (*panel 25A*) and magnetic resonance (*panel 25B*) scans in a 35-year-old man with fever and nose bleeds in the setting of acute graft rejection. Two years previously the patient had undergone liver transplantation. Opacification of the left maxillary sinus was found to be due to *Aspergillus fumigatus*. Tissue-invasive fungal infection in the transplant recipient requires surgical debridement, reduction of immunosuppressive therapy, and aggressive antifungal therapy. Successful antifungal therapy required four surgical debridements to clean margins and > 4 g of intravenous amphotericin B over a period of 4 months. (*Courtesy of* M. Joseph, MD, S. Salman, MD, and M. Goodman, MD.)

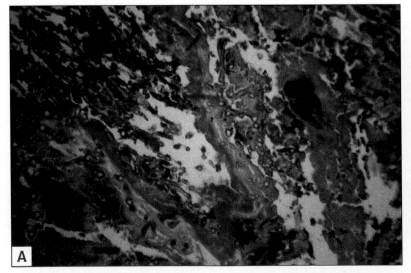

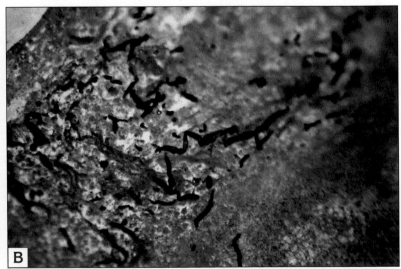

FIGURE 11-26 Biopsy of sinus infected with *Aspergillus*. **A**, Hematoxylin-eosin stain. **B**, Methenamine silver stain. (*Courtesy of* M. Joseph, MD, S. Salman, MD, and M. Goodman, MD.)

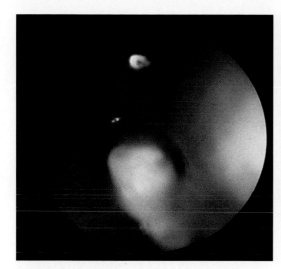

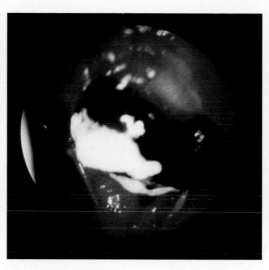

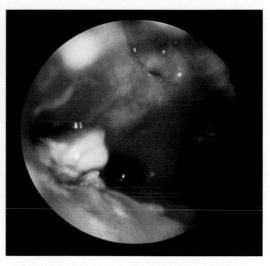

FIGURE 11-27 Nasal endoscopic view of an allergic polyp in a patient infected with *Aspergillus.* Chronic bacterial sinusitis is often associated with the development of fungal infection. The presence of polyps and/or allergic disease may provide the anatomic niche needed for the development of rhinosinusitis and/or mastoiditis. The presentation may be benign or similar to that of bacterial infection. However, epistaxis, swelling, and facial erythema are common with invasive disease. (*Courtesy of* M. Joseph, MD, S. Salman, MD, and M. Goodman, MD.)

FIGURE 11-28 Nasal endoscopic view of an *Aspergillus*-infected blood clot. Following debridement, irrigation is a useful adjunct to antifungal therapy to promote healing and reduce fungal load. (*Courtesy of* M. Joseph, MD, S. Salman, MD, and M. Goodman, MD.)

FIGURE 11-29 *Aspergillus* growing out of a maxillary sinus ostium as seen via sinus endoscopy. (*Courtesy of* M. Joseph, MD, S. Salman, MD, and M. Goodman, MD.)

Mucormycosis

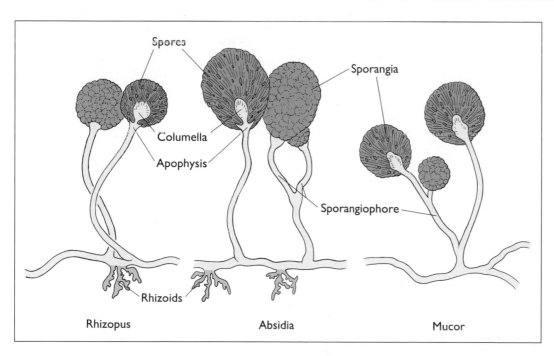

FIGURE 11-30 Pathogenic species in mucormycosis. The Zygomycetes fungi cause significant infection (zygomycosis, mucormycosis, phycomycosis) in the immunocompromised host in association with anatomic abnormalities of the sinuses, lungs, skin, or other mucosal surfaces. Diabetics, patients with neutropenia, and transplant recipients are the most common targets of these infections. All of the agents of the order Mucorales have broad hyphae with few septae without an eosinophilic sheath and can cause infection in compromised individuals. Members of the order Entomophthorales of the Zygomycetes rarely cause such opportunistic infections. Most of the agents of mucormycosis have been associated with infection in the transplant recipient. (*From* Sugar [4]; with permission.)

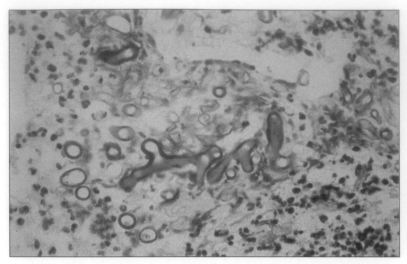

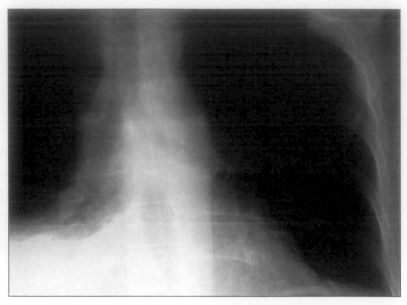

FIGURE 11-31 Hematoxylin-eosin stain of sinus tissue in invasive mucormycosis. Infections due to the Mucoraceae occur most often in diabetic patients but are prominent causes of infection in neutropenic and transplant patients. The presentation of sinusitis may include orbital cellulitis, proptosis, or ophthalmoplegia, cavernous sinus or carotid artery thrombosis, or cerebral abscess. In immunocompromised patients, infection is due to the inhalation of spores or inoculation by intravenous catheters, tape, and other breaks in the mucosa and skin. Cultures are often negative, and histopathologic specimens are required for diagnosis. Surgical debridement of infected sites is critical for successful treatment of these infections.

FIGURE 11-32 Chest radiograph of 48-year-old woman 4 years after liver transplantation with pulmonary cavity due to mucormycosis. The clinical presentation of pulmonary mucormycosis is not distinguishable from that of pulmonary infection due to *Aspergillus*. However, rapid enlargement and cavitation of pulmonary lesions (in 1–2 days) is more common with the agents of mucormycosis. Because the agents of mucormycosis are relatively resistant to antifungal therapy, surgical debridement is often essential to successful cure of these infections.

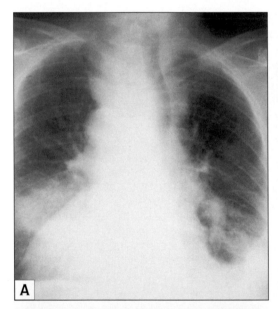

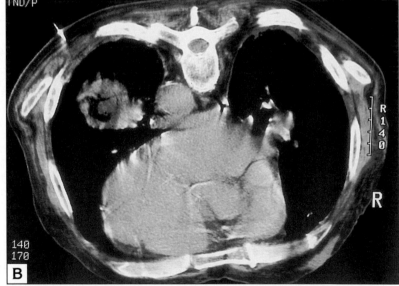

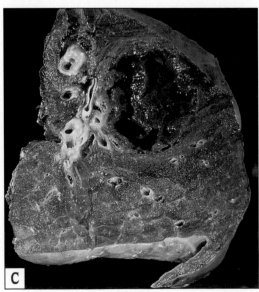

FIGURE 11-33 Pulmonary mucormycosis presenting as a rapidly progressive, solitary abscess. A 65-year-old man 5 years after cadaveric kidney transplantation presented with a cough and low-grade fever. **A,** Initial chest radiograph was read as consistent with a new lingular infiltrate, probable pneumonia. Bronchoscopy and examination of bronchoalveolar lavage fluid were unremarkable. **B,** Computed tomography scan evaluation showed the lung abscess had doubled in size over 36 hours, despite therapy with broad-spectrum antibiotics and amphotericin B. Examination of an aspirate obtained by percutaneous needle aspiration was negative. However, the clinical appearance was consistent with mucormycosis, and the patient was taken to surgery for resection. **C,** At surgery, the lingula and adjacent tissue were friable and gray in appearance and resected en bloc. The resected lung contained a single large abscess cavity containing necrotic tissue and blood. No organisms were detected within the necrotic tissues on frozen section evaluation. *Mucor circinelloides* was found by histopathologic techniques in the perivascular areas of the ischemic lung tissue.

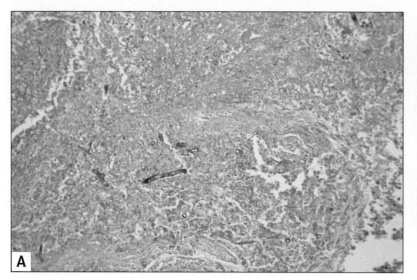

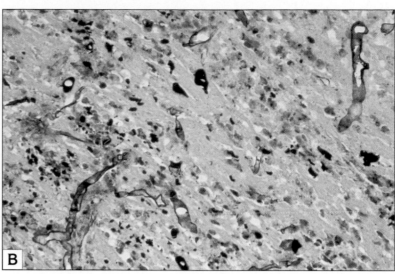

FIGURE 11-34 Histopathologic examinations of lung tissue in pulmonary mucormycosis. **A**, Hematoxylin-eosin stain of the cavity wall seen in Figure 11-33 showed broad, nonseptate hyphal elements. An inflammatory vasculitis was appreciated with extensive tissue necrosis. Thrombosis of the small arteries and pulmonary veins was notable. **B**, Methenamine silver stain revealed hyphae with right-angle branching and occasional septae, consistent with a Mucoraceae species.

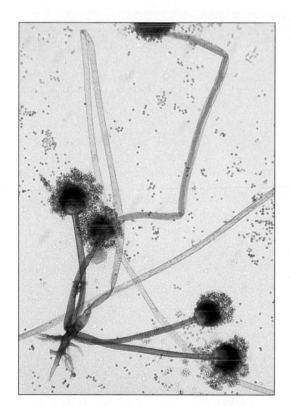

FIGURE 11-35 Cultured *Mucor* showing right-angle branching of hyphae and septae. Two days after the resection of tissues (*see* Figs. 11-33 and 11-34), a single colony of *Mucor* species was isolated from fungal cultures from the original percutaneous lung aspirate. This information at that time was not useful in the clinical management of the immuno-compromised host. Fatal pulmonary hemorrhage is a complication of rapidly expanding areas of tissue necrosis, which may be associated with mucormycosis. Prompt, invasive diagnosis and debridement are essential.

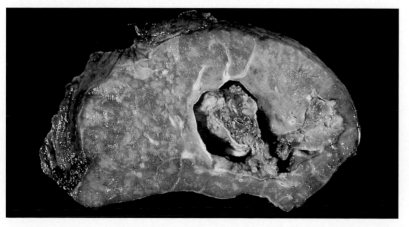

FIGURE 11-36 Gross specimen showing invasive pulmonary mucormycosis in a 68-year-old diabetic renal transplant recipient. Patients receiving chelation therapy with deferoxamine, with renal failure and dialysis, are at increased risk for the development of mucormycosis.

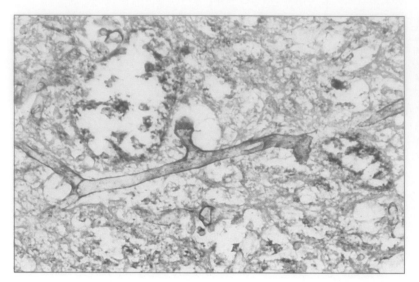

FIGURE 11-37 Methenamine silver stain of *Rhizopus orzyae* in a biopsy specimen from a transplanted lung. Sparse septae, broad hyphae, and right-angle branching are seen. The *Rhizopus* species belong to the Mucoraceae and are agents of mucormycosis. These fungi grow as hyphae both in nature and tissues. *R. orzyae* is ubiquitous but usually causes disease only in the immunocompromised host, particularly in diabetic individuals or transplant recipients receiving corticosteroids. Macrophage dysfunction or anatomic disease (*eg,* undrained sinuses) is most often associated with disease due to the Mucoraceae. (*Courtesy of* T.F. Patterson, MD.)

Pneumocystosis

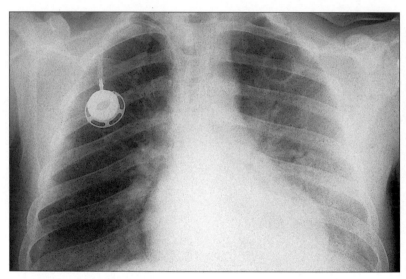

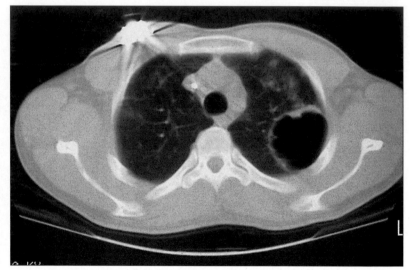

FIGURE 11-38 Chest radiograph of 27-year-old diabetic after kidney transplantation, showing a pulmonary cavity discovered during taper of corticosteroid therapy. The cavity contained *Aspergillus* and *Pneumocystis carinii*. Dual infections are not uncommon in the lungs of transplant recipients. Failure to respond to optimal therapy for one infection should suggest the presence of a second process (infectious or noninfectious). Cytomegalovirus often coinfects the lungs in bone marrow and lung transplant recipients. Histopathologic documentation of infection should be considered in all immunocompromised patients, particularly those failing to respond to therapy.

FIGURE 11-39 Chest computed tomography (CT) scan of the patient in Figure 11-38 with dual infection by *Pneumocystis* and *Aspergillus*. The chest CT is useful to distinguish interstitial processes from invasive disease. Disease masked by corticosteroids or immunosuppression is often seen by CT.

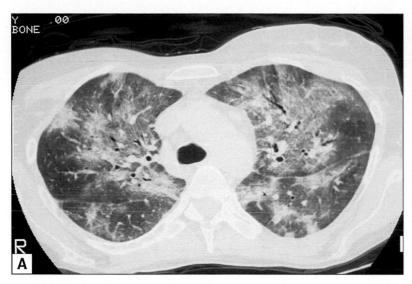

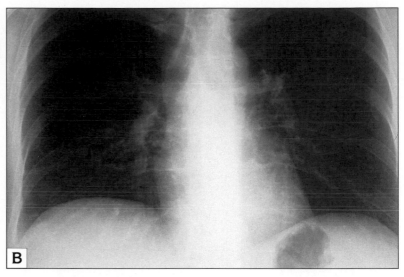

FIGURE 11-40 *Pneumocystis* pneumonia in a 44-year-old woman after liver transplantation. **A,** Chest computed tomography (CT) scan shows inhomogeneous and diffuse interstitial infiltrates in contrast with the relatively mild pattern observed on a routine chest radiograph. **B,** The chest radiograph shows minimal bilateral, bibasilar interstitial infiltrates, despite marked hypoxemia and extensive disease observed by CT scan.

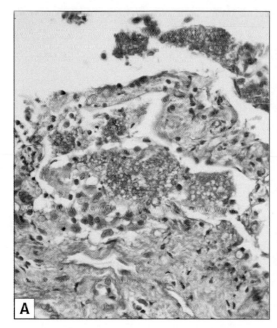

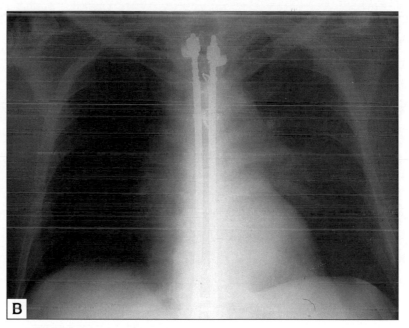

FIGURE 11-41 *Pneumocystis* pneumonia in a renal transplant recipient. **A,** Lung biopsy specimen stained for fungi with periodic acid–Schiff (PAS) stain. *Pneumocystis carinii* stains with PAS, revealing the frothy intra-alveolar infiltrate containing organisms and debris with inflammatory exudate seen in this section. Hematoxylin-eosin or silver stains also can demonstrate the typical pattern of pulmonary pneumocystosis. The diagnosis of *Pneumocystis* pneumonia can be made noninvasively using fluorescent antibody staining on induced sputum specimens. However, the yield of induced sputum specimens is reduced by the use of prophylaxis (*eg,* pentamidine), and bronchoalveolar lavage may be necessary in the susceptible host. The evaluation of polymerase chain reaction methodology may improve the diagnosis of *Pneumocystis* infection if issues regarding the sensitivity of this assay can be resolved. **B,** Chest radiograph from the patient. (Panel 41A *courtesy of* R. Kradin, MD.)

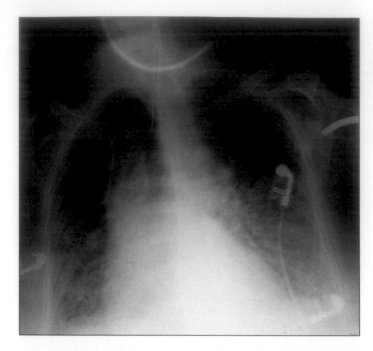

FIGURE 11-42 Chest radiograph of a patient with dual *Pneumocystis* and cytomegalovirus pneumonia during treatment for acute hepatic allograft rejection. Both infections, and others requiring cell-mediated immunity for clearance, are enhanced by acute changes in the level of immune suppression: pulse steroids, antilymphocyte antibodies, and irradiation. The documentation of cytomegalovirus (CMV) infection in the lungs should not rely solely on culture data, as many patients secrete CMV in the absence of significant parenchymal disease. CMV antigenemia assays or biopsy specimens may be needed to demonstrate pulmonary infection.

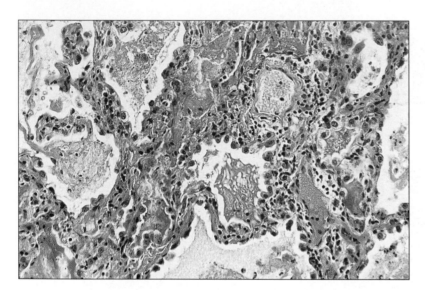

FIGURE 11-43 Hematoxylin-eosin stain showing prominent interstitial infiltrates and alveolar exudates typical of *Pneumocystis* infection. The patient was a bone marrow transplant recipient who developed *Pneumocystis* pneumonia following intensive chemotherapy for breast cancer.

Clinical presentation of *Pneumocystis* pneumonia

Feature	Non-AIDS	AIDS
Presentation	Acute illness	Subacute
Signs and symptoms	Dyspnea, fever, cough, few physical findings	
Chest radiograph	Bilateral interstitial infiltrates, nodules, variable	
Blood gases	Hypoxemia with respiratory alkalosis	
Organism burden	Moderate	High
Diagnostic yield	Good	Excellent
Prognosis	Good	Good
Relapse	Uncommon	Always without prophylaxis
Adverse reactions to:		
TMP/SMX	Uncommon	Common
Pentamidine (intravenously)	Uncommon	Common

TMP-SMX—trimethoprim-sulfamethoxazole.

FIGURE 11-44 Clinical presentation of *Pneumocystis carinii* pneumonia (PCP) in patients with and without AIDS. The replication of *Pneumocystis carinii* occurs over 7 to 12 days *in vitro*, but the development of clinical symptoms with PCP is delayed in the setting of immunosuppression. Patients receiving corticosteroid therapy and patients with AIDS manifest symptoms later than other susceptible hosts. As a result, the organism burden in these patients may be greater at the time of diagnosis, even though the clinical manifestations may remain muted. Diagnosis by induced sputum examination is enhanced in these patients, but response to treatment may be less rapid than in other hosts. Patients developing PCP while on prophylactic antibiotics may require bronchoscopy for the demonstration of organisms.

Cryptococcosis

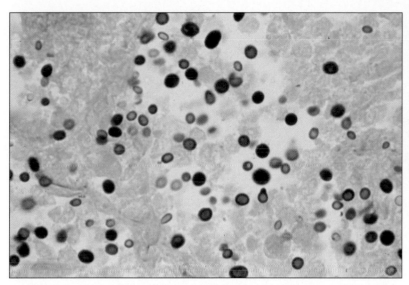

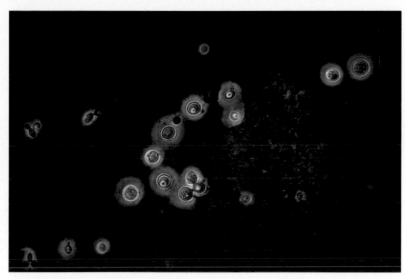

FIGURE 11-45 Methenamine silver stain in a lung transplant recipient with pulmonary cryptococcosis. Alternative stains include the periodic acid–Schiff (PAS) or mucicarmine stains. *Cryptococcus* infection is assumed to be a disseminated infection at the time of diagnosis. Preferred sites for infection include the central nervous system, lungs, and skin. Detection of the polysaccharide capsular antigen of *Cryptococcus neoformans* in blood is useful in both the diagnosis and assessment of the success of therapy for this infection. Cutaneous involvement begins as small papules or ulcerative areas, often under taper, and may progress to deep and necrotic lesions. Biopsy is necessary to distinguish these lesions from those of atypical bacteria, *Nocardia asteroides*, or *Aspergillus* infections. The portal of entry is assumed to be the lungs. However, there are generally few pulmonary symptoms, and involvement of the lungs is often established in retrospect.

FIGURE 11-46 India ink preparation showing *Cryptococcus neoformans* bronchoalveolar lavage fluid. *C. neoformans* is a major cause of infection in the neutropenic host. The portal of entry is generally the respiratory tract. In cryptococcal meningitis, demonstration of the organism by India ink preparation is possible in up to half of infected individuals. The details of internal structure are critical to the separation from other artifacts. The capsule is thick and distinctly outlined, the cell wall is doubly refractile, and the cytoplasm contains refractile inclusions. Narrow-based budding of the organism may also be seen in some preparations or histopathologic examination. (*Courtesy of* M.J. Rosen, MD.)

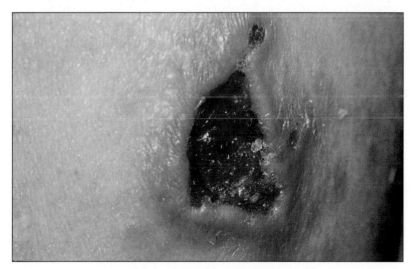

FIGURE 11-47 Nonspecific lesion of cutaneous cryptococcosis. An unusual ulcerated lesion is seen, although other lesions may appear as papules, pustules, plaques, or subcutaneous masses. Cryptococcal infection may affect skin lesions or cause metastatic infection via the bloodstream. Cultures of blood and urine and serum and cerebrospinal fluid cultures and cryptococcal antigen studies should be performed. Any suspicious skin lesions require urgent biopsy. (*Courtesy of* G.J. Raugi, MD.)

Histoplasmosis

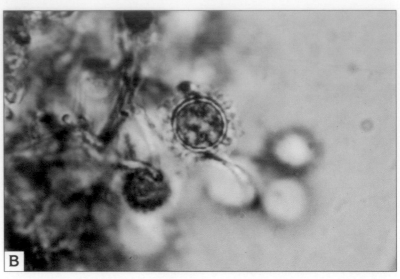

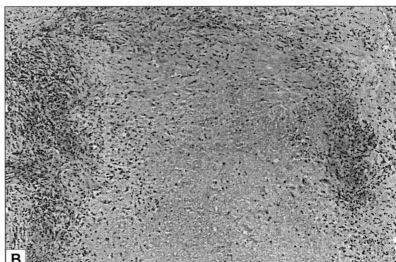

FIGURE 11-48 Dimorphic presentations of *Histoplasma capsulatum*. **A**, Tuberculated macroconidia and small oval microconidia of the mycelial form. **B**, Yeast forms in human tissue. (Lactophenol cotton blue; original magnification, × 1000.) (*Courtesy of* E.J. Bottone, PhD.)

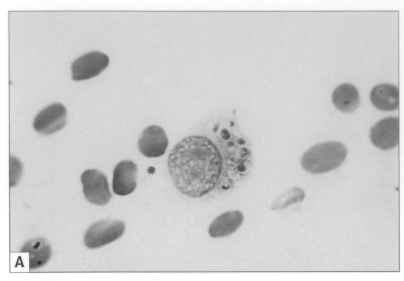

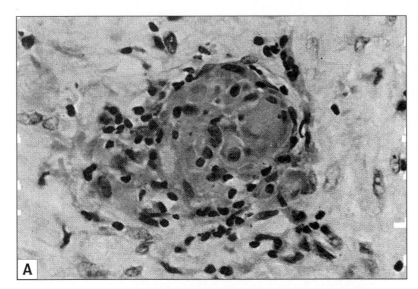

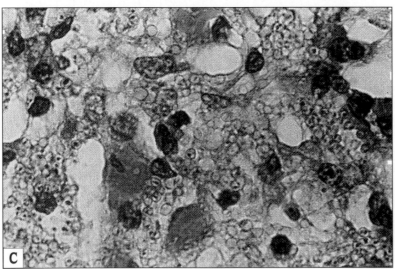

FIGURE 11-49 Immunohistopathologic spectrum of histoplasmosis. **A**, Sarcoidal-type granuloma. (Original magnification, × 480.) **B**, Granulomatous inflammation with caseation necrosis. (Original magnification, × 120.) **C**, Diffuse infiltrate of foamy macrophages containing very large numbers of yeast forms in an AIDS patient with acute progressive disseminated histoplasmosis. (Original magnification, × 320.) (*From* Bullock [5]; with permission.)

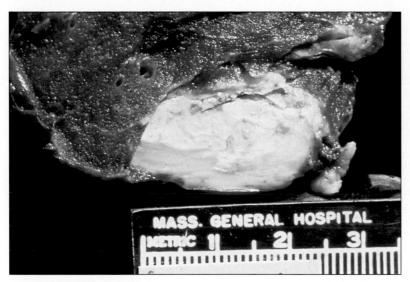

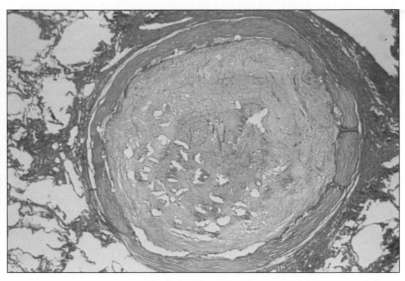

FIGURE 11-50 Resected native lung from a lung transplant recipient showing pulmonary histoplasmosis. Like cryptococcosis, infection due to *Histoplasma capsulatum* is generally disseminated at the time of detection in the immunocompromised patient. The clinical presentation is usually nonspecific, and pulmonary disease may be asymptomatic. The chest radiograph is normal in up to 50% of patients. Many patients present with hepatic or splenic involvement. Infection is usually due to new primary exposure in endemic geographic regions, although reactivation disease has occurred in transplant recipients.

FIGURE 11-51 Old granuloma in pulmonary histoplasmosis. Reactivation disease may occur in immunosuppressed or malnourished individuals. Serologic testing is usually positive in patients from endemic areas but may be negative in the immunosuppressed individual. Both immunodiffusion and complement fixation tests are positive in the majority of infected persons, but antigen detection tests are useful in the acute setting

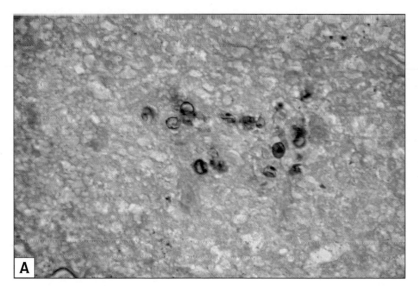

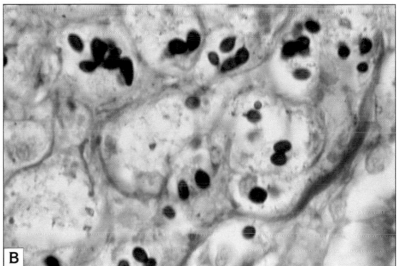

FIGURE 11-52 A and **B**, Methenamine silver staining in pulmonary histoplasmosis.

BACTERIAL INFECTIONS

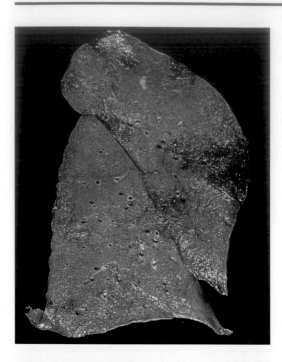

FIGURE 11-53 Pulmonary infarction following *Pseudomonas* bacteremia in a bone marrow transplant recipient. Bacteremia during neutropenia is generally due to endogenous organisms (*ie*, from gastrointestinal or oropharyngeal colonization). The return of normal immune function may be delayed after marrow engraftment, particularly in the presence of viral infection such as that with cytomegalovirus or hepatitis viruses. The risk of bacterial infection is related to the type of chemotherapy and duration of neutropenia, preexisting infections, breaks in mucosal and skin integrity (*eg*, intravenous or urinary catheters), and intensity of nosocomial exposure.

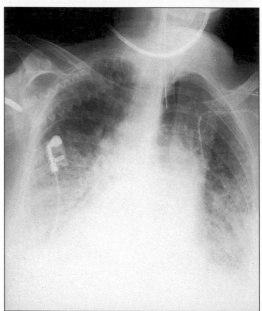

FIGURE 11-54 Chest radiograph from renal transplant recipient with candidal and enterococcal bacteremia. Dual infections are common in transplant recipients. In this patient, the organisms suggested a gastrointestinal source, and a diverticular abscess was detected. Cultures of the peritoneum grew both *Candida* and *Streptococcus faecalis*.

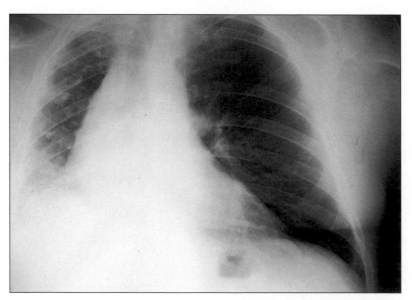

FIGURE 11-55 Left-lung transplant recipient with aspiration pneumonitis of the residual right lung. Anatomic defects and foreign bodies (bronchial stents) are most often associated with infections of the transplanted lung in the immediate postoperative period. However, persistence of the underlying disease or diminished blood flow in the residual lung will increase the risk of infection in this lung.

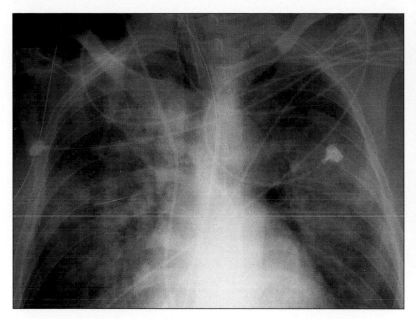

FIGURE 11-56 Chest radiograph of a patient who developed *Staphylococcus aureus* pneumonia during pentamidine treatment for *Pneumocystis* pneumonia. Intubated patients who are colonized with nosocomial pathogens are at increased risk for bacterial superinfection. Suctioned specimens from the endotracheal tube may reflect only colonization. Bronchoscopic samples are valuable in the detection of secondary infection [6].

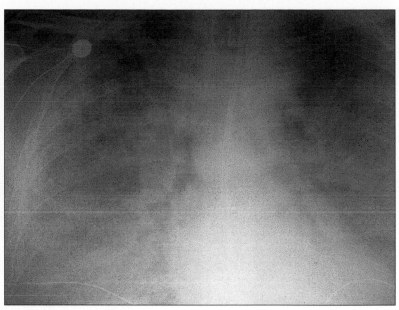

FIGURE 11-57 Chest radiograph in an hepatic transplant recipient with adult respiratory distress syndrome and *Klebsiella* sepsis due to a biliary anastomotic leak. Diffuse pulmonary infiltrates obscure the observation of free air under the right hemidiaphragm. In the first month following transplantation, infection is often associated with "technical" complications: anastomotic leaks, lymphocele, urinary tract infections associated with catheters, drug interactions, infections carried from the donor, and aspiration pneumonitis. Infections after the first month are more often due to reactivation of latent infection or community-acquired infection.

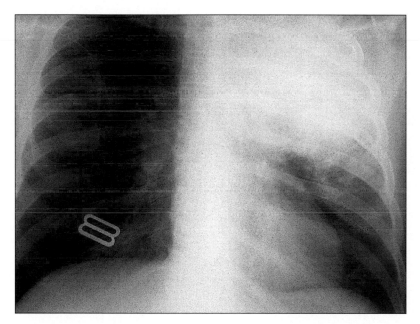

FIGURE 11-58 Chest radiograph showing *Legionella pneumophila* pneumonia in a renal transplant recipient. The broad defect in cellular immunity seen in transplant recipients predisposes to infection with intracellular pathogens. Because erythromycin may increase serum cyclosporine levels, close follow-up of such levels is advisable during macrolide therapy. Controlled trials have not been completed with newer macrolide agents (azithromycin, clarithromycin), rifampin (in combination with macrolide), trimethoprim-sulfamethoxazole, quinolines, or tetracyclines. *Legionella* urinary antigen detection tests identify approximately 80% of *L. pneumophila* infections, but not infections due to other *Legionella* species. Culture on buffered charcoal yeast extract supplemented with dyes and antibiotics is advantageous. The yield of cultures from good sputum samples is generally equivalent to those of induced or bronchoscopic specimens. Direct fluorescent antibody testing is highly specific (up to 99%) but may miss infections with small numbers of organisms. DNA probes and polymerase chain reaction tests are also available, having high levels of sensitivity and specificity (for the ribosomal messenger RNA of the *Legionella* family).

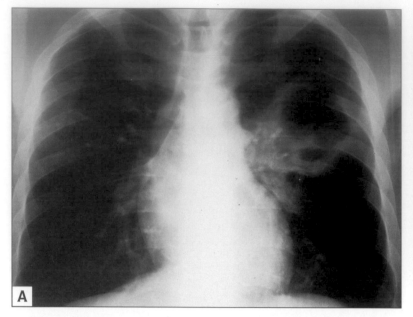

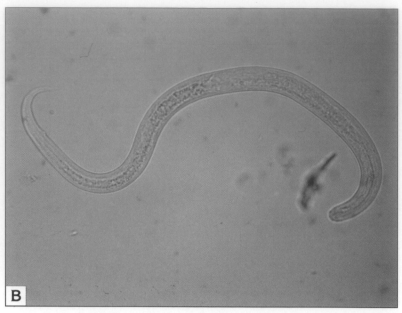

FIGURE 11-59 Bacterial lung abscess with coinfection by Strongyloides stercoralis in a Vietnamese kidney transplant recipient. **A**, Chest radiograph shows a lung abscess due to *Enterobacter* species. Bronchoscopic examination revealed simultaneous *Pneumocystis carinii* and *S. stercoralis* infections. *Strongyloides* is capable of completing its life cycle within the human host but is usually limited to the gastrointestinal tract by the intact immune system. During immunosuppression, infectious complications may be observed in locations through which the nematode passes during acute infection, including the skin, bloodstream, lungs, and gastrointestinal tract. Migration across the wall of the gastrointestinal tract during immunosuppression (hyperinfection) is associated with systemic signs of "sepsis" and central nervous system infection (parasitic and bacterial). **B**, *Strongyloides stercoralis* from the lung of the patient with bacterial lung abscess. Preventative therapy for strongyloidiasis may be useful in patients from endemic regions who are being evaluated for organ transplantation. The activation of systemic infection (hyperinfection) due to *Strongyloides* migrating from the gastrointestinal tract or the anatomic obstruction produced by migration through the lung parenchyma may contribute to life-threatening bacterial infection. The immune mechanisms responsible for the control of *Strongyloides* infection are under investigation.

VIRAL INFECTIONS

Cytomegalovirus

Clinical effects of cytomegalovirus infection in organ transplant recipients

Early manifestations (1–6 mos after transplantation)
  Fever
  Lymphadenopathy (mononucleosis syndrome)
  Pneumonia (lung and marrow transplant)
  Hepatitis, pancreatitis, nephritis (allograft injury)
  Gastrointestinal ulcerations, with bleeding and/or perforation
  Leukopenia and thrombocytopenia
  Encephalitis (rare)
  Transverse myelitis (rare)
  Cutaneous vasculitis (rare)
  Allograft rejection
  Immunosuppression
Late manifestations (> 6 mos after transplantation)
  Progressive chorioretinitis (possibly underdiagnosed)
  Primary disease in seronegative recipient (rare)

FIGURE 11-60 Clinical effects of cytomegalovirus (CMV) infection in organ transplant recipients. CMV has the greatest impact on the transplanted organ. Patients may present with altered graft function or rejection or with systemic evidence of "viral" disease.

Effect of types of immunosuppression on incidence of cytomegalovirus pneumonia in kidney recipients

Transplant center	Immunosuppression	Patients, *n*	Cytomegalovirus pneumonia, *n (%)*
Pittsburgh	Azathioprine-prednisone	138	3 (2.2)
Pittsburgh	Cyclosporine-prednisone	131	3 (2.0)
Minnesota	Azathioprine-prednisone-antithymocyte globulin	349	29 (8.3)*
Minnesota	Cyclosporine-prednisone	76	2 (2.6)

*Significantly different.

FIGURE 11-61 Effect of types of immunosuppression on incidence of cytomegalovirus (CMV) pneumonia in kidney transplant recipients. The activation of CMV in the transplant recipient is related to the nature, dose, and duration of immunosuppressive therapies, status of host immunity to CMV, and dose of CMV associated with the allograft. (*From* Peterson *et al.* [7]; with permission.)

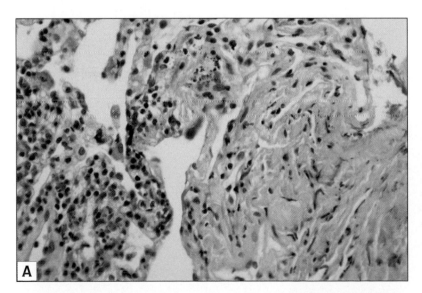

FIGURE 11-62 Chest radiograph of a 52-year-old man with cytomegalovirus (CMV) pneumonitis 2 months after allogeneic bone marrow transplantation. Both infectious (CMV) and idiopathic pneumonitis syndromes generally occur up to 100 days following bone marrow engraftment. Pneumonitis associated with CMV appears to be associated with immune reactivity to CMV antigens but does not require active replication of the virus. Prophylactic antiviral agents have been effective in preventing 25% to 50% of this form of pneumonitis following bone marrow transplantation. Risk factors for CMV pneumonitis include graft-vs-host disease, mismatched (especially allogeneic) transplantation, patient age, CMV seropositivity, and pulmonary irradiation. Other infectious etiologies must be excluded in the evaluation of the patient.

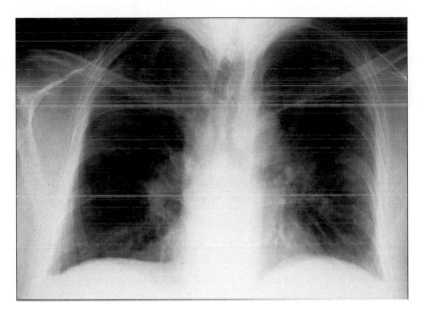
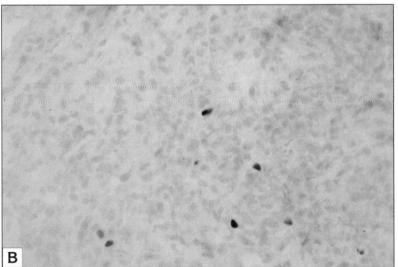

FIGURE 11-63 Histopathologic evaluation of a specimen from a bronchoscopic biopsy specimen from a lung transplant recipient with fever and diffuse pulmonary infiltrates on chest radiography. **A,** Hematoxylin-eosin stain shows occasional intranuclear and intracytoplasmic inclusion bodies in tissue. **B,** Antibody staining of lung tissue with monoclonal antibody against human cytomegalovirus (CMV) and a horseradish peroxidase–coupled second antibody. Brown precipitate labels cells infected with CMV and expressing CMV antigens. Transplantation of a lung from a CMV-seropositive donor into a seronegative recipient is associated with a high incidence of CMV pneumonitis and coinfection. Routine use of antiviral therapy may limit the impact of CMV infection in this population. Presentation of CMV disease may include pulmonary superinfection (*eg, Pneumocystis*, bacterial, fungal), systemic "flulike" illness, allograft rejection, or progressive hypoxemia.

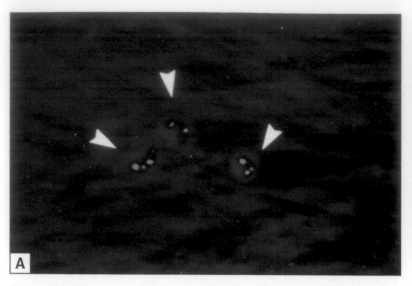

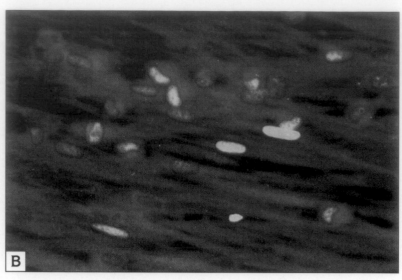

FIGURE 11-64 Immunofluorescent assays for cytomegalovirus (CMV). **A,** Detection of CMV in the clinical laboratory includes rapid stains for CMV antigens expressed in centrifuged shell vial cultures. CMV early antigen is expressed in the nuclei of human fibroblasts *in vitro* and is detected by immunofluorescence using monoclonal antibodies directed against CMV immediate early antigens. **B,** Blood buffy coat has been used to infect fibroblasts with CMV. The preparation is stained with monoclonal antibody directed against the early antigen of CMV. (*Courtesy of* A. Caliendo, MD.)

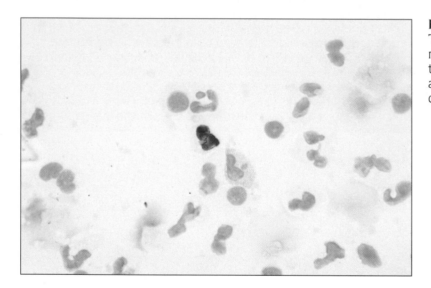

FIGURE 11-65 Detection of cytomegalovirus (CMV) antigenemia. The detection of CMV matrix protein gp65 within circulating neutrophils allows preemptive therapy of CMV infection in organ transplant recipients. The number of neutrophils stained with this antibody (brown peroxidase label in the central cell in this figure) correlates with the intensity of infection [8].

Respiratory Syncytial Virus

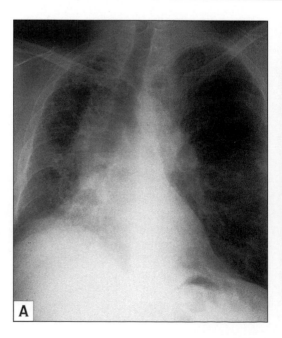

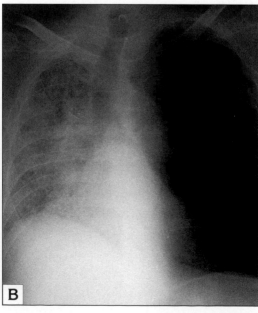

FIGURE 11-66 A, Chest radiograph of a 49-year-old man with bilateral pneumonitis due to respiratory syncytial virus (RSV) following single left-lung transplantation. RSV is a common cause of pediatric pneumonitis, and the virus is frequently shed in the lungs of immunosuppressed children. In lung and bone marrow transplant recipients, RSV may be a cofactor in the pathogenesis of pneumonia or graft dysfunction (rejection). Some adult lung transplant recipients have benefited from treatment of RSV pneumonia in the absence of other etiologies for pulmonary deterioration, but the role of RSV and antiviral therapy for RSV in the general population of immunocompromised adults remains controversial. Mortality in the bone marrow transplant recipient prior to marrow engraftment is high. **B,** The patient also had simultaneous *Klebsiella* pneumonia in the residual (native) right lung.

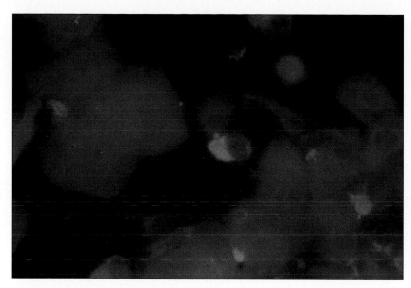

FIGURE 11-67 Nasal washings stained with bovine antibody to human respiratory syncytial virus. Positive staining results in the green color seen in the cytoplasm of infected mononuclear cells.

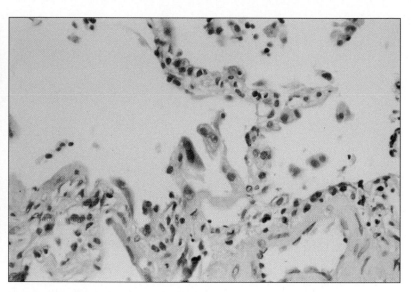

FIGURE 11-68 Transbronchial biopsy from an adult bilateral lung transplant recipient with respiratory syncytial virus pneumonia. All other viral, bacterial, fungal, and parasitic studies done on this patient were unrevealing. Lymphocytic peribronchial inflammation with edema, some early hyaline membrane formation, and epithelial injury with sloughing are observed. (Hematoxylin-eosin stain.) (Courtesy of B. Kradin, MD.)

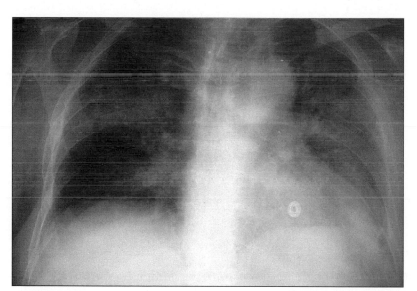

FIGURE 11-69 Chest radiograph of a 79-year-old man 18 years after renal transplantation, showing pneumonia due to primary varicella-zoster virus (VZV) infection. The patient was known to be seronegative for VZV. VZV causes a broad range of visceral disease in the immunocompromised patient. Noncutaneous infection may present as central nervous system disease with cerebral angiitis, encephalitis, or cerebellar ataxia (usually in children), as well as myocarditis or hepatitis. Pulmonary disease in the immunocompromised adult is life threatening. Symptoms (dyspnea, cough, fever, tachypnea) may begin 3 to 5 days after cutaneous eruption or in the presence or absence of skin rash.

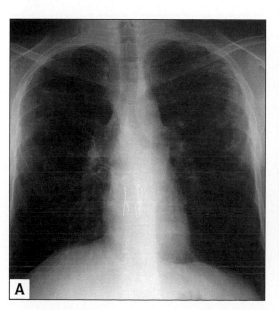

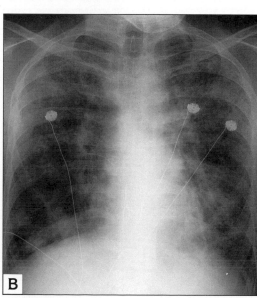

FIGURE 11-70 A, Chest radiograph at baseline in a 23-year-old man who received bilateral lung transplantation for cystic fibrosis. **B,** Chest radiograph shows development of respiratory syncytial virus pneumonia. The patient had negative viral, fungal, bacterial, and parasitic evaluations on multiple bronchoscopies, including biopsies. Treatment with aerosolized ribavirin resulted in clinical and symptomatic improvement over 5 days.

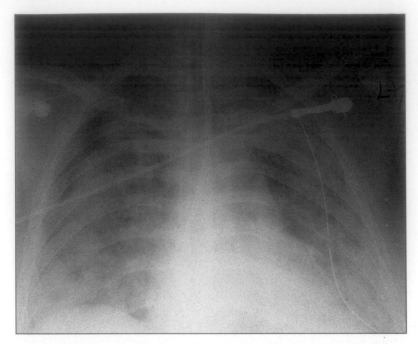

FIGURE 11-71 Chest radiograph of a 44-year-old woman after renal transplantation, with respiratory syncytial virus (RSV) pneumonia and congestive heart failure. The diagnosis of RSV was made by shell vial viral culture of swabs of the throat and nasopharynx combined as one specimen. Cytopathic effect was observed on day 4 of culture, and the identification of RSV was confirmed by immunofluorescent staining. Rapid antigen detection of nasal swab specimens was negative. The use of α-interferon and antibody therapy remains investigative.

REFERENCES

1. Rubin RH, Wolfson JS, Cosimi AB, *et al.*: Infection in the renal transplant recipient. *Am J Med* 1981, 70:405–411.

2. Kusne S, Dummer JS, Ho M, *et al.*: Infections after liver transplantation: An analysis of 101 consecutive cases. *Medicine* 1988, 67:132–143.

3. Wheat J: Fungal infections. *In* Rubin R, Young LS (eds.): *Clinical Approach to Infection in the Compromised Host.* New York: Plenum Medical Press; 1994:211–237.

4. Sugar AM: Agents of mucomycosis and related species. *In* Mandell GL, Bennett JE, Dolin R (eds.): *Principles and Practice of Infectious Diseases,* 4th ed. New York: Churchill Livingstone; 1995:2312.

5. Bullock WE: *Histoplasma capsulatum. In* Mandell GL, Bennett JE, Dolin R (eds.): *Principles and Practice of Infectious Diseases,* 4th ed. New York: Churchill Livingstone; 1995:2340–2353.

6. Jourdain B, Novara A, Joly-Guillou M, *et al.*: Role of quantitative cultures of endotracheal aspirates in the diagnosis of nosocomial pneumonia. *Am J Respir Crit Care Med* 1995, 152:241–246.

7. Peterson PK, Balfour HH Jr, Fryd DS, *et al.*: Risk factors in the development of cytomegalovirus-related pneumonia in renal transplant recipients. *J Infect Dis* 1983, 148:1121.

8. Mazzuli T, Rubin RH, Ferraro MJ, *et al.*: Cytomegalovirus antigenemia: Clinical correlates in transplant patients and in persons with AIDS. *J Clin Microbiol* 1993, 31:2824–2877.

SELECTED BIBLIOGRAPHY

Fishman JA: Pneumocystis and parasitic infection in the transplant recipient. *Annu Rev Infect Dis* 1995, (in press).

Ho M, Dummer JS: Infections in transplant recipients. *In* Mandell GL, Bennett JE, Dolin R (eds.) *Principles and Practice of Infectious Diseases* 4th ed. New York: Churchill Livingstone; 1995:2709–2716.

Horvath J, Dummer JS, Lloyd J, *et al.*: Infections in the transplanted and native lung after single lung transplantation. *Chest* 1993, 104:681–685.

Rubin RH: Infectious disease complications of renal transplantation. *Kidney Int* 1993, 44:221–236.

Rubin RH, Young LS (eds.): *Clinical Approach to Infection in the Immunocompromised Host.* New York: Plenum Medical Press; 1994.

CHAPTER 12

Pulmonary Manifestations of Extrapulmonary Infection

James J. Herdegen
Roger C. Bone

Extrapulmonary infections with pulmonary manifestations	

Bacteria
 Gram-positive (*Staphylococcus aureus*)
  Septic emboli
  Sepsis/ARDS
 Gram-negative (*Escherichia coli*)
  Sepsis/ARDS
 Anaerobic
  Ludwig's angina (mediastinitis)
 Syphilis
  Aortitis
  Syphylitic gumma
 Rocky Mountain spotted fever
 	
Viruses
 Varicella-zoster virus
 Hanta virus
	Ebola virus
	 Cytomegalovirus
	
	Fungi
	 Cryptococcosis
	 Actinomycosis
	 Blastomycosis
	 Mucormycosis
	
	Parasites
	 Paragonimiasis
	 Echinococcosis (hydatid cyst)
	 Strongyloidiasis
	 Filariasis

ARDS—acute respiratory distress syndrome.

FIGURE 12-1 Extrapulmonary infections with pulmonary manifestations. A wide variety of infectious agents is capable of causing a systemic illness with pulmonary manifestations.

BACTERIAL INFECTIONS

Tertiary Syphilis

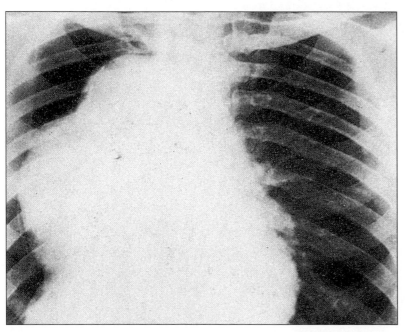

Figure 12-2 Syphilitic aortitis. A 40-year-old man presented with a history of an irritating cough and hoarse voice for the previous 6 months. The chest radiograph demonstrates a large aortic aneurysm involving the ascending part, arch, and descending thoracic aorta. A strongly positive result on treponemal serologic testing confirmed the diagnosis of tertiary syphilis. Syphilitic involvement of the main pulmonary artery has also been reported and is similar in appearance to syphilitic aortitis. Macroscopically, there is aneurysmal dilatation accompanied by irregular intimal scarring and luminal thrombus formation. Histologic examination reveals medial fibrosis, disruption of elastic tissue, adventitial endarteritis, and perivascular plasma cell infiltration. Organisms are rarely identified. (*From* Edmond and Rowland [1]; with permission.)

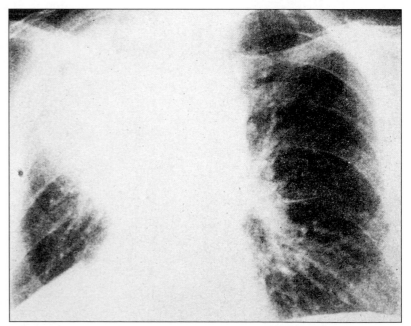

FIGURE 12-3 Syphilitic gumma of the lung. Routine chest radiograph of a 70-year-old man admitted with symptoms of benign prostatic hypertrophy. Serologic testing for syphilis was positive, and open lung biopsy confirmed fibroblastic proliferation that is characteristic of gummas. Prolonged treatment with penicillin G benzathine resulted in some clearing, with residual retraction and fibrotic scarring of the left upper lobe. (*From* Danemann *et al.* [2]; with permission.)

Mycotic Aortic Aneurysm

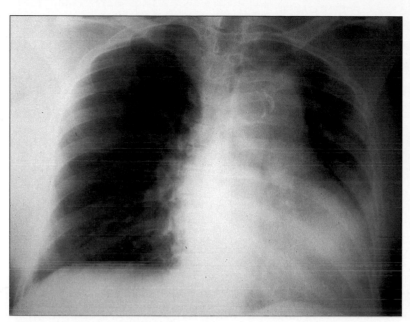

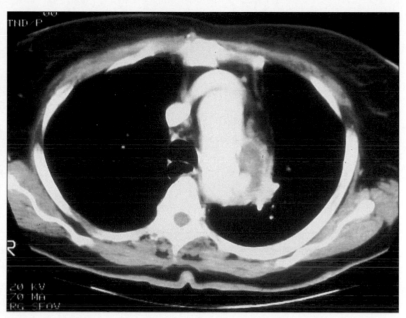

Figure 12-4 Admitting chest radiograph demonstrating a widened upper mediastinum in a 73-year-old woman recently placed on hemodialysis via a Quentin catheter. The catheter had become infected with *Staphylococcus aureus*, prompting its removal 1 month before this admission. The patient's presenting complaints included episodic nausea, vomiting, and pain in the left upper chest. The soft-tissue density extending beyond the calcification of the aortic knob can be noted in this radiograph.

Figure 12-5 Computed tomographic (CT) evaluation of mycotic aortic aneurysm. A CT scan at the level of the aortic arch demonstrates a soft-tissue and fluid density mass extending from the aortic arch and descending aorta. This mass is in direct contact with the aortic arch but is clearly extraluminal. Blood cultures performed at admission were positive for *Staphylococcus aureus*. Mycotic aneurysms typically develop as the result of staphylococcal, streptococcal, or salmonellal infections of the aorta, usually at an atherosclerotic plaque. Blood cultures are usually positive for one of these pathogens.

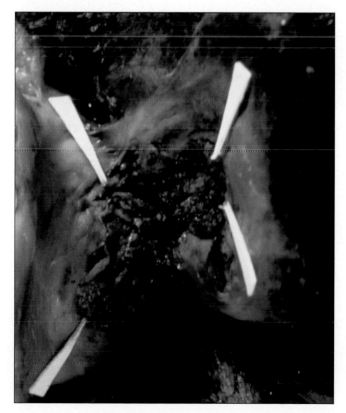

FIGURE 12-6 Gross pathology findings demonstrating intrapulmonary hemorrhage secondary to rupture of a mycotic aortic aneurysm. The development of an aortico-bronchial fistula secondary to a mycotic aneurysm has been rarely described in the literature.

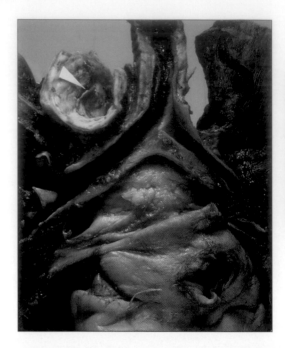
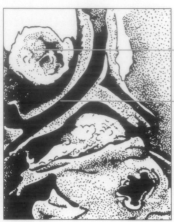

- Aortic aneurysm

- Left mainstream and trachea hemorrhage

FIGURE 12-7 Gross pathology findings at autopsy demonstrating the extensive intra-pulmonary hemorrhage and resultant left-sided bronchial and tracheal thrombus. The section of transverse aorta also demonstrates the aortic aneurysm.

Septic Emboli

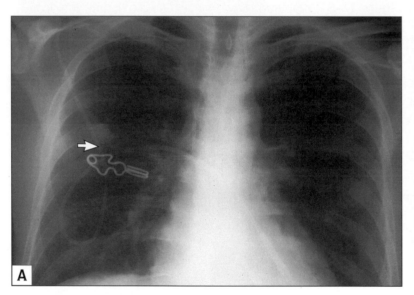
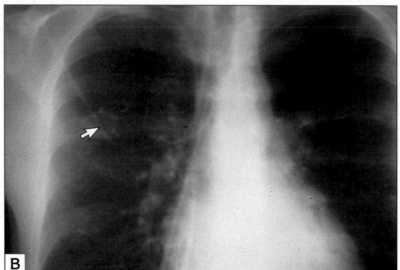

FIGURE 12-8 Cavitary lung infarction from septic emboli secondary to indwelling catheter infection. **A**, Chest radiograph demonstrating a 2-cm nodule in the right midlung field (*arrow*) in a febrile patient with HIV infection. Hyperalimentation via a Hickman catheter had been started because of intractable diarrhea (20–25 stools/day) and abdominal pain secondary to both cytomegalovirus-induced colitis and cryptosporidiosis. Slight erythema at the catheter site was noted. **B**, Despite administration of broad-spectrum antibiotics, the patient continued to be febrile and developed hemoptysis. A follow-up chest radiograph demonstrates cavitation of the right midlung nodule (*arrow*). Fiberoptic bronchoscopy with protected brushing yielded *Staphylococcus aureus* on culture, which had identical antibiotic resistance to cultures of specimens from blood and the tip of the Hickman catheter. Cavitary lung infarction from septic embolism is commonly associated with *S. aureus*, various anaerobes, and *Candida* spp. Successful treatment of an indwelling catheter infection without removing the catheter is difficult once the entrance site becomes infected.

Acute Respiratory Distress Syndrome and Systemic Inflammatory Response Syndrome

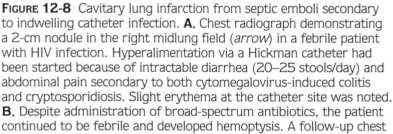

Infectious causes of ARDS
Bacterial pneumonia
Fungal and *Pneumocystis carinii* pneumonia
Gram-negative sepsis
Tuberculosis
Viral pneumonia
ARDS—acute respiratory distress syndrome.

FIGURE 12-9 Infectious causes of acute respiratory distress syndrome (ARDS). A wide variety of infectious agents that cause either systemic or localized illness can predispose patients to developing ARDS.

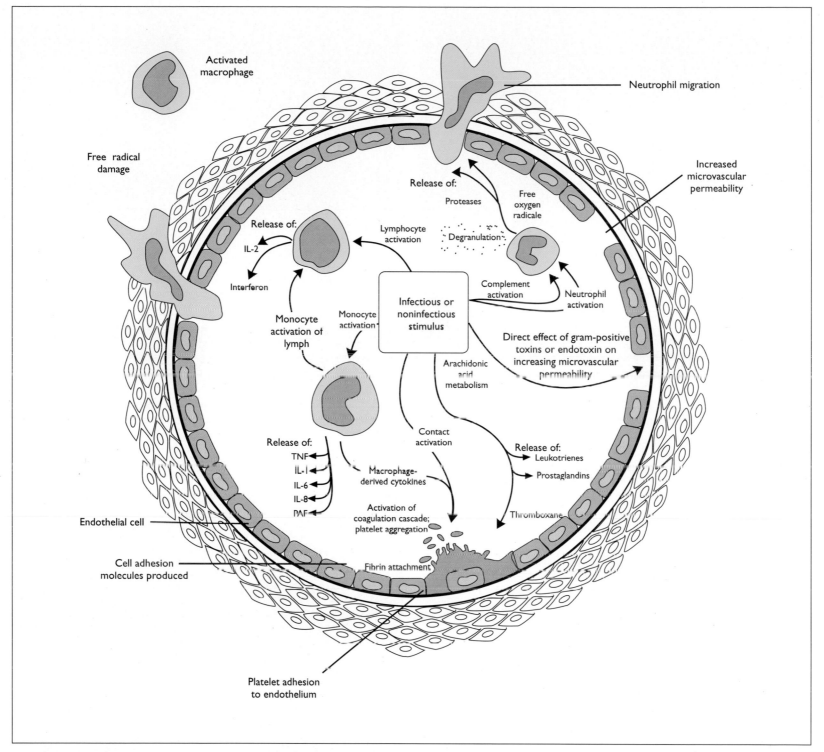

FIGURE 12-10 Inflammatory mediators associated with the systemic inflammatory response syndrome. The uncontrolled release of mediators, even at sites distant to the lung, can lead to disruption of the pulmonary endothelial barrier, increased vascular permeability, and diffuse alveolar damage. The clinical definition of acute respiratory distress syndrome includes the uniform finding of impaired oxygenation (PaO$_2$:FIO$_2$ ratio $\leq$ 200), regardless of the level of positive end-expiratory pressure being used; the presence of bilateral pulmonary infiltrates; and a pulmonary-artery occlusion (wedge) pressure $\leq$ 18 mm Hg or no clinical evidence of elevated left atrial pressure on the basis of the chest radiograph and other clinical data. (IL—interleukin; PAF—platelet-activating factor; TNF—tumor necrosis factor.)

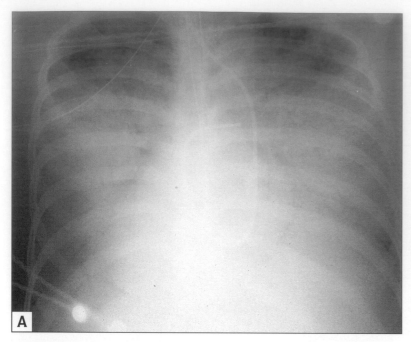

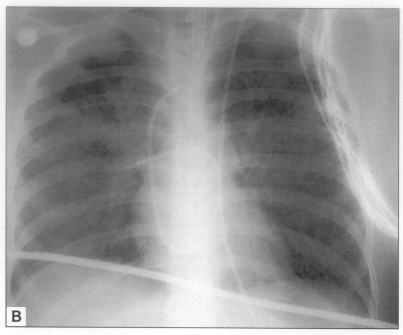

FIGURE 12-11 Chest radiographic patterns in acute respiratory distress syndrome (ARDS). A 35-year-old hispanic woman initially presented with a 6- to 9-month prodrome of constitutional symptoms, including rash, weight loss, arthralgias, and night sweats. A collagen vascular work-up was consistent with systemic lupus erythematosus. Several weeks after an emperic trial of high-dose steroids, a transaminitis developed, prompting a liver biopsy. The biopsy demonstrated acid-fast organisms, which were also demonstrated in her sputum, and culture grew *Mycobacterium tuberculosis*. **A**, Her chest radiograph rapidly progressed to a pattern of diffuse, bilateral, alveolar infiltrates. As alveolar filling progresses in ARDS, more of the lung parenchyma becomes involved, occasionally progressing to a near-total "whiteout" of both lung fields, as seen here. **B**, A chest radiograph taken soon after the patient began high-frequency jet ventilation, shows increased lucency bilaterally, which is likely a result of redistributed lung water from her ARDS process.

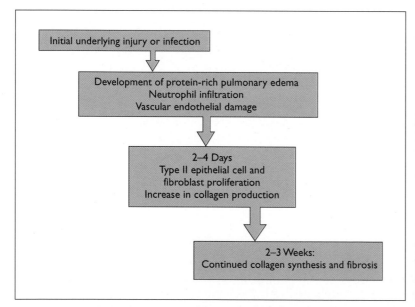

FIGURE 12-12 Four-stage process in the pathogenesis of acute respiratory distress syndrome (ARDS). In the initial stage, there are often no clinical or radiographic findings of ARDS. In the second stage, the patient may hyperventilate, and infiltrates may appear on the chest radiograph. The third stage is characterized by respiratory insufficiency and chest radiographic evidence of edematous changes within the lung as well as alveolar and interstitial infiltrates. The fourth, or terminal, stage is characterized by severe hypoxemia, even when pure oxygen is breathed.

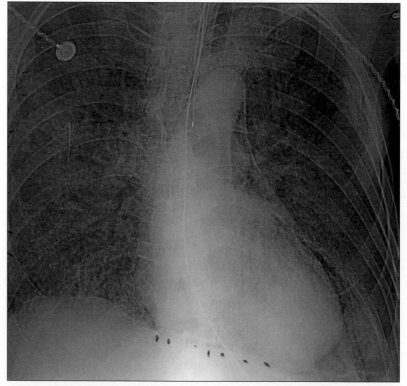

FIGURE 12-13 Pulmonary barotrauma associated with acute respiratory distress syndrome. In addition to diffuse alveolar damage and increased vascular permeability, high airway pressures are present as a result of impaired lung compliance and increased airway resistance. Peak airway pressures > 40 to 45 cm of water are associated with a significantly higher risk of pulmonary barotrauma, including pneumothorax and pneumomediastinum, as demonstrated in this patient (*dashed lines*).

Mediastinal Abscess

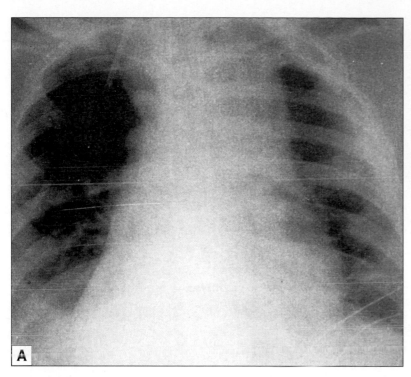

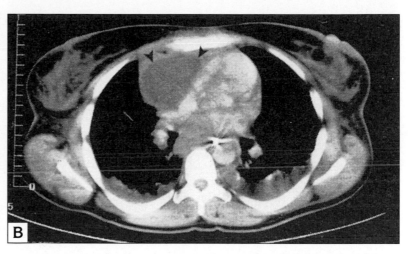

FIGURE 12-14 Mediastinal abscess from upper respiratory infection. A 34-year-old woman presented with a 3-day history of sore throat and fever. The initial examination demonstrated pharyngitis, odynophagia, trismus, and neck swelling. **A,** A chest radiograph showed a widened mediastinum. Several days after admission the patient developed stridor, increased pain, and marked neck swelling. **B,** The computed tomography scan demonstrated an abscess in the superior and anterior mediastinum and bilateral pleural effusions. Organisms associated with suppurative mediastinitis complicating upper airway infections are typically mixed and include β-hemolytic streptococci, nonhemolytic streptococci, and various anaerobes. (*From* Isaacs *et al.* [3]; with permission.)

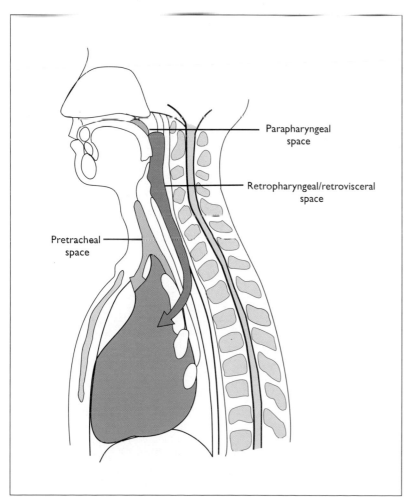

FIGURE 12-15 Anatomic sites with potential for spread to the superior mediastinum. Cervical spaces that can be sites of abscess, with potential spread of infection to the superior mediastinum, include the parapharyngeal space, retropharyngeal/retrovisceral space, and pretracheal space. (*Adapted from* Isaacs *et al.* [3]; with permission.)

Zoonotic Infections

Zoonotic pathogens causing pneumonia

Agent	Disease	Epidemiologic associations
Bacillus anthracis	Inhalation anthrax	Imported animal hides, raw wool, sick domestic animals
Brucella spp	Brucellosis	Food animals and product handling, ingestion, inhalation
Chlamydia psittaci	Psittacosis, ornithosis	Bird exposure (pet and pet shops, veterinarians, turkey farmers)
Coxiella burnetti	Q fever	Inhaled endospores from animal-contaminated soil; cat afterbirth, ticks
Francisella tularenisis	Tularemia	Aerosol from dead birds, animals; bacteremic spread from bubo; ticks and biting flies
Leptospira interrogans spp	Leptospirosis	Domestic and wild animals, contaminated water, veterinarians, farmers
Pasteurella multocida	Pasteurellosis	Underlying respiratory disease; contact with cat, dog in home
Pseudomonas pseudomallei	Melioidosis	Penetrating injury in endemic area in rodent-contaminated soil or water
Rickettsia rickettsii	Rocky Mountain spotted fever	Tick associated, typical rash
Toxoplasma gondii	Toxoplasmosis	Contact with domestic food animals and pets, ingestion cysts, pneumonia in immunocompromised persons
Yersinia pestis	Plague	Contact with mammals and fleas; veterinarians; and outdoor activities in endemic area; cats

FIGURE 12-16 Zoonotic pathogens causing pneumonia. A variety of the community-acquired organisms are associated with vertebrate or arthropod vectors and can cause atypical pneumonias. The clinical presentation and exposure history often provide clues to the diagnosis.

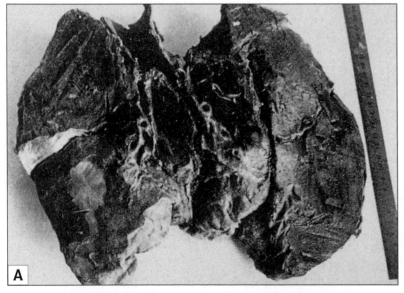

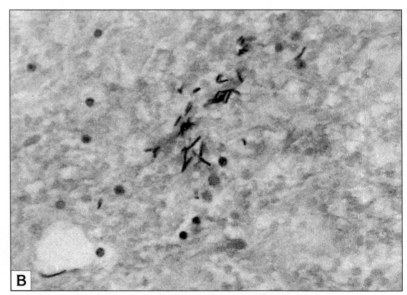

FIGURE 12-17 Inhalational anthrax. **A**, Gross anatomic findings in anthrax. This 29-year-old man was one of a number of cases of fatal anthrax bacteremia and toxemia that mysteriously developed in the former Soviet Union in 1979. The cut surface of the lungs, trachea, and hilar lymph nodes reveals massive hemorrhagic enlargement of the peribronchial and carinal lymph nodes, with extension of the hemorrhage into the adjacent tissues including the submucosa of the bronchi and trachea. **B**, Microscopic analysis demonstrating *Bacillus anthracis* organisms. A photomicrograph shows a cluster of gram-positive *B. anthracis* in a hemorrhagic area of the mediastinum, from a 25-year-old man with fatal anthrax. (Brown-Brenn stain; original magnification, × 375.) (*From* Abramova *et al.* [4]; with permission.)

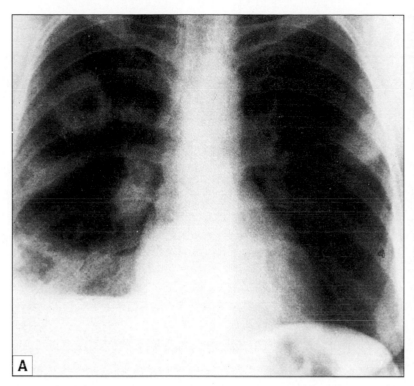
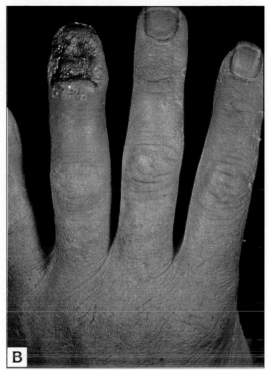

FIGURE 12-18 *Francisella tularenisis* is a gram-negative, pleomorphic coccobacillary organism that grows poorly on artificial media unless fortified with serum, glucose, and cystine. The organism is associated with a large number of wild animals, especially squirrels and rabbits. The infection is spread among animals via deerflies or ticks or by bites from infected animals. Most human cases are acquired from contact with infected animals, via deerfly or tick bites, or through ingestion of contaminated meat. **A,** Chest radiograph of a 51-year-old woman who presented with acute onset of chills, fever, nausea, malaise, myalgia, and headache several days after being bitten by numerous ticks. Respiratory disease often begins with a poorly productive cough, chest pain, and dyspnea. Radiologic changes characteristically include evidence of parenchymal and pleural disease. The pattern is diffuse bronchopneumonia, often with hilar adenopathy. Pleural effusions are not unusual, as demonstrated in this patient. **B,** Irregular ulcer due to infection with *F. tularenisis*. When tularemia is contracted through insect or animal bites, the initial sites of infection demonstrate necrosis, granuloma formation, and local abscesses. Ingestion of infected meat may result in pharyngeal and intestinal involvement with ulceration. Pulmonary infection causes pneumonitis features with mediastinal lymph node enlargement. (Panel 18A *from* Rubin [5]; with permission: panel 18B *courtesy of* E.D. Everett, MD.)

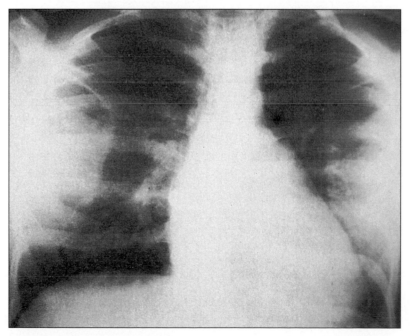
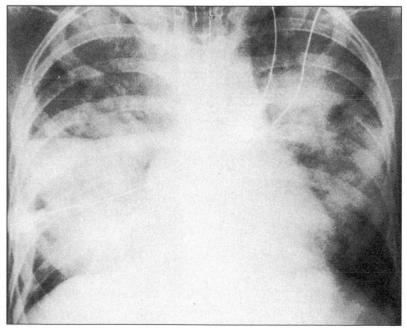

FIGURE 12-19 Rocky Mountain spotted fever. A chest radiograph demonstrated bilateral infiltrates that progressed to an acute respiratory distress syndrome pattern. The typical presentation of Rocky Mountain spotted fever is that of an acute febrile illness with headache, malaise, myalgia, and a maculopapular rash that begins on the extremities and spreads centrally. In severe cases, there can be multiple organ involvement. (*From* Sacks *et al.* [6]; with permission.)

FIGURE 12-20 Pneumonic plague. A chest radiograph demonstrates large nodular and bilateral alveolar infiltrates in a 14-year-old boy. Plague, caused by *Yersinia pestis*, is endemic in rock squirrels, prairie dogs, and other ground animals in areas west of the Rocky Mountains. Pneumonic plague is highly contagious, and organisms have the potential to spread from one person to many persons (*From* Alsofrom *et al.* [7]; with permission.)

VIRAL INFECTIONS

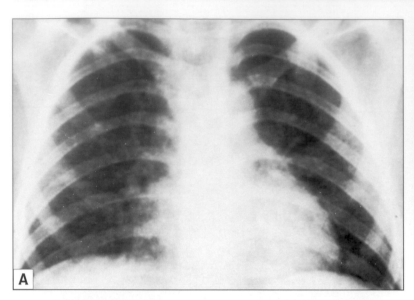

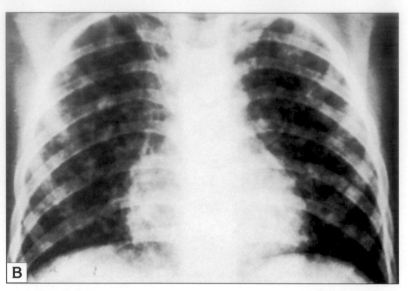

FIGURE 12-21 Acute varicella-zoster pneumonia in a 6-year-old boy with acute leukemia. **A** and **B**, The characteristic radiographic pattern is patchy, diffuse airspace consolidation. Minute, widespread foci of calcification throughout both lungs has also been described in adults with a previous history of chickenpox in adulthood. (*From* Fraser *et al.* [8]; with permission.)

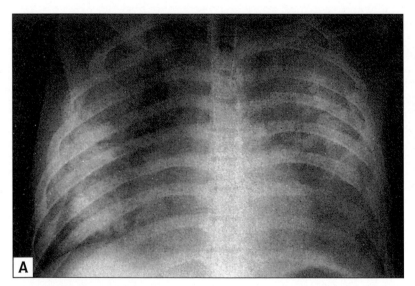

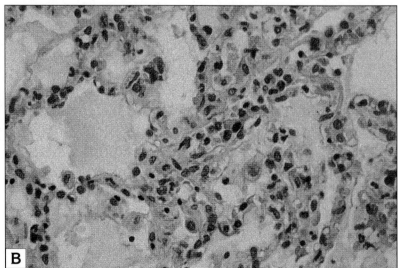

FIGURE 12-22 Hantavirus pulmonary syndrome. **A**, Chest radiograph demonstrates the characteristic diffuse interstitial and alveolar infiltrates. The hantavirus family is included in a group of viruses causing disorders with clinical features of hematologic abnormalities (hemorrhagic fever), renal involvement, and increased vascular permeability. Severe disease is characterized by five phases: febrile, hypotensive, oliguric, diuretic, and convalescent. Respiratory symptoms are generally not pronounced, and pulmonary involvement has not been a prominent feature of the known hantaviral syndromes. **B**, Lung-tissue sample from a patient with hantavirus-associated interstitial pneumonitis. The specimen shows minimal to moderate interstitial lymphoid cell infiltrates, congestion, and intra-alveolar edema. (Hematoxylin-eosin stain; original magnification, $\times$ 285.) (*From* Duchin *et al.* [9]; with permission.)

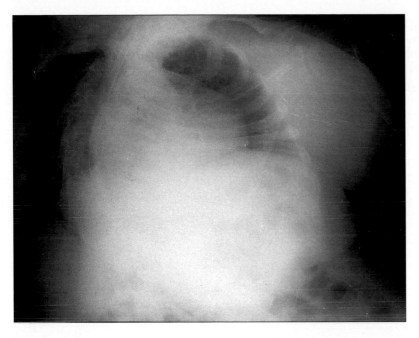

FIGURE 12-23 Postpolio syndrome leading to chronic respiratory failure. A latent manifestation of acute poliomyelitis is progressive respiratory muscle fatigue. This patient, who had polio as a child, had residual motor weakness leading to immobilization and the development of severe kyphoscoliosis. In addition, a mild upper respiratory infection led to worsening respiratory muscle strength and acute on chronic hypercapneic respiratory failure.

FUNGAL INFECTIONS

Cryptococcosis

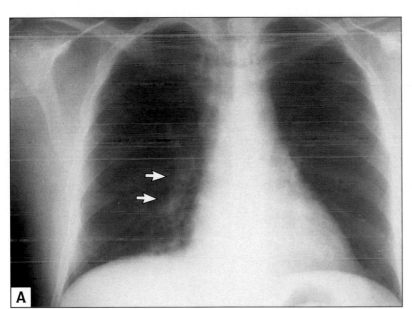

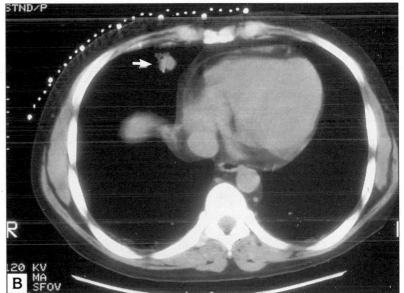

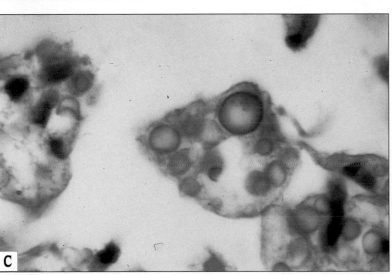

FIGURE 12-24 Pulmonary cryptococcosis. A renal transplant patient presented with a history of low-grade fever and nonproductive cough for 2 weeks. **A,** The chest radiograph demonstrates a subtle infiltrate in the right mid and lower lung fields (*arrows*). The patient had a prior history of malaria, hepatitis B, and exposure to active tuberculosis. The patient was receiving azathioprine, prednisone, and clonidine. The leukocyte count was 2.8/mm^3 on admission. **B,** Computed tomography scan confirming a nodular-appearing infiltrate in the right middle lobe (*arrow*). **C,** Cytopathology specimen demonstrating numerous, irregularly sized organisms (5–10 µm in diameter) consistent with *Cryptococcus neoformans*, which was subsequently confirmed by fungal culture. Pulmonary cryptococcosis can appear in several distinct forms, including well-defined, solitary or multiple nodules; ill-defined areas of parenchymal consolidation; and widely disseminated parenchymal nodules measuring 1 to 2 mm, representing miliary hematogenous spread. In immunocompromised patients, a predominantly interstitial pattern accompanied by minimal cellular inflammation and no granuloma formation is often seen.

Actinomycosis

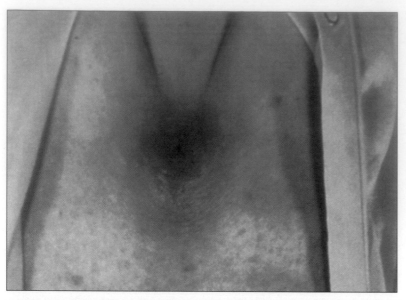

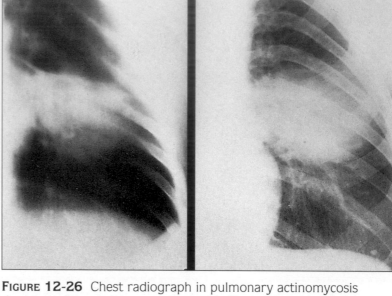

FIGURE 12-25 Persistent upper sternum erythema due to actinomycosis in a patient with coronary artery bypass graft. Actinomycosis was demonstrated by culture. Before the use of antibiotics, actinomycosis was the most commonly diagnosed "fungal" disease of the lungs, characteristically presenting as an empyema with sinus tracts in the chest wall. Currently, actinomycosis occurs most commonly as a disease of the cervicofacial region following dental extraction, usually in the form of osteomyelitis of the mandible or as a soft-tissue abscess that often drains spontaneously through the skin. Gastrointestinal infection is next in frequency, followed by thoracopulmonary disease.

FIGURE 12-26 Chest radiograph in pulmonary actinomycosis demonstrating an intraparenchymal infiltrate that frequently extends to the chest wall. The typical radiographic pattern of acute actinomycosis consists of airspace pneumonia, without recognizable segmental distribution, commonly in the periphery of the lung and with a predilection for the lower lobes. With appropriate antibiotic therapy, the infection is usually resolved without complications. Without therapy, a lung abscess may develop, or the infection may extend into the pleura and chest wall, with osteomyelitis of the ribs and abscess formation in these areas. (*From* Fraser *et al.* [8]; with permission.)

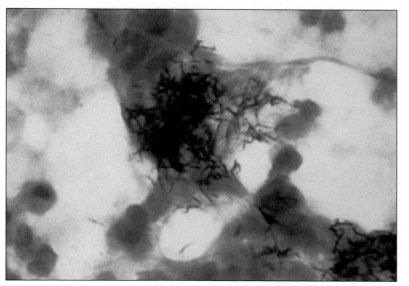

FIGURE 12-27 Aspirated sputum demonstrating *Actinomyces* organisms, which are characterized by pleomorphic branching filaments 0.2 to 0.3 μm in diameter. Within tissue, mycelial (sulfur) granules are characteristic, although similar structures can develop in other bacterial infections. These sulfur granules are so named because of their yellow color, although their actual sulfur content is minimal. The organisms are normal inhabitants of the human oropharynx and are frequently found in the crypts of surgically excised tonsils, in dental caries, and at the gingival margins of persons with poor oral hygiene. Penicillin and ampicillin remain the antibiotics of choice.

Sporotrichosis

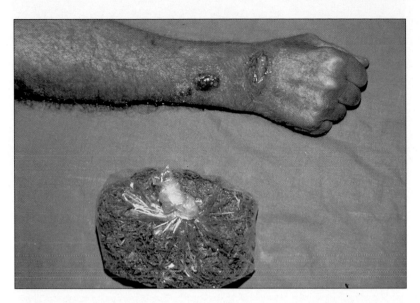

FIGURE 12-28 Open skin wound of sporotrichosis in a gardener working with sphagnum peat moss. Sporotrichosis is caused by *Sporothrix (Sporotrichum) schenckii*, a common saprophyte of worldwide distribution isolated from soil, sphagnum moss, peat moss, decaying vegetable matter, thorns, and a variety of other substances. The disease is usually acquired by direct inoculation into the skin through a scratch from thorns, splinters, grasses, or other contaminated objects. Farmers, laborers, florists, and horti-culturalists are especially vulnerable. (*From Infections of the Skin* [slide series] [10]; with permission.)

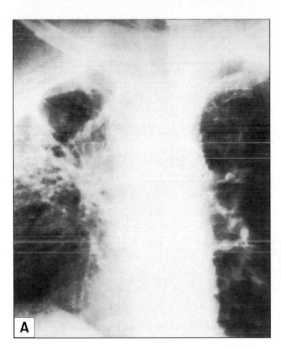

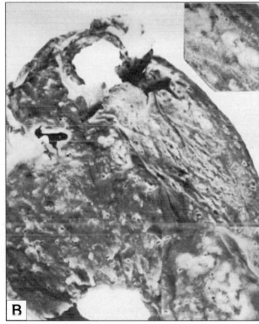

FIGURE 12-29 Primary pulmonary sporotrichosis. **A**, Chest radiograph of a patient presenting with a history of cough, fever, and weight loss and found to be infected with *Sporothrix schenckii*. Radiographically, primary pulmonary sporotrichosis closely resembles postprimary tuberculosis. Findings include isolated nodular masses that may cavitate, hilar lymph node enlargement, and, occasionally, a diffuse reticulonodular pattern. The prognosis tends to be poor in the chronic cavitary and disseminated forms of the disease but good when the disease is confined to the bronchopulmonary and mediastinal nodes. **B**, Gross pathologic specimen from the lung demonstrates the apical cavity and the granulomatous foci in the superior portion of the lingula and superior segment of the lower lobe. (*From* McGarran *et al.* [11]; with permission.)

Blastomycosis

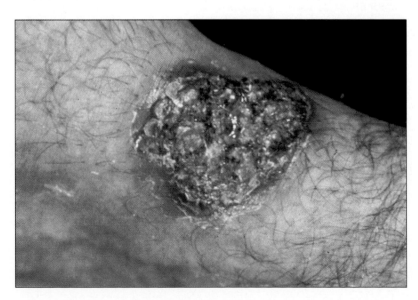

Figure 12-30 Ulcerative skin lesion on dorsum of hand in a patient with blastomycosis. Skin disease is common in patients with chronic pulmonary blastomycosis and may occur without evidence of infection elsewhere. The characteristic lesions are raised and crusted with irregular borders. They frequently occur on the face or extremities and may mimic basal cell carcinoma; one distinguishing feature is the finding of small microabscesses at the periphery of the lesions.

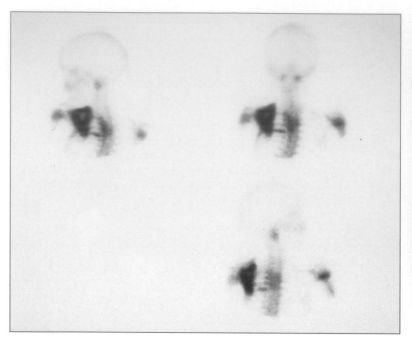

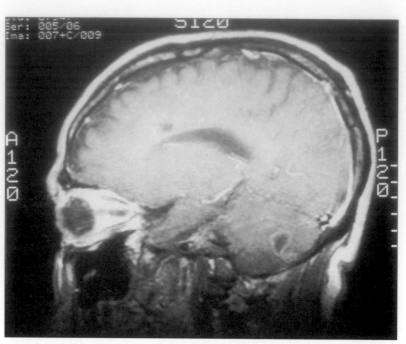

FIGURE 12-31 Bone scan of a patient with right scapular pain due to blastomycosis. Bone is the second most common distant site of infection in blastomycosis. The spine is most frequently involved, followed by the ribs, skull, and long bones. Involvement of the spine mimics tuberculosis, with involvement of adjacent vertebrae and destruction of the intervening disc space. Osteolytic and osteoblastic processes may be seen on radiographs. Long bones are involved near the epiphysis, and the infection can extend directly to an adjacent joint space.

FIGURE 12-32 Cranial magnetic resonance image of a patient with blastomycosis demonstrating multiple intraparenchymal ring-enhancing lesions. Brain abscess is a less common manifestation of disseminated blastomycosis; the more common sites of spread are to the skin, bone, and prostate.

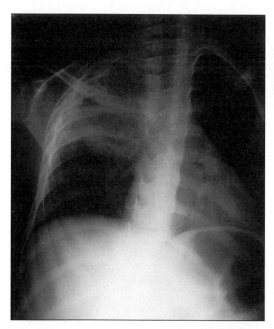

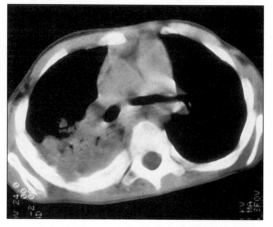

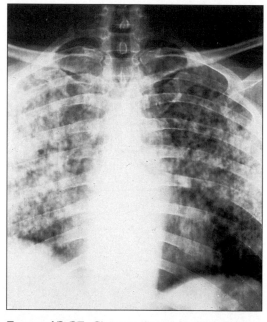

FIGURE 12-34 Computed tomography scan demonstrating a dense apical infiltrate in the right upper lobe in a patient with blastomycosis. This patient presented with symptoms of an acute febrile illness unresponsive to conventional antibiotic therapy. In blastomycosis, unlike histoplasmosis, infections that produce symptoms tend to demonstrate less healing, thus requiring specific antifungal therapy in a greater proportion of patients.

FIGURE 12-33 Chest radiograph showing a consolidating right upper lobe infiltrate in an 8-year-old boy with pulmonary blastomycosis. In contrast with histoplasmosis and coccidioidomycosis, direct, intimate exposure to an infected site (such as an area of construction) is probably necessary for infection with *Blastomyces dermatitidis*. When a person is exposed to a contaminated site, microconidia of the fungus can be inhaled. If infection occurs, an intense neutrophilic response develops. A specific cell-mediated immunologic response occurs within 7 to 14 days. Blastomycosis occurs most frequently in rural areas among individuals with outdoor jobs or interests.

FIGURE 12-35 Chest radiograph of a patient demonstrating diffuse pulmonary infiltrates secondary to blastomycosis. Inhalation of microconidia results in patchy areas of alveolar consolidation as exudation occurs and neutrophils are recruited. Pulmonary involvement may be bilateral, and it is common for the lower lobes to be affected. Hilar adenopathy may occur with primary infection, but pleural effusion and cavitation of infiltrates are uncommon. Symptoms, if present, are those of an acute pneumonia and include high fever, productive cough, pleuritic chest pain, and myalgias.

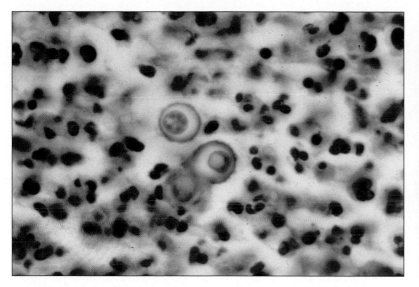

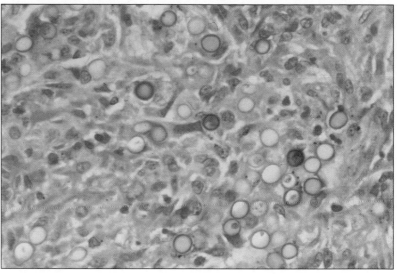

FIGURE 12-36 Hematoxylin-eosin stain demonstrating several *Blastomyces dermatitidis* organisms surrounded by an intense inflammatory reaction. The diagnosis of blastomycosis can often be confirmed by demonstrating the characteristic yeast forms (broad-necked single buds) in sputum. Growth of *B. dermatitidis* on primary isolation is slow, often requiring a month or more. The complement fixation test is not sensitive—it is positive in < 10% of cases of acute pulmonary blastomycosis and < 50% of chronic pulmonary and extrapulmonary infections. The test is also not specific, as many patients with histoplasmosis yield a positive test.

FIGURE 12-37 Periodic acid–Schiff stain demonstrating the thick-walled capsule of *Blastomyces dermatitidis* organisms.

Mucormycosis

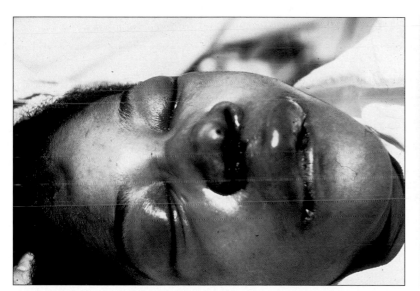

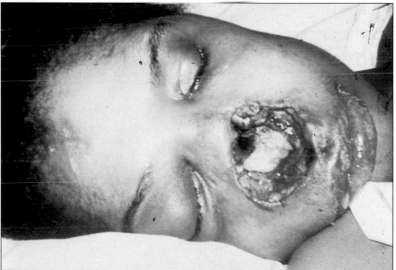

FIGURE 12-38 Diabetic patient with rhinocerebral mucormycosis. Rhinocerebral mucormycosis is a fulminant disease that involves the nose and paranasal sinuses and frequently extends into the orbits and cranium, where it causes orbital cellulitis and meningoencephalitis. Patients at risk for mucormycosis include those with diabetes mellitus, renal failure, burns, or immunocompromise for other reasons. Mucormycosis can be divided into rhinocerebral, pulmonary, cutaneous and subcutaneous, and gastrointestinal forms. Usually there is only local progression of disease at these sites, although dissemination occasionally results in multiorgan involvement. Once established, the organisms appear to grow well in tissue and are frequently seen extending along natural surfaces such as nerves, musculofascial planes, and the walls of arteries and veins.

FIGURE 12-39 Residual sinus infection after surgical debridement of mucormycosis. Mucormycosis can be a rapidly progressive disease, leading to death within 1 week; thus, aggressive care is always warranted. Although the overall prognosis of patients with this disease is grave, conservative debridement and drainage, correction of diabetic acidosis, and fungicidal therapy (with amphotericin B) can result in cure.

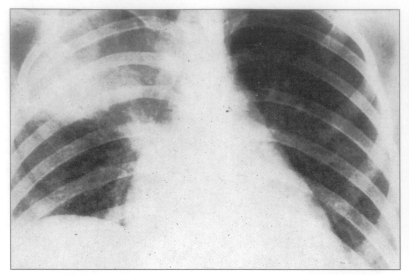

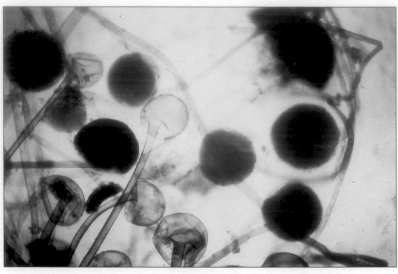

FIGURE 12-40 Chest radiograph of an 18-year-old woman with mucormycosis presenting with a neutropenic fever, cough, and generalized weakness. Subsequent autopsy found fungi of order Mucorales throughout the lung. Pulmonary mucormycosis is characterized by parenchymal hemorrhage or infarction with or without cavitation, depending on the time course of the disease. The tendency for the organism to invade blood vessels is illustrated by reports of occlusion of coronary arteries with resultant myocardial infarction and of fatal massive pulmonary hemorrhage caused by erosion of a pulmonary artery. Infrequent complications include bronchopleural fistula, superior vena caval obstruction, empyema, mediastinitis, and upper airway obstruction caused by tracheal disease. (*From* Bartrum *et al.* [12]; with permission.)

FIGURE 12-41 Microscopic findings of *Mucor* organisms grown in culture. In tissue, the organisms appear as broad (5–20 µm), frequently irregular, nonseptate hyphae that branch at varying angles up to 90°. In culture and in nature, the hyphae produce large sporangia (as seen here) that liberate sporangiospores into the air. It is believed that most human infections are acquired by inhalation of the sporangiospores. (Methylene blue [vital] stain.)

PARASITIC INFECTIONS

Paragonimiasis

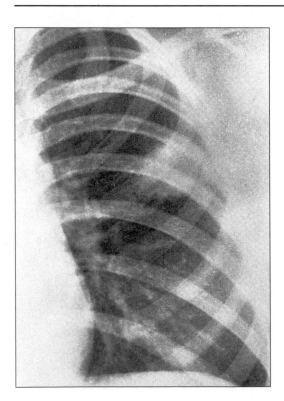

Figure 12-42 Chest radiograph of a 13-year-old Nigerian boy with paragonimiasis demonstrating a homogeneous density in the right midlung. *Paragonimus* ova were present in the patient's sputum. Paragonimiasis is seen most frequently in southeast Asia, South and Central America, and western Africa. In North America, wild and domestic animals can harbor the parasites, although the disease is uncommon. (*From* Ogakwu and Nwokoló [13]; with permission.)

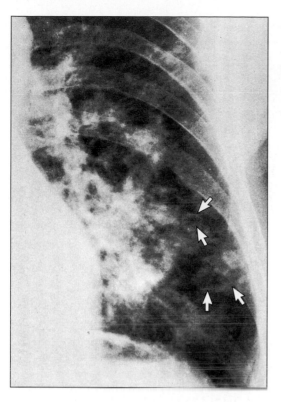

FIGURE 12-43 Chest radiograph in paragonimiasis demonstrating an infiltrate in the left lower lung field. Aspiration biopsy of the left lower lobe demonstrated *Paragonimus westermani*. Radiographic manifestations of paragonimiasis are varied. The chest radiograph is normal in 20% of patients in whom *Paragonimus* eggs are identified in the sputum. Abnormal radiographic patterns include 1) a poorly defined, somewhat hazy, inhomogeneous shadow; 2) shadows of homogeneous density with better-defined margins; 3) one to four smoothly outlined cystic areas (*arrows*); and 4) a similar type of shadow as described in 1 and 2 but with linear streaks. (*From* Fraser *et al.* [8]; with permission.)

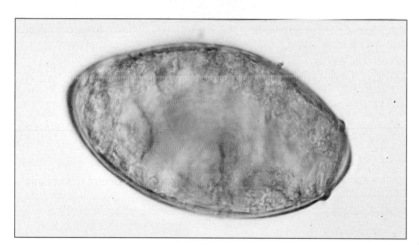

FIGURE 12-44 Egg with multiple *Paragonimus* organisms found in stool. The diagnosis of paragonimiasis is readily made in most patients by identifying the typical golden-brown, operculated eggs in the sputum, stool, or pleural fluid.

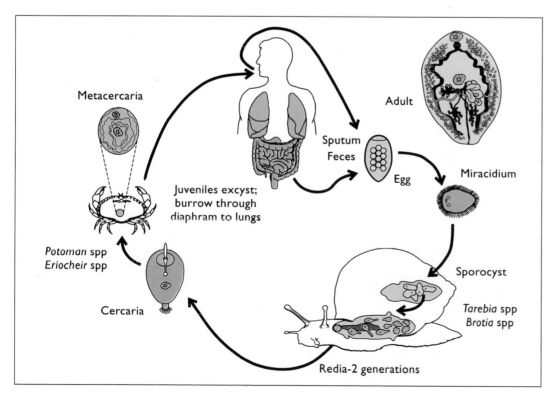

FIGURE 12-45 Life cycle of *Paragonimus westermani*. Humans acquire the disease by ingesting raw or undercooked crabs or crayfish or by drinking water contaminated by them. When ingested by the definitive host, *Paragonimus metacercariae* are liberated in the jejunum, from which they penetrate the wall of the small bowel into the peritoneal cavity, burrow through the diaphragm into the pleural space, and, finally, invade the lung. Within the lungs of humans or animals, the larval forms develop into adult flukes, which deposit eggs in burrows in lung parenchyma. The eggs are coughed up, swallowed, and excreted in the feces.

Echinococcosis (Hydatid Disease)

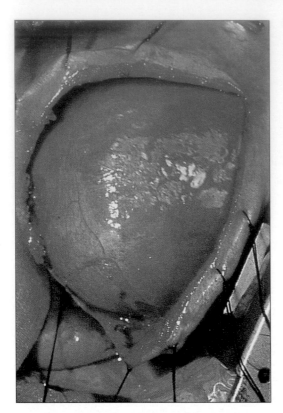

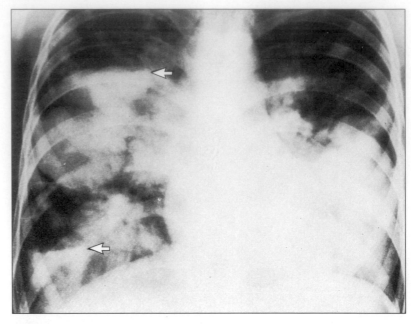

FIGURE 12-46 Large hydatid cyst of the liver. Approximately 65% to 70% of *Echinococcus granulosus* cysts occur in the liver and 15% to 30% in the lungs; the remaining 3% to 5% can be found virtually anywhere in the body but most commonly in the spleen, kidney, brain, or bones. (*From* Edmond and Rowland [1]; with permission.)

FIGURE 12-47 Chest radiograph of a 14-year-old Iranian girl with multiple hydatid cysts of the lung. The majority of these cysts are intact, but at least four have ruptured into the tracheobronchial tree and show prominent air–fluid levels (*arrows*). The irregular configuration of the air–fluid interface is a result of floating membranes (water-lily sign). Pulmonary echinococcal cysts characteristically present as solitary, sharply circumscribed masses surrounded by normal lung, predominantly in the lower lobes. (*From* Fraser *et al.* [8]; with permission.)

Characteristics of *Echinococcus granulosus*

Eggs	Diagnosis	Pathogenesis of hydatid disease
31–43 µm, spherical Nonoperculate Embryonated (hexacanth) shell very thick with many tiny pores giving it a striated look like eggs of *Taenia* spp	Radiographs Computed tomography scan Ultrasonography	Uniocular hydatid cysts occur in any tissue and provoke inflammatory responses and pressure necrosis. Most common sites are liver (jaundice, cirrhosis), lung (chest pain, dyspnea), and central nervous system. Cysts grow 1–5 mm in diameter annually but may rupture spilling: 1. Highly antigenic fluid that precipitates anaphylactic shock 2. Scolices that initiate formation of new cysts

FIGURE 12-48 Characteristics of *Echinococcus granulosus*. *E. granulosus* causes most cases of human hydatid disease, which occurs in two forms, pastoral and sylvatic. The more common pastoral variety occurs in rural settings where sheep, cows, or pigs are the intermediate hosts and dogs the usual definitive hosts. Humans usually acquire the disease by direct contact with infested dogs or by ingestion of egg-contaminated water, food, or soil; humans therefore become accidental intermediate hosts. The disease is particularly common in the sheep-raising Mediterranean regions and in Argentina, Chile, Uruguay, Australasia, and portions of Africa. The sylvatic variety of echinococcosis is likely caused by a different species of the tapeworm, *E. multilocularis*, with the definitive hosts being several species of the Canidae family, including the dog, wolf, arctic fox, and coyote. It produces multilocular hydatid cysts. (*From Parasitology Medical Slide Series* [14]; with permission.)

Strongyloidiasis

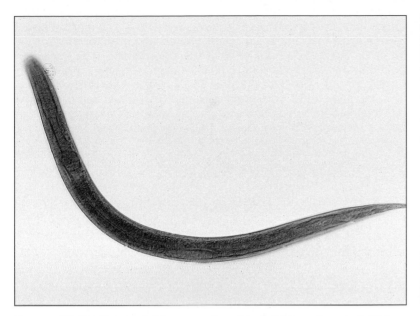

FIGURE 12-49 *Strongyloides* organism (rhabditiform larva). Initial infection with *Strongyloides stercoralis* occurs when filariform larvae, present in fecally contaminated soil, penetrate human skin and sequentially pass hematogenously to the lungs, penetrate into alveolar air sacs, and ascend the tracheobronchial tree to be swallowed. Eggs are produced that hatch within the lumen of the gut to release rhabditiform larvae. The diagnosis of uncomplicated strongyloidiasis usually is made by detecting rhabditiform larvae in concentrates of multiple stools.

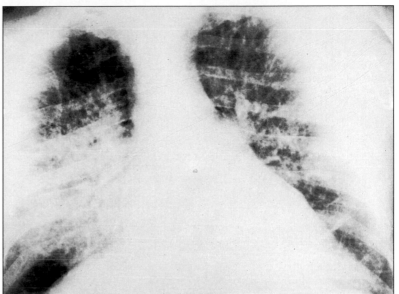

FIGURE 12-50 Chest radiograph of a patient with *Strongyloides* infection. Pulmonary infiltrates typically consist of foci of hemorrhage, pneumonitis, and edema. In disseminated strongyloidiasis, filariform larvae can be found in the stool as well as sputum, pleural fluid, peritoneal fluid, and surgical drainage fluid. (*From* Fraser *et al.* [8]; with permission.)

Tropical Eosinophilia (Filariasis)

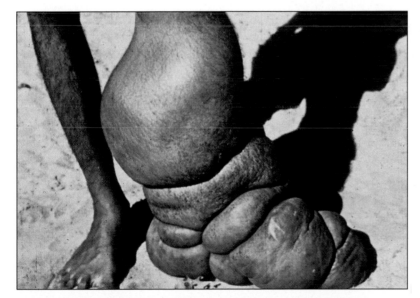

FIGURE 12-51 Chronic lymphedema of the leg secondary to Bancroft's filariasis. The syndrome of tropical filarial pulmonary eosinophilia is characterized by marked blood eosinophilia, paroxysmal nonproductive cough, wheezing, weight loss (in some cases), lymphadenopathy, and low-grade fever. The syndrome represents a peculiar immunologic reaction to infection with filarial parasites. (*Courtesy of* the Indian Commission on Filariasis.)

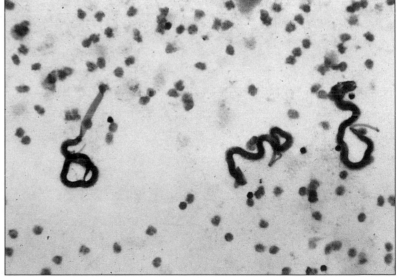

FIGURE 12-52 Giemsa-stained blood smear showing *Wuchereria bancrofti*. Diagnosis of Bancroft's filariasis is made by finding the sheathed microfilaria of *W. bancrofti* in a stained blood smear. The cardinal laboratory finding is an elevation in blood eosinophils, usually above 3000/mm³. Total serum IgE levels are elevated, often above 1000 U/mL. Filarial antibody levels are detectable in high titers. However, microfilariae usually cannot be found circulating in peripheral blood. (*Courtesy of* G.B. Craig, Jr, MD.)

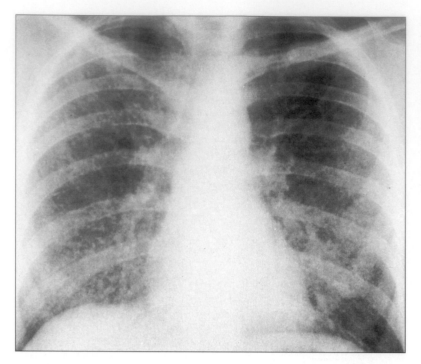

FIGURE 12-53 Chest radiograph of a patient with tropical eosinophilia demonstrating multiple discrete and confluent nodular opacities throughout both lungs. In classic filarial disease such as Bancroft's filariasis, humans are infected by mosquito bite, which introduces filariform larvae into the skin. The larvae mature into adult worms in draining lymphatic vessels and there produce microfilariae that eventually reach the bloodstream. The main pulmonary symptom is cough, usually producing small amounts of mucoid or mucopurulent material. Coughing is frequently worse at night, sometimes associated with blood-streaked sputum, with paroxysms of coughing and dyspnea so severe as to suggest status asthmaticus. (*From* Fraser *et al.* [8]; with permission.)

REFERENCES

1. Edmond RTD, Rowland HAK: *Diagnostic Picture Tests in Infectious Diseases*, 2nd ed. Ipswich, UK: Year-Book Medical Publishers; 1987:83.

2. Danemann HA, Cohen DB, Snider GL: Syphilitic gumma of the lung. *Arch Intern Med* 1961, 108:141–146.

3. Isaacs LM, Kotton B, Peralta MM, *et al.*: Fatal mediastinal abscess from upper respiratory infection. *Ear Nose Throat J* 1993, 72:620–631.

4. Abramova FA, Grinberg LM, Yampolskaya OV, Walker DH: Pathology of inhalational anthrax in 42 cases from the Sverdlovsk outbreak of 1979. *Proc Natl Acad Sci U S A* 1993, 90:2291–2294.

5. Rubin SA: Radiographic spectrum of pleuropulmonary tularemia. *AJR* 1978, 131:277–281.

6. Sacks HS, Lyons RW, Lahiri B: Adult respiratory distress syndrome in Rocky Mountain spotted fever. *Am Rev Respir Dis* 1981, 123:547–549.

7. Alsofrom DJ, Mettler FA, Mann JM, Radiographic manifestations of plague in New Mexico, 1975–1980. *Radiology* 1981, 139:561–565.

8. Fraser RG, Paré JAP, Paré PD, *et al.*: *Diagnosis of Diseases of the Chest*, 3rd ed. Philadelphia: W.B. Saunders; 1989.

9. Duchin JS, *et al.* Hantavirus pulmonary syndrome: A clinical description of 17 patients with a newly recognized disease. *N Engl J Med* 1994, 330:949–955.

10. *Infections of the Skin* [slide series]. Evanston, IL: American Academy of Dermatology; 1977: Fig. 30.

11. McGarran MH, Koboyaski G, Newmark L, *et al.*: Pulmonary sporotrichosis. *Dis Chest* 1969, 56:547–549.

12. Bartrum RJ Jr, Watnick M, Herman PG: Roentgenographic findings in pulmonary mucormycosis. *AJR* 1973, 117:810–815.

13. Ogakwu M, Nwokolo C: Radiological findings in pulmonary paragonimiasis as seen in Nigeria: A review based on one hundred cases. *Br J Radiol* 1973, 46:699–705.

14. *Parasitology Medical Slide Series*. Tallahassee, FL: Teach America; 1991: Fig. 7.10.

SELECTED BIBLIOGRAPHY

Barrett-Connor E: Parasitic pulmonary disease. *Am Rev Respir Dis* 1982, 126:558–563.

Pennington JE: *Respiratory Infections: Diagnosis and Management*, 2nd ed. New York: Raven Press; 1989.

Perfect JR: Cryptococcosis. *Infect Dis Clin North Am* 1989, 3:77–102.

Pressler V, McNamara JJ: Aneurysm of the thoracic aorta: Review of 260 cases. *J Thorac Cardiovasc Surg* 1985, 89:50–54.

CHAPTER 13

Acute and Chronic Bronchitis and Bronchiolitis

Herbert Y. Reynolds
Michael S. Simberkoff

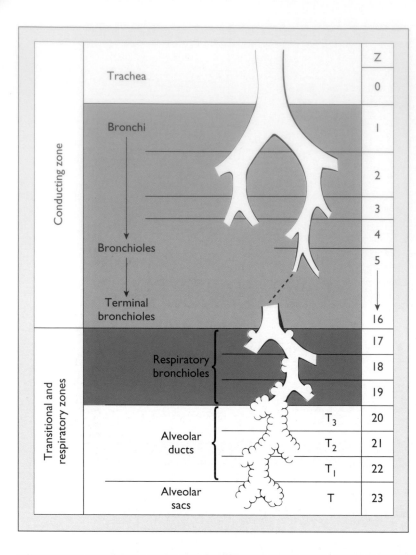

FIGURE 13-1 Airway branching in human lungs. Bronchitis, defined as irritation or infection of the mucosal and epithelial surfaces of the conducting airways, causes inflammation, excessive secretions, and mucosal edema in the large cartilaginous portion of the tracheobronchial tree. Bronchiolitis is a similar inflammatory response at the level of the respiratory bronchioles, which is a transition area between the terminal conducting airways and the alveolar unit where actual air exchange occurs. Both conditions occur as a result of inhaled airborne irritants (gases, smoke) or infection by bacterial or viral microbes. There are numerous components of the respiratory host defenses spaced along the conducting airways down to the alveolar air-exchange surface. These filter and purify inhaled ambient air and remove dust and smaller particulates and bacteria (0.5–3 µm size) that are inhaled, aspirated in secretions from the naso-oropharynx, or refluxed with gastric contents. The junction between the terminal conducting airways and the alveolar unit, the respiratory bronchioles, is an important anatomic landmark because host defenses change dramatically at this level from largely mechanical and barrier-type mechanisms to cellular and phagocytic ones on the alveolar surface. (*Adapted from* Weibel and Taylor [1].)

NORMAL AIRWAY HOST DEFENSES AND MICROBIAL PATHOGENIC MECHANISMS

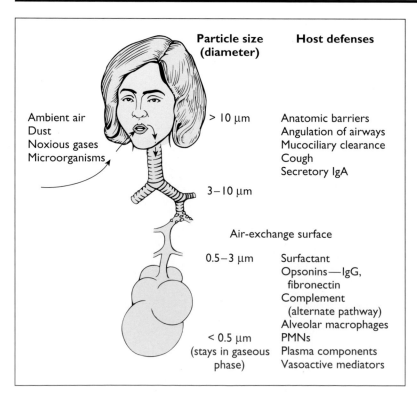

FIGURE 13-2 Host defenses along the airways. Ambient air, along with its impurities, is filtered in the naso-oropharynx and in the conducting airways, where large particulates and most microbes are prevented from entering by action of the glottis and laryngeal structures or are impacted against the mucosa and removed by sneezing, coughing, and mucociliary clearance. Aspirated secretions are handled in a similar manner. A few smaller particles and bacteria may escape clearance and reach the alveolar surface. As air velocity and flow have ceased at this level in the alveolar ducts, other defense mechanisms are required to cleanse the alveolar surface. These consist of opsonins, immune and nonimmune components, phagocytic cells (especially macrophages and polymorphonuclear leukocytes [PMNs]), and various components of systemic immunity that can enter the alveoli if inflammation occurs to alter permeability of the air–blood interface. (*Adapted from* Reynolds [2].)

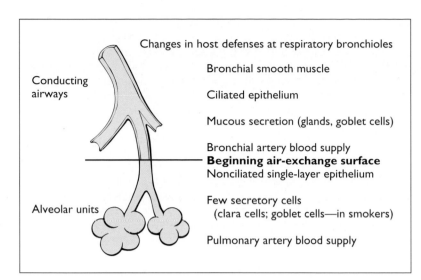

Changes in host defenses at respiratory bronchioles

Conducting airways

Bronchial smooth muscle

Ciliated epithelium

Mucous secretion (glands, goblet cells)

Bronchial artery blood supply
Beginning air-exchange surface
Nonciliated single-layer epithelium

Few secretory cells
(clara cells; goblet cells—in smokers)

Alveolar units

Pulmonary artery blood supply

FIGURE 13-3 Host defenses in respiratory bronchioles. As the conducting airways terminate at the respiratory bronchioles, a number of important host defenses disappear—ciliated epithelial cells, secretions that may act as a barrier, certain immunoglobulins such as secretory IgA or those that provide lubrication for the airway surface. Also, as the inhaled air velocity has ceased and diffusion of molecules into the alveoli causes gas exchange, different host mechanisms are required to capture microbes and particles such as phagocytic cells (alveolar macrophages). At this junction in the airways, the lymphatic channels begin, which drain the alveoli and lung interstitium into the hilar lymph nodes. The blood supply for the conducting airways and for the alveolar units is from different sources.

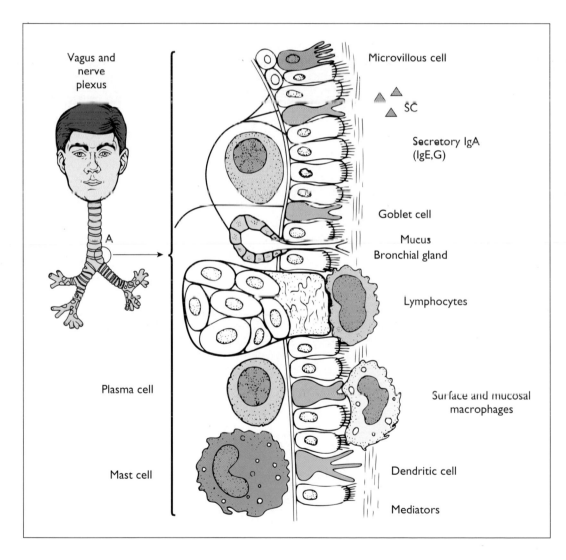

Vagus and nerve plexus

A

Microvillous cell

SC

Secretory IgA (IgE,G)

Goblet cell

Mucus
Bronchial gland

Lymphocytes

Plasma cell

Surface and mucosal macrophages

Mast cell

Dendritic cell

Mediators

FIGURE 13-4 Mucosa and submucosal structures of the conducting airway surface. The pseudostratified ciliated epithelium has a covering layer of mucus (produced by goblet cells and bronchial glands) and fluid that contains various proteins, including immunoglobulins (secretory IgA, IgG, and trace amounts of IgE) and secretory component (SC). A few surface cells may be present, such as lymphocytes (from bronchial-associated lymphoid aggregates) and macrophages. Among the epithelial cells are absorptive microvillous cells and dendritic (macrophage) cells whose cellular processes do not reach to the mucosal surface. In addition, the epithelial cells can produce arachidonic acid metabolites that influence mucosal swelling and permeability. In the submucosa below the basement membrane, plasma cells and mast cells reside that secrete local immunoglobulins (such as IgA) and mediators (such as histamine). Joining all of these glandular and cellular networks together are nerves, perhaps exerting their control through neuropeptides and by adrenergic and cholinergic nerve fibers. A rich vascular supply exists also. (*Adapted from* Reynolds [3].)

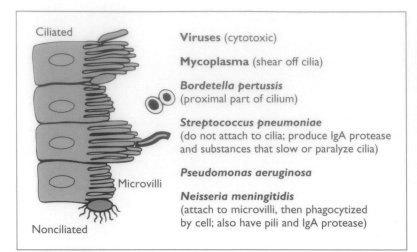

FIGURE 13-5 Interactions of respiratory epithelium and microbes. The respiratory epithelium of the conducting airways consists principally of ciliated cells that are interspersed with goblet cells,

ducts leading from bronchial glands, and some absorptive cells that have microvilli instead of cilia. For the interaction with microbes, the ciliated and microvillous cells are most involved. Viruses have the property of invading the cell to integrate into the nuclear apparatus for replication, eventually causing cytotoxicity and death of the epithelial cell. A variety of bacteria attack the cellular appendages. *Mycoplasma pneumoniae* bind to receptors on cilia and can shear them off, whereas *Bordetella pertussis* do the same thing but attack at a more proximal location on the cilium. Bacteria usually have several weapons to overcome the host defenses in the area, *ie*, ciliary motion and secretory immunoglobulin A (S-IgA). Pili and adhesion substances on bacteria increase their attachment sites, proteolytic enzymes can selectively degrade S-IgA$_1$, or cilotoxic factors, secreted by *Pseudomonas aeruginosa*, can slow or paralyze ciliary motion, perhaps allowing attachment to occur more readily. *Streptococcus pneumoniae*, *Haemophilus influenzae*, *Neisseria meningitidis*, and some gram-negative bacilli such as *Pseudomonas aeruginosa* can secrete IgA proteases. Certain *Neisseria* species attach to the microvilli of these absorptive cells. (*Adapted from* Reynolds [4].)

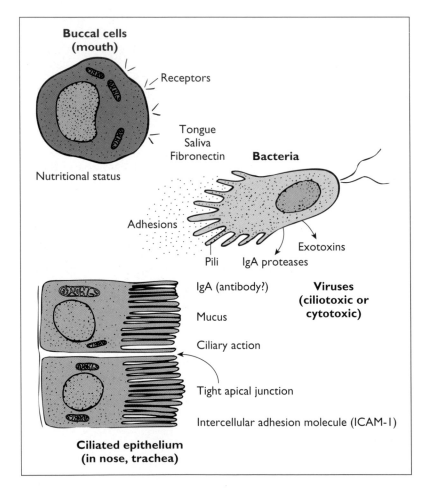

FIGURE 13-6 Mechanisms of microbial attachment and host resistance. Bacteria have various mechanisms for attaching to mucosal cells, which include surface adhesions that fit into cell receptors (various sugar or glycosamine receptors) or special microbial adaptations such as pili that promote contact. To reach these receptors, it may be necessary to clear away surface secretions such as IgA, and specific proteases or exotoxins can be produced by some bacteria to accomplish this. Other microbes, such as *Mycoplasma* and *Bordetella pertussis*, attach specifically to portions of the protruding cilia on the ciliated epithelial cells. In other circumstances, virus are cilotoxic and infect ciliated cells directly. Counterbalancing the adaptive strategies of microbes, the host has many mechanisms to resist them, and these form part of the defense apparatus of the respiratory tract. Mechanical mechanisms (sneezing, coughing, motion of the tongue, and ciliary action) resist microbial attachment, and surface secretions are interspersed also to impede adherence (salivary protease, immunoglobulins, fibronectin, and mucus). Undoubtedly, the nutritional status of the host, which may determine cellular rate of mitotic renewal and regeneration, is an important factor, too. Integrity of the tight apical junctions between the ciliated epithelial cells and the squamous epithelial surface in parts of the mouth is important as a mechanical barrier that prevents microbes from penetrating into the submucosa. (*Adapted from* Reynolds [5].)

Common causes of chronic bronchitis

Bacteria	~60%–80%
Haemophilus influenzae	
Streptococcus pneumoniae	
Moraxella catarrhalis	
Chlamydia psittaci	
Viruses	18%–41%
Rhinovirus	
Influenza A and B virus	
Coronavirus	
Herpes simplex virus	
Respiratory syncytial virus	
Adenovirus	
Mycoplasma pneumoniae	2%–9%

FIGURE 13-7 Common causes of chronic bronchitis. *Haemophilus influenzae* is the most common bacterial organism associated with exacerbations of chronic bronchitis. Viruses account for 18% to 41% of exacerbations, with rhinoviruses being the most frequently isolated. *Mycoplasma pneumoniae* accounts for 2% to 9% of cases. (*Adapted from* Kronenberg and Griffith [6].)

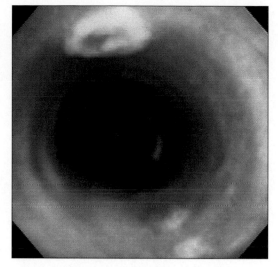

FIGURE 13-8 Bronchoscopic view of tracheobronchial tree showing white plaques due to *Aspergillus* infection. The infectious causes include bacteria, predominantly *Streptococcus pneumoniae*, *Haemophilus influenzae*, *Moraxella catarrhalis*, and *Legionella*; *Mycobacterium tuberculosis*; *Chlamydia* (TWAR strain); *Mycoplasma pneumoniae*; fungi, such as *Candida* spp, *Histoplasma capsulatum*, and *Aspergillus* spp; and a number of viruses. The photograph shows a bronchoscopic view of the tracheobronchial tree of a patient with AIDS. The white plaques proved to be due to *Aspergillus* infection. (*Courtesy of* J. Jagirdar, MD.)

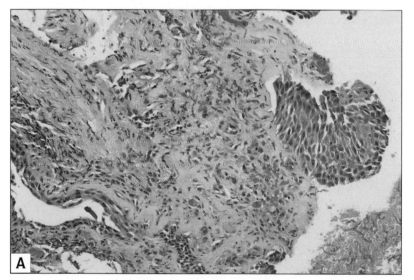
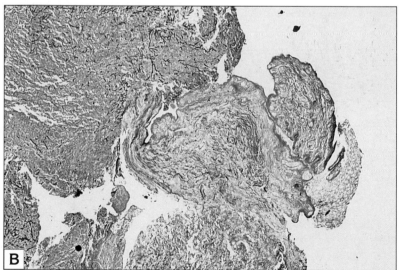

FIGURE 13-9 Histopathologic examination in acute tracheobronchitis due to *Aspergillus*. **A**, Low-power view of a tracheobronchial biopsy specimen obtained from the patient described in Figure 13-8 and stained with hematoxylin-eosin. Squamous metaplasia is seen, and there are cells with intranuclear inclusions characteristic of cytomegalovirus infection. **B**, Gomori methenamine silver stain demonstrates the branched septated hyphae characteristic of *Aspergillus* infection. (*Courtesy of* J. Jagirdar, MD.)

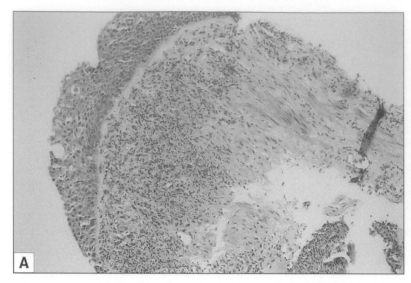

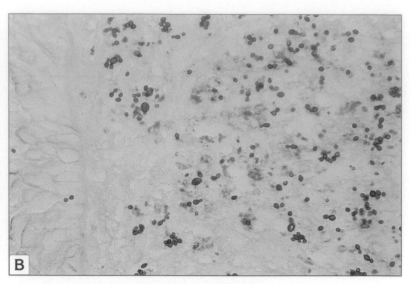

FIGURE 13-10 Histopathologic specimen demonstrating *Histo-plasma* tracheobronchitis. Transbronchial biopsy was performed on a Puerto Rican man with AIDS plus cough and shortness of breath. **A**, Hematoxylin-eosin staining reveals intense inflamma-tion beneath the bronchial mucosa. **B**, High-power view of the biopsy specimen stained with Gomori methenamine silver shows budding yeasts. Cultures grew *Histoplasma capsulatum*. (*Courtesy of* J. Jagirdar, MD.)

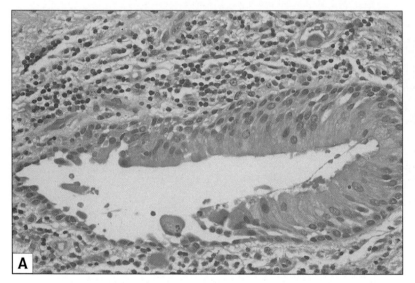

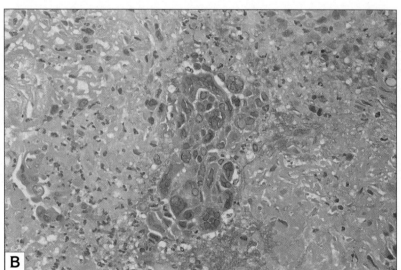

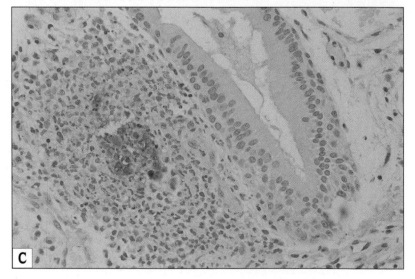

FIGURE 13-11 Histopathologic examination in viral tracheobron-chitis. Transbronchial biopsy was performed on a 50-year-old Chinese woman with polymyositis who was treated with pred-nisone and developed a cough and shortness of breath. An initial biopsy had shown atypical cells suspicious of malignancy, prompt-ing a sleeve resection. **A**, On hematoxylin-eosin staining, there is inflammation in the submucosa and cells with inclusions suggest-ing that both cytomegalovirus and herpes simplex virus (HSV) infection are present. **B**, Another area of the biopsy specimen, also stained with hematoxylin-eosin, demonstrates many cells with intranuclear inclusions suggestive of HSV infection, including multinucleated cells with the characteristic ballooning inclusions. **C**, Immunohistochemical staining proved that the infection was caused by HSV-1. (*Courtesy of* J. Jagirdar, MD.)

Nonantibiotic treatment of chronic bronchitis
Smoking cessation
Bronchodilators
Steroids
Oxygen
Pulmonary rehabilitation
Mucolytics
Chest physiotherapy

FIGURE 13-12 Nonantibiotic treatment of chronic bronchitis. Although use of antibiotics in the treatment of chronic bronchitis remains controversial, various nonantibiotic measures can be helpful, the foremost of which is smoking cessation. Smoking is a major irritant to the airways and one of the predisposing causes of chronic bronchitis. Accumulation and clearance of secretions can be a problem for some patients, and nonantibiotic treatment can be directed to help improve clearance of secretions [6].

Causes of acute febrile tracheobronchitis

Infectious causes

Respiratory syncytial virus	Parainfluenza virus
Influenza virus	Coronavirus
Rhinovirus	Adenovirus
Herpes simplex virus	Cytomegalovirus
Mycoplasma pneumoniae	*Chlamydia* (TWAR strain)
Haemophilus influenzae	*Streptococcus pneumoniae*
Moraxella catarrhalis	*Legionella*
Mycobacterium tuberculosis	

Noninfectious causes

Industrial gases
Ozone

FIGURE 13-13 Causes of acute febrile tracheobronchitis. Acute febrile tracheobronchitis is a common clinical syndrome characterized by cough and the increased production of sputum. It is part of a continuum that includes nasopharyngeal infection and bronchitis, with the inflammatory process extending from large airways to involve small airways (*ie*, bronchiolitis). The presence of serum antibody to bacterial pathogens and the antibiotic response support a possible infectious cause of these exacerbations. In children and otherwise healthy adults, viruses are the most common pathogens. In addition, inhalation of irritating and toxic substances as a result of air pollution or occupational exposure can induce this condition. Examples of noxious gases include ammonia, chlorine, sulfur dioxide, and ozone [6].

Agents causing bronchiolitis

Agent	Cases, %	Epidemiology
Respiratory syncytial virus	45–75	Yearly epidemics winter to spring
Parainfluenza viruses		
Type 3	8–15	Predominantly spring to fall
Type 1	5–12	Epidemics in the fall every other year
Type 2	1–5	Fall
Rhinoviruses	3–8	Endemic, all seasons
Adenoviruses	3–10	Endemic, all seasons
Influenza viruses	5–8	Epidemic, winter to spring
Mycoplasma pneumoniae	1–7	Endemic, all seasons
Enteroviruses	1–5	Summer to fall

FIGURE 13-14 Agents causing bronchiolitis. Bronchiolitis, an acute respiratory tract illness usually due to a viral infection, most often affects infants and young children. It involves the medium and small airways down to the alveoli, presenting clinical findings of cough, wheezing, and hyperaeration. Viral agents and a number of situations involving proliferation of lymphocytes that can present as aggregates in the vicinity of the respiratory bronchioles (minor graft versus host reactions after bone marrow or lung transplantation or infection with HIV) can promote airway obstruction that is troublesome to treat in the affected patient. This portion of the airway is a bottleneck and a natural place for constriction to develop. With chronic inflammation, a bronchiolitis obliterans can develop, as seen with certain forms of organizing pneumonia (BOOP) or in a number of chronic interstitial lung diseases. (*From* Hall and Hall [7].)

REFERENCES

1. Weibel ER, Taylor CR: Design and structure of the human lung. *In* Fishman AP (ed.): *Pulmonary Diseases and Disorders*, 2nd ed. New York: McGraw-Hill; 1988:13.

2. Reynolds HY: Host defense impairments that may lead to respiratory infections. *Clin Chest Med* 1987, 8:339–358.

3. Reynolds HY: Pulmonary host defense–state of the art. *Chest* 1989, 95:223S–230S.

4. Reynolds HY: Integrated host defense against infections. *In* Crystal RG, West JB, *et al.* (eds.): *The Lung: Scientific Foundations*. New York: Raven Press; 1991:1899–1911.

5. Reynolds HY: Bacterial adherence to respiratory tract mucosa–a dynamic interaction leading to colonization. *Semin Respir Infect* 1987, 2:8–19.

6. Kronenberg RS, Griffith DE: Bronchitis and acute febrile tracheobronchitis. *In* Niederman MS, Sarosi GA, Glassroth J (eds.): *Respiratory Infections: A Scientific Basis for Management*. Philadelphia: W.B. Saunders; 1994:95.

7. Hall CB, Hall WJ: Bronchiolitis. *In* Mandell GL, Bennett JE, Dolin R (eds.): *Principles and Practice of Infectious Diseases*, 4th ed. New York: Churchill Livingstone; 1995:612–619.

SELECTED BIBLIOGRAPHY

Reynolds HY: Immunologic system in the respiratory tract. *Physiol Rev* 1991, 71:1117–1133.

Reynolds HY: Pulmonary host defenses–state of the art. *Chest* 1989, 95:223S–230S.

Robinson GR, Canto RG, Reynolds HY: Host defense mechanisms in respiratory infection. *Immunol Allergy Clin North Am* 1993, 13:1–25.

Sibille Y, Reynolds HY: Macrophages and polymorphonuclear neutrophils in lung defense and injury. *Am Rev Respir Dis* 1990, 141:471–501.

INDEX